Emergency Department Resuscitation of the Critically Ill

Michael E. Winters, MD, FACEP, FAAEM
Editor-in-Chief
Assistant Professor of Emergency Medicine and Medicine
Director, Critical Care Education
Co-Director, Combined Emergency Medicine/Internal Medicine/Critical Care
Department of Emergency Medicine
University of Maryland School of Medicine
Baltimore, Maryland

Peter DeBlieux, MD, FACEP
Associate Editor

LSUHSC Professor of Clinical Medicine
Director of Resident and Faculty Development
Section of Emergency Medicine
Section of Pulmonary and Critical Care Medicine
Louisiana State University School of Medicine
New Orleans, Louisiana

Evie G. Marcolini, MD, FAAEM
Associate Editor

Assistant Professor of Emergency Medicine and
   Critical Care
Department of Emergency Medicine
Yale University School of Medicine
New Haven, Connecticut

Michael C. Bond, MD, FACEP, FAAEM
Associate Editor

Assistant Professor
Assistant Residency Program Director
Department of Emergency Medicine
University of Maryland School of Medicine
Baltimore, Maryland

Dale P. Woolridge, MD, PhD, FACEP
Associate Editor

Associate Professor
Department of Emergency Medicine and Pediatrics
University of Arizona
Tucson, Arizona

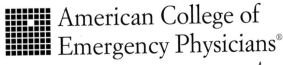

American College of Emergency Physicians®

ADVANCING EMERGENCY CARE

Additional copies of this publication can be ordered from the ACEP Bookstore, PO Box 619911, Dallas, TX 75261-9911; toll-free 800-798-1822, extension 4, or 972-550-0911; www.acep.org/bookstore.

The computed tomography image of intracranial hemorrhage on the cover was provided courtesy of Joshua S. Broder, MD, FACEP.

First printing June 2011

ISBN 978-0-9834288-0-0

Mary Anne Mitchell, Managing Editor

Jessica Hamilton, Publications Assistant

Mike C. Goodwin, Creative Services Manager

Emma Kiewice, Publications Marketing Manager

Lexi Schwartz, Sales and Service Representative

Marta Foster, Director, Educational Publications

Thomas S. Werlinich, Associate Executive Director, Educational Products

Indexing: Hughes Analytics, Chicago, Illinois

Printing: United Book Press, Inc.

About the Editors

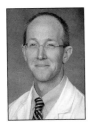

Michael E. Winters, MD, FACEP, FAAEM. Dr. Winters is an assistant professor of emergency medicine and medicine at the University of Maryland School of Medicine. He is the Associate Director of the Combined Emergency Medicine/Internal Medicine Residency Program and the founder and Co-Director of the Combined Emergency Medicine/Internal Medicine/Critical Care Residency Program. Dr. Winters has received numerous teaching awards, including the National Emergency Medicine Faculty Teaching Award from the American College of Emergency Physicians and the Young Educators Award from the American Academy of Emergency Physicians. He has lectured nationally and internationally, authored numerous articles and textbook chapters, and hosts a monthly podcast on the management of the critically ill emergency department patient. Dr. Winters completed a combined emergency medicine/internal medicine residency at the University of Maryland, after which he completed a teaching fellowship with a special focus on emergency critical care.

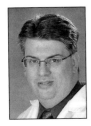

Michael C. Bond, MD, FACEP, FAAEM. Dr. Bond is an assistant professor and the Assistant Residency Program Director for the Department of Emergency Medicine at the University of Maryland. Dr. Bond received the Future Academician Award from his residency class and the 2009 University of Maryland Department of Emergency Medicine's Outstanding Teaching Attending Award. Dr. Bond has a strong interest in critical care medicine and orthopedics and recently was guest editor of an *Emergency Medicine Clinics of North America* edition on orthopedic emergencies. He has also written several book chapters on cardiology emergencies, specifically, pericarditis, myocarditis, Wolff-Parkinson-White syndrome, and temporary pacing, in addition to being a co-author on several cardiology literature summaries. In July 2010, Dr. Bond completed the combined emergency medicine/internal medicine residency program at Allegheny General Hospital, where he always volunteered to be the senior resident covering the medical intensive care unit. He found it very rewarding to care for the most critical of patients while teaching brand new interns to do the same.

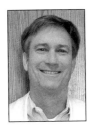

Peter DeBlieux, MD, FACEP. Dr. DeBlieux is an attending physician in emergency medicine and the medical intensive care unit of Louisiana State University Health Sciences Center Charity Hospital. He is Director of the LSUHSC Medical Student Skills Lab and Director of Emergency Medicine Services at the LSUHSC Interim Hospital. He holds appointments with LSUHSC as clinical professor of medicine and with Tulane University Medical School as clinical professor of surgery. He was Program Director of the LSUHSC Charity Hospital Emergency Medicine Residency for 10 years and is currently the Director of Resident and Faculty Development. He completed medical school at LSUHSC, an internship in internal medicine at LSUHSC Department of Medicine, residency and chief residency in emergency medicine at LSUHSC Charity Hospital, and a pulmonary critical care fellowship in the LSUHSC Section of Pulmonary and Critical Care Medicine at LSUHSC Charity Hospital.

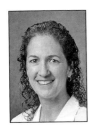

Evie G. Marcolini, MD, FAAEM. Dr. Marcolini is an assistant professor in emergency medicine and critical care at Yale University School of Medicine. She completed a fellowship in surgical critical care at the R Adams Cowley Shock Trauma Center at the University of Maryland. At the University of Maryland Medical Center, she was an attending physician in emergency medicine and surgical critical care and received a faculty award for outstanding teaching. Now at Yale, she divides her time between the emergency department, the surgical intensive care unit, and the neuroscience intensive care unit. Dr. Marcolini has presented lectures on trauma and critical care issues in medical forums in Egypt, India, and Argentina. An avid mountaineer, she teaches for Wilderness Medical Associates and has been an invited lecturer for the Wilderness Medical Society.

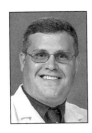

Dale P. Woolridge, MD, PhD, FACEP. Dr. Woolridge is an associate professor of emergency medicine and pediatrics at the University of Arizona. He has received multiple awards for his teaching efforts in medical school and residency training and is Director of the University of Arizona's Pediatric and Emergency Medicine Combined Residency Training Program. He has lectured throughout the state of Arizona and nationally in pediatric emergency medicine. He is Medical Director of the Southern Arizona Children's Advocacy Center, the primary referral center for all children in southern Arizona subjected to abuse and neglect. His statewide activities include serving as committee chair for the Arizona State Health Department's Pediatric Advisory Council for Emergency Services (PACES), and he is the pediatric representative on the Arizona State EMS Advisory Council. He has published two books on pediatric emergency care and has been a co-author on an additional three.

DEDICATIONS

To Erika, Hayden, Emma, and Taylor, for your endless love and support; you are my world and my inspiration for everything. To the emergency medicine residents and faculty at the University of Maryland, it is a privilege to be your colleague. – MEW

To Karen, Joshua, and Zachary for patience, love, and understanding. You are the joy in my life. To my emergency medicine and critical care colleagues at LSUHSC New Orleans, thanks for your inspiration, education, and support. – PD

To my husband, Paul, whose support made my participation possible and whose love and inspiration help me accomplish my dreams. To my past, present, and future residents, who constantly teach and inspire me. – EGM

I would like to thank my wife, Ginger, and my three children, Gabbi, Emily, and Zachary, for all of their support, and for keeping life fun and interesting. – MCB

To my family, Michelle, Anna, and Garrett, for being there. For my residents who continue to teach me daily. – DW

ACKNOWLEDGMENTS

We wish to acknowledge all those who care for the critically ill emergency department patient. Your tireless efforts in caring for these challenging patients serve as an inspiration to all. We also wish to acknowledge and thank Linda J. Kesselring, ELS, MS, the technical editor/writer for the Department of Emergency Medicine at the University of Maryland, for her outstanding contributions and assistance in preparing this textbook.

Michael E. Winters

Peter DeBlieux

Evie G. Marcolini

Michael C. Bond

Dale P. Woolridge

Contributors

Richard Amini, MD
Assistant Professor
Department of Emergency Medicine
University of Arizona
Tucson, Arizona
Chapter 24, Pediatric Trauma Updates

Fermin Barrueto, Jr, MD, FACEP, FAAEM, FACMT
Chair, Department of Emergency Medicine
Upper Chesapeake Health Systems
Clinical Assistant Professor
University of Maryland School of Medicine
Baltimore, Maryland
Chapter 14, The Critically Ill Poisoned Patient

Alan Bedrick, MD
Professor of Pediatrics
University of Arizona
Tucson, Arizona
Chapter 22, Resuscitation of the Critically Ill Neonate

Dale S. Birenbaum, MD, FACEP
Academic Chairman
Program Director
Emergency Medicine Residency Program
Florida Hospital
Clinical Assistant Professor
University of Central Florida College of Medicine
Florida State University College of Medicine
Orlando, Florida
Chapter 17, Intracerebral Hemorrhage

Michael C. Bond, MD, FACEP, FAAEM, Associate Editor
Assistant Professor
Assistant Residency Program Director
Department of Emergency Medicine
University of Maryland School of Medicine
Baltimore, Maryland
Chapter 6, Post-Cardiac Arrest Management

Eduardo Borquez, MD
Assistant Professor of Clinical Emergency Medicine
USC Keck School of Medicine
Assistant Program Director
LAC USC Emergency Medicine Residency
Los Angeles, California
Chapter 11, The Unstable Patient with Gastrointestinal Hemorrhage

William J. Brady, MD, FACEP
Professor of Emergency Medicine & Medicine
University of Virginia School of Medicine
Operational Medical Director, Charlottesville
Albemarle Rescue Squad & Albemarle County Fire Rescue
Charlottesville, Virginia
Chapter 7, Deadly Arrhythmias: Recognition and Resuscitative Management

Justin O. Cook, MD, FACEP
Attending Physician
Department of Emergency Medicine
Legacy Good Samaritan and Emanuel Hospitals
Portland, Oregon
Clinical Faculty
Department of Emergency Medicine
Alameda County Medical Center-Highland Campus
Oakland, California
Affiliate Assistant Professor
Department of Emergency Medicine
Oregon Health and Sciences University
Portland, Oregon
Chapter 20, Bedside Ultrasonography in the Critically Ill Patient

Jonathan E. Davis, MD, FACEP, FAAEM
Associate Program Director
Associate Professor of Emergency Medicine
Department of Emergency Medicine
Georgetown University Hospital
Washington Hospital Center
Washington, District of Columbia
Chapter 19, The Crashing Anaphylaxis Patient

Peter DeBlieux, MD, FACEP, Associate Editor
LSUHSC Professor of Clinical Medicine
Director of Resident and Faculty Development
Section of Emergency Medicine
Section of Pulmonary and Critical Care Medicine
Louisiana State University School of Medicine
New Orleans, Louisiana

Timothy J. Ellender, MD
Assistant Professor of Clinical Emergency Medicine
Department of Emergency Medicine
Indiana University
Emergency Medicine and Critical Care
Indiana University Health–Methodist Hospital
Indianapolis, Indiana
Chapter 10, The Unstable Patient with Pulmonary Embolism

Lillian L. Emlet, MD, MS, FACEP
Assistant Professor, Department of Critical Care Medicine & Emergency Medicine
Program Director, EM-CCM Fellowship of the MCCTP
University of Pittsburgh Medical Center
Pittsburgh, Pennsylvania
Chapter 13, The Unstable Patient with Asthma or Chronic Obstructive Pulmonary Disease

Carl A. Germann, MD, FACEP
Assistant Professor
Tufts University School of Medicine
Department of Emergency Medicine
Maine Medical Center
Portland, Maine
Chapter 18, Status Epilepticus

Michael A. Gibbs, MD, FACEP
Professor of Emergency Medicine
Tufts University School of Medicine
Chief, Department of Emergency Medicine
Maine Medical Center
Portland, Maine
Chapter 2, The Difficult Airway in the Critically Ill Patient
Chapter 15, The Crashing Trauma Patient

Alan C. Heffner, MD
Director, Medical Intensive Care Unit
Pulmonary and Critical Care Consultants
Department of Internal Medicine
Department of Emergency Medicine
Carolinas Medical Center
Charlotte, North Carolina
Chapter 4, Fluid Management in the Critically Ill Patient
Chapter 12, Severe Sepsis and Septic Shock

Benjamin J. Lawner, DO, EMT-P
Assistant Professor
Department of Emergency Medicine
University of Maryland School of Medicine
Baltimore, Maryland
Chapter 5, Cardiac Arrest Updates

Aaron Leetch, MD
Third-Year Resident
Department of Emergency Medicine and Pediatrics
University of Arizona
Tucson, Arizona
Chapter 22, Resuscitation of the Critically Ill Neonate

Daniel M. Lugassy, MD
Assistant Professor
Department of Emergency Medicine
New York University/Bellevue Hospital Center
New York City Poison Control Center
New York, New York
Chapter 14, The Critically Ill Poisoned Patient

Daniel R. Mantuani, MD, MPH
Ultrasound Fellow
Department of Emergency Medicine
Alameda County Medical Center–Highland Campus
Oakland, California
Chapter 20, Bedside Ultrasonography in the Critically Ill Patient

Evie G. Marcolini, MD, FAAEM, Associate Editor
Assistant Professor of Emergency Medicine & Critical Care
Department of Emergency Medicine
Yale University School of Medicine
New Haven, Connecticut
Chapter 6, Post-Cardiac Arrest Management

Amal Mattu, MD, FACEP, FAAEM
Professor of Emergency Medicine
Program Director, Emergency Medicine Residency
Department of Emergency Medicine
University of Maryland School of Medicine
Baltimore, Maryland
Chapter 8, Cardiogenic Shock

Jehangir Meer, MD, RDMS, FACEP
Assistant Professor of Emergency Medicine
Department of Emergency Medicine
University of Maryland School of Medicine
Baltimore, Maryland
Chapter 8, Cardiogenic Shock

Jenny S. Mendelson, MD
Fourth-Year Resident
Department of Emergency Medicine/Pediatrics
University of Arizona
Tucson, Arizona
Chapter 23, Pediatric Resuscitation

Chad M. Meyers, MD
Director of Emergency Critical Care
Department of Emergency Medicine
Bellevue Hospital Center
Assistant Professor of Clinical Emergency Medicine
NYU School of Medicine
New York, New York
Chapter 1, The Patient with Undifferentiated Shock

Ryan G.K. Mihata, MD
Fellow, Multidiscipline Emergency Medicine/Critical Care
  Fellowship
Indiana University Health–Methodist Hospital
Indianapolis, Indiana
Chapter 10, The Unstable Patient with Pulmonary Embolism

Lisa D. Mills, MD, FACEP
Associate Professor
Department of Emergency Medicine
UC Davis School of Medicine
Sacramento, California
Chapter 20, Bedside Ultrasonography in the Critically Ill Patient

Peter Philip Monteleone, MD
Chief Resident
Department of Internal Medicine
University of Virginia Medical Center
Charlottesville, Virginia
Chapter 7, Deadly Arrhythmias: Recognition and Resuscitative Management

Robert L. Norris, MD, FACEP, FAAEM
Professor, Department of Surgery
Chief, Division of Emergency Medicine
Stanford University Medical Center
Palo Alto, California
Chapter 19, The Crashing Anaphylaxis Patient

Andrew D. Perron, MD, FACEP, FACSM
Professor
Tufts University School of Medicine
Residency Program Director
Department of Emergency Medicine
Maine Medical Center
Portland, Maine
Chapter 18, Status Epilepticus

Jennifer V. Pope, MD
Assistant Residency Director
Department of Emergency Medicine
Beth Israel Deaconess Medical Center
Clinical Instructor of Medicine
Harvard Medical School
Boston, Massachusetts
Chapter 21, The Difficult Emergency Delivery

Joshua C. Reynolds, MD
Third-Year Resident
Department of Emergency Medicine
The University of Maryland School of Medicine
Baltimore, Maryland
Chapter 5, Cardiac Arrest Updates

Matthew T. Robinson, MD, FACEP
Assistant Professor of Clinical Emergency Medicine
Department of Emergency Medicine
University of Missouri Hospitals and Clinics
Columbia, Missouri
Chapter 4, Fluid Management in the Critically Ill Patient

Robert L. Rogers, MD, FACEP, FAAEM, FACP
Associate Professor of Emergency Medicine and Medicine
Director of Undergraduate Medical Education
Department of Emergency Medicine
The University of Maryland School of Medicine
Baltimore, Maryland
Chapter 9, Aortic Catastrophes

Jairo I. Santanilla, MD
Clinical Assistant Professor of Medicine
Section of Emergency Medicine
Section of Pulmonary/Critical Care Medicine
Louisiana State University Health Sciences Center
Department of Pulmonary/Critical Care Medicine
Ochsner Medical Center
New Orleans, Louisiana
Chapter 3, The Crashing Ventilated Patient

Joseph R. Shiber, MD, FACEP, FACP
Associate Professor
Director, Emergency Medicine Critical Care
Baylor College of Medicine
Houston, Texas
Chapter 16, Emergency Transfusions

J. C. Skinner, MD
Intensivist
Instructor, Emergency Medicine/Critical Care Medicine
    Fellowship
Critical Care Medicine
Indiana University Health Physicians
Indiana University Health–Methodist
Indianapolis, Indiana
Chapter 10, The Unstable Patient with Pulmonary Embolism

Mark R. Sochor, MD, MS, FACEP
Associate Professor and Research Director
Department of Emergency Medicine
University of Virginia Medical Center
Charlottesville, Virginia
*Chapter 7, Deadly Arrhythmias: Recognition and
    Resuscitative Management*

Stuart P. Swadron, MD, FACEP, FAAEM
Associate Professor
Department of Emergency Medicine
Los Angeles County/USC Medical Center
Keck School of Medicine of the University of Southern
    California
Los Angeles, California
*Chapter 11, The Unstable Patient with Gastrointestinal
    Hemorrhage*

Carrie D. Tibbles, MD
Associate Residency Director
Department of Emergency Medicine
Beth Israel Deaconess Medical Center
Assistant Professor of Medicine
Harvard Medical School
Boston, Massachusetts
Chapter 21, The Difficult Emergency Delivery

Chad D. Viscusi, MD
Assistant Professor
Department of Emergency Medicine and Pediatrics
University of Arizona
Tucson, Arizona
Chapter 23, Pediatric Resuscitation

Robert J. Vissers, MD, FACEP
Medical Director, Emergency Department
Associate CMO and Quality Director
Legacy Emanuel Medical Center
Adjunct Associate Professor
Oregon Health Sciences University
Portland, Oregon
Chapter 2, The Difficult Airway in the Critically Ill Patient

Scott D. Weingart, MD, RDMS, FACEP
Assistant Professor
Director, Division of Emergency Critical Care
Department of Emergency Medicine
Mount Sinai School of Medicine
New York, New York
Chapter 1, The Patient with Undifferentiated Shock

George C. Willis, MD
Clinical Instructor
Department of Emergency Medicine
University of Maryland School of Medicine
Baltimore, Maryland
Chapter 9, Aortic Catastrophes

Robert J. Winchell, MD
Associate Professor of Surgery
Tufts University School of Medicine
Chief, Division of Trauma
Department of Surgery
Maine Medical Center
Portland, Maine
Chapter 15, The Crashing Trauma Patient

Michael E. Winters, MD, FACEP, FAAEM, Editor-in-Chief
Assistant Professor of Emergency Medicine and Medicine
Director, Critical Care Education
Co-Director, Combined Emergency Medicine/Internal
    Medicine/Critical Care
Department of Emergency Medicine
University of Maryland School of Medicine
Baltimore, Maryland

Dale P. Woolridge, MD, PhD, FACEP, Associate Editor
Associate Professor
Department of Emergency Medicine and Pediatrics
University of Arizona
Tucson, Arizona
Chapter 24, Pediatric Trauma Updates

Foreword

Emergency medicine came of age as a specialty through mastery of the emergency airway, both in "routine" and in difficult clinical situations. Airway management is a clear differentiator between emergency medicine and all other specialties: the ability to provide acute care for a patient with any emergent condition, even if the severity or trajectory of the patient's presentation requires immediate, active airway management.

But, that was then, and this is now. Emergency physicians routinely and expertly manage emergency airways, an expectation that is taken for granted, deeply embedded in everyday practice, training programs, and clinical research. Without a doubt, the incorporation of this skill and cognitive set into the ethos of every emergency physician has saved lives and prevented disability. No longer do we think that "good enough" is good enough. We hold ourselves and our colleagues to the highest standards: excellent assessment skills with sound, reproducible decision-making and precise execution of the associated technical tasks. Why is this so? Why is a once esoteric skill, solidly in the domain of another specialty, now considered an essential, defining aspect of our practice? The answer lies in patient safety, outcomes, and expectations.

When the physicians staffing emergency departments decades ago attempted a clumsy intubation using a poor choice of pharmacologic agents, the ensuing bad outcome invariably was attributed to the illness or injury, not to the inadequate care. This no longer is the case. Every patient rightfully has come to expect that preventable morbidity or mortality will, indeed, be prevented, that the practitioner will be well trained and practiced and will make good, evidence-based decisions.

This is true with respect to airway management and it is true with respect to providing care to the critically ill patient. Critical illness breaks down traditional care paradigms, both their content and their timelines. It challenges practitioners to recognize the (often subtle) grave threats to the patient and to intervene the right way in the right time. Initial care of the critically ill patient is as central to the practice of emergency medicine as is airway management.

Equally importantly, on-going care, including weighing the risks and benefits of various pressor agents, titrating ventilator settings as precisely as intravenous fluids, and making key decisions to optimize the patient's outcome, occurs in the emergency department, managed by the emergency physician. The patient, whether physically located in an ICU or an ED, deserves the same expertise and level of care. Emergency physicians must be expert not only in the "golden hour" of care, but in the "golden 12 hours," or the "golden day." Pressure on inpatient resources has brought this challenge to the forefront more rapidly, but it is a challenge we must embrace. Equality and partnership with critical care services foster excellent patient management, seamless transitions, and optimal outcome.

This book, by some of the true leaders in the emerging area of "critical care emergency medicine," fills a great void by picking up where conventional textbooks leave off and facing squarely the unique issues related to acute critical care. It heralds the next great advance of the specialty of emergency medicine, the fulfillment of our promise to provide care for every acutely ill and injured patient in our society, with a standard not just of "good enough," but of "right, right now."

Ron M. Walls, MD
Professor and Chair
Department of Emergency Medicine
Brigham and Women's Hospital
Harvard Medical School
Boston, Massachusetts

Preface

As emergency care providers, we rise to our professional best when evaluating, diagnosing, and providing life-sustaining therapies to critically ill patients. Whether performing rapid sequence intubation, initiating and adjusting mechanical ventilation, titrating vasoactive medications, or simply administering intravenous fluids, the emergency physician must be expert at resuscitation. In recent years, it has become common for critically ill patients to remain in the ED for exceedingly long periods of time. During these crucial initial hours of critical illness, many pathologic processes begin to take hold—processes that, if not recognized and reversed, will undoubtedly lead to poor outcomes. During this time, lives can be saved… or lost!

With these urgent scenarios in mind, we have prepared this textbook for the acute health care provider working in an ED, urgent care center, or ICU. Rather than discuss general medical conditions, we have focused on those conditions in which a patient is "crashing" before your eyes. We have focused on caring for the sickest of the sick: the crashing ventilated patient; the severely injured trauma patient; the unstable patient with undifferentiated shock, pulmonary embolism, or gastrointestinal hemorrhage; the patient who has been revived after cardiac arrest. What physiologic possibilities must you consider immediately? What steps should you take now to save the patient's life?

The authors of these chapters were selected based on their expertise in critical care and emergency medicine. Within each chapter, critical information is emphasized in tables, figures, "key points," and "pearls." Many chapters contain flow diagrams that can be referenced quickly during a shift in the ED or ICU.

It is our hope that acute health care providers will refer to this text frequently to broaden their knowledge base for the delivery of rapid, efficient, and appropriate critical care to the moribund patient. Quite simply, we believe this text will help you save lives!

Michael Winters
March 2011

Contents

CHAPTER 1

The Patient with Undifferentiated Shock

Scott D. Weingart and Chad M. Meyers

IN THIS CHAPTER

Initial approach to the patient in shock

Performing the initial stabilization

Making a definitive diagnosis

Introduction

The treatment of a patient in shock is one of the defining roles of our specialty. Sometimes the cause of the shock state is apparent from the first contact with the patient. The hypotensive patient with a gunshot wound to the abdomen does not present a diagnostic dilemma, even though the resuscitation may not be as easy. Many patients who present with shock do not allow as quick a diagnosis. Often emergency physicians must start resuscitation simultaneously with gathering the information necessary to find the cause.

KEY POINT

Shock is a time-dependent disorder. If left to languish, many of these patients will have a worse outcome than if they had received rapid, aggressive care.

When reduced to the simplest description, shock is inadequate tissue perfusion. In the early stages, patients in shock may have a benign physical examination and normal vital signs. At this stage, the shock state can be said to be *cryptic* and will be found only by examining biomarkers such as lactate or by using tissue perfusion monitors. For many emergency physicians, shock is almost synonymous with hypotension. This conflation usually leads to late recognition of the shock state and a more difficult treatment course.

At times, even a low blood pressure is not enough to spur action. When assessing an otherwise well-looking patient, it is tempting to discount borderline or transient hypotension; however, even a single episode of systolic blood pressure lower than 100 mm Hg has been associated with increased mortality in emergency department patients.[1] The lower the blood pressure observed, the higher the associated risk of death.[1] A pattern witnessed in severe sepsis consists of transient, self-limited dips of the blood pressure.

KEY POINT

Instead of reassurance, intermittent low blood pressures should inspire trepidation and a diligent search for a cause.

Initial Assessment

In addition to the standard history and physical examination that are obtained on every sick patient in the emergency department, the following simple evaluations should be performed immediately on a patient with undifferentiated shock:

- Blood glucose measurement to screen for hypoglycemia
- Pregnancy test in female patients of child-bearing age for suspected ectopic pregnancy
- ECG to identify arrhythmia and ischemia
- Assessment of feet and hands for abnormal vasodilation

- Examination of the neck veins as an indicator of paradoxically increased central venous pressure
- Rectal examination for melena/gastrointestinal blood for occult bleeding
- Chest radiograph to evaluate for pneumonia, pneumothorax or hemothorax, and pulmonary edema

Initial Stabilization

After a patent airway and adequate oxygenation are ensured, establishing access to the circulation is crucial. Short, large-bore intravenous lines represent the first line for venous access. In the critically ill patient, if peripheral access is difficult to obtain, an immediate shift to central access, using a percutaneous introducer catheter or a dialysis catheter, provides a reliable means of fluid resuscitation. New devices allow access to the intraosseous space; they may provide a quickly established route of medication administration, although they are not suitable for rapid volume loading.

Empiric fluid administration will help almost every cause of hypotension. Even the patient with undiagnosed cardiogenic shock will not have deleterious effects from 1 or 2 liters of crystalloid, even if the fluid is unlikely to help. The one exception is the patient with hemorrhagic shock. In these patients, crystalloid will further dilute their hemoglobin, platelets, and clotting factors. Hemorrhaging patients derive more benefit from blood products such as packed red blood cells, plasma, and platelets.

The goal of fluid loading is to achieve a mean arterial pressure (MAP) of more than 65 mm Hg. Values lower than this can lead to poor organ perfusion as well as further worsening of cardiac output secondary to poor cardiac perfusion. Raising the MAP significantly higher than 65 mm Hg with exogenous medications or aggressive fluid loading predisposes the patient to complications without any added benefit.[2]

It is common for patients with septic shock to require more than 6 liters of crystalloid during their emergency department stay to obtain adequate vascular loading. Although empiric fluid loading may be used, assessing volume status and titrating fluid administration using ultrasonography could provide more precise guidance (see page 4).

Some patients will have a MAP so low (<40–50 mm Hg) that it could be dangerous to wait to see the effects of fluid loading. In these patients, vasopressors should be given while fluid loading is underway. Although a continuous infusion of any of the agents shown in Table 1-1 will suffice for this purpose, push-dose pressors (Table 1-2) are another option during the initial stages of patient evaluation/stabilization.[3]

PEARL

The Trendelenburg position will have only transient effects on blood pressure; it has no value as a resuscitation position during shock.[4-6]

TABLE 1-1.

Conventional vasoactive medications

Dopamine	Initial dose: 5 mcg/kg/min
	Titrate by: 5-10 mcg/kg/min
	Maximum dose: 20 mcg/kg/min
Norepinephrine	Initial dose: 0.5-1 mcg/kg/min
	Titrate by: 1-2 mcg/min
	Maximum dose: 30 mcg/min
Dobutamine	Initial dose: 2.5 mcg/kg/min
	Titrate by: 2.5 mcg/kg/min
	Maximum dose: 20 mcg/kg/min
Epinephrine	Initial dose: 1 mcg/min
	Titrate by: 1 mcg/min
	Maximum dose: 10 mcg/min
Phenylephrine	Initial dose: 100-180 mcg/min
	Titrate by: 100 mcg/min
	Maximum dose: 10 mcg/kg/min
Vasopressin	Initial dose: 0.01 units/min
	Titrate by: 0.01 units
	Maximum dose: 0.04 units/min

TABLE 1-2.

Push-dose pressors (may be administered through peripheral lines)

Phenylephrine is a pure α agent, so it has no intrinsic inotropy, but the increase in heart perfusion that it induces from normalizing the MAP can improve cardiac output.

    Onset: 1 minute
    Duration: 20 minutes
    Mixing instructions:
        Into a 3-mL syringe, draw up 1 mL of phenylephrine from a vial of phenylephrine, 10 mg/mL.
        Inject this amount into a 100-mL bag of normal saline.
        This gives 100 mL of phenylephrine with a concentration of 100 mcg/mL.
        Draw some solution into a syringe; each milliliter in the syringe contains 100 mcg.
    Dose: 0.5–2 mL every 2–5 minutes (50–200 mcg)

Epinephrine has α-, β_1-, and β_2-effects, so it is an inopressor.
    Onset: 1 minute
    Duration: 5–10 minutes
    Mixing instructions:
        Draw 9 mL of normal saline into a 10-mL syringe.
        Into this syringe, draw up 1 mL of epinephrine from the cardiac epinephrine ampule. (A cardiac ampule contains 10 mL of epinephrine at a concentration of 100 mcg/mL or 1:10,000.)
        This yields 10 mL of epinephrine at a concentration of 10 mcg/mL (1:100,000).
    Dose: 0.5–2 mL every 2–5 minutes (5–20 mcg)

PEARL

Hypocalcemia can cause decreased blood pressure. Administration of calcium chloride, 500–1,000 mg, preferably through a central line or into a large antecubital vein, will lead to increases in inotropy and vasoconstriction in any patient, but especially in patients with hypocalcemia.

Differential Diagnosis

The causes of shock can be conceptualized by an analogy to a simple water pumping system (Figure 1-1).[7] The four components of the system are a reservoir, a pump, and the pump's inflow and outflow pipes. Shock results from an empty reservoir, pump failure, inflow obstruction, or leaky, enlarged pipes (Figure 1-1).

Clues to the Diagnosis

The following concepts, although not foolproof, can provide hints as to the cause of undifferentiated shock:

- Warm extremities in a patient with hypotension point to abnormal vasodilation from conditions such as sepsis, anaphylaxis, pancreatitis, and overdose or poisoning.[8]

PEARL

Although patients with cirrhosis have abnormal vasodilation and therefore low baseline MAPs, they are predisposed to infections and could have septic shock. Have a high degree of suspicion for sepsis in these patients.

- Conversely, cold extremities and hypotension can indicate hemorrhagic, hypovolemic, or cardiogenic causes. Cold extremities are indicative of endogenous sympathetic compensation for the hypotension.
- Cardiogenic shock from myocardial infarction is extremely unlikely with an ECG that shows no signs of ischemia. It is virtually impossible to have cardiogenic shock with completely clear lungs, unless a right ventricular infarction is the cause of the hypotension.

PEARL

In suspected cardiogenic shock patients, carefully auscultate the heart for new murmurs. Valve rupture and ischemic pump failure require very different treatments.

- In patients in anaphylactic shock, skin findings (urticaria, angioedema), facial swelling, and respiratory compromise usually (not always) accompany the hypotension.
- Undifferentiated shock in a female patient of child-bearing age should be assumed to be from a ruptured ectopic pregnancy until a negative pregnancy test is returned.
- Jugular vein distention in the setting of hypotension should prompt consideration of an obstruction (pulmonary embolism, tension pneumothorax, or pericardial tamponade) or pump failure.

FIGURE 1-1.

Schematic of the circulatory system by analogy to a water pump. Image reproduced with permission from EMCrit.org.

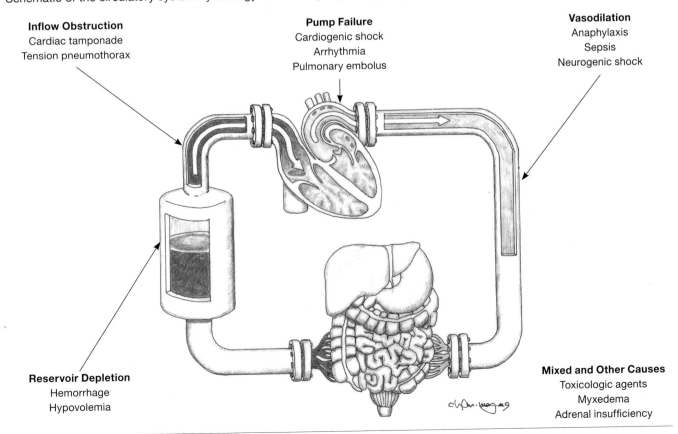

Inflow Obstruction
Cardiac tamponade
Tension pneumothorax

Pump Failure
Cardiogenic shock
Arrhythmia
Pulmonary embolus

Vasodilation
Anaphylaxis
Sepsis
Neurogenic shock

Reservoir Depletion
Hemorrhage
Hypovolemia

Mixed and Other Causes
Toxicologic agents
Myxedema
Adrenal insufficiency

Ultrasonography for Further Delineation of the Shock State

Although the history and physical examination offer clues to the cause of the shock state, ultrasonography offers a more precise and sensitive determination of the source. Rapid Ultrasound for Shock and Hypotension (RUSH) allows quick determination of the cause and extent of many hypotensive states.[9] A similar protocol, Rapid Ultrasound for SHock, also offers a path to rapid diagnosis.[10] Many other protocols can be found in the literature.[11-14]

The sequencing of the RUSH examination is shown in Figure 1-2. A more detailed description of the examination and images and videos that have been produced by it can be found at http://rush.emcrit.org. The entire examination can be completed in less than 2 minutes using readily available portable machines. The HI-MAP acronym indicates the steps, in order:

H Examine the **heart: parasternal long** and then **four-chamber cardiac views,** with the general purpose or cardiac probe.

I Obtain an **inferior vena cava (IVC) view** with the same probe.

M Scan the **Morison pouch and splenorenal views** with **thorax** images and then examine the **bladder window** using a general purpose abdominal probe.

A Increase the depth, and find the **aorta** with four views: just below the xiphoid, above and below the renal artery, and at the bifurcation of the aorta to the iliac arteries.

P Scan both sides of the chest for **pneumothorax.** It may be beneficial to switch to a small-parts, high-frequency transducer, but the general purpose probe will often supply sufficient views of the pleural interface.

FIGURE 1-2.

Sequencing of the RUSH examination. Image reproduced with permission from EMCrit.org.

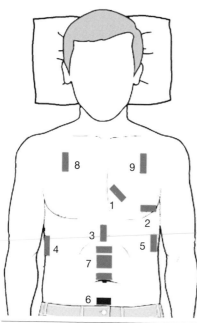

RUSH exam sequencing

1. Parasternal long cardiac view
2. Apical four-chamber cardiac view
3. Inferior vena cava view
4. Morison with hemothorax view
5. Splenorenal with hemothorax view
6. Bladder view
7. Aortic slide view
8. Pneumothorax view
9. Pneumothorax view

Use curvilinear array for 1 through 7.
Use high-frequency array for 8 and 9.

The RUSH examination protocol will give the following information:

- Identification or exclusion of pericardial tamponade (cardiac windows)
- Hints as to the presence of pulmonary embolism or right ventricular infarction (cardiac windows)
- A rough evaluation of cardiac output (cardiac windows)
- Assessment of whether the patient's cardiac output will increase with fluid administration (dynamic IVC assessment)
- Intraperitoneal bleeding or ascites (Focused Assessment with Sonography for Trauma [FAST] views)
- Pleural effusions or hemothoraces (FAST views)
- Abdominal aortic aneurysm (AAA views)
- Pneumothorax (lung windows)

Conclusion

Undifferentiated shock requires rapid recognition and aggressive empiric treatment to reestablish perfusion. Once the patient is stabilized, a search for the cause of the shock state can proceed with bedside assessments, laboratory testing, and ultrasonography. Once the type of shock is discovered, the individual cause will dictate specific treatments. Further details on each of these causes will be presented in the chapters that follow.

References

1. Jones AE, Yiannibas V, Johnson C, et al. Emergency department hypotension predicts sudden unexpected in-hospital mortality: a prospective cohort study. *Chest.* 2006;130:941-946.

2. Bourgoin A, Leone M, Delmas A, et al. Increasing mean arterial pressure in patients with septic shock: effects on oxygen variables and renal function. *Crit Care Med.* 2005;33:780-786.

3. Weingart S. Push-dose pressors. *ACEP News.* 2010;29(3):4.

4. Bivins HG, Knopp R, dos Santos PA. Blood volume distribution in the Trendelenburg position. *Ann Emerg Med.* 1985;14:641-643.

5. Johnson S, Henderson SO. Myth: the Trendelenburg position improves circulation in cases of shock. *CJEM.* 2004;6:48-49.

6. Taylor J, Weil MH. Failure of the Trendelenburg position to improve circulation during clinical shock. *Surg Gynecol Obstet.* 1967;124:1005-1010.

7. Wood KE. Major pulmonary embolism: review of a pathophysiologic approach to the golden hour of hemodynamically significant pulmonary embolism. *Chest.* 2002;121:877-905.

8. Melo J, Peters JI. Low systemic vascular resistance: differential diagnosis and outcome. *Crit Care.* 1999;3:71-77.

9. Weingart SD, Duque D, Nelson B. Rapid ultrasound for shock and hypotension. [online] At www.emedhome.com. 2009.

10. Perera P, Mailhot T, Riley D, et al. The RUSH exam: Rapid Ultrasound in SHock in the evaluation of the critically ill. *Emerg Med Clin North Am.* 2010;28:29-56.

11. Weekes AJ, Zapata RJ, Napolitano A. Symptomatic hypotension: ED stabilization and the emerging role of sonography. *Emerg Med Pract.* 2007;9:1-28.

12. Rose JS, Bair AE, Mandavia D, et al. The UHP ultrasound protocol: a novel ultrasound approach to the empiric evaluation of the undifferentiated hypotensive patient. *Am J Emerg Med.* 2001;19:299-302.

13. Jones AE, Tayal VS, Sullivan DM, et al. Randomized, controlled trial of immediate versus delayed goal-directed ultrasound to identify the cause of nontraumatic hypotension in emergency department patients. *Crit Care Med.* 2004;32:1703-1708.

14. Hernandez C, Shuler K, Hannan H, et al. C.A.U.S.E.: Cardiac arrest ultra-sound exam—a better approach to managing patients in primary non-arrhythmogenic cardiac arrest. *Resuscitation.* 2008;76:198-206.

CHAPTER 2

The Difficult Airway in the Critically Ill Patient

Robert J. Vissers and Michael A. Gibbs

IN THIS CHAPTER

Assessing the difficult airway

Predicting difficult laryngoscopy and intubation

Managing the difficult airway

Techniques to improve the success of laryngoscopy

Rescue devices

Introduction

Emergency airway management is one of the most challenging aspects of emergency care. Time is usually limited, and the priority of managing the airway can preclude complete patient assessment, diagnosis, and stabilization. When the patient's condition is critical or an airway fails, the potential for significant morbidity or death is heightened. Furthermore, in the critically ill patient, the acute condition itself could predispose the individual to physiologic insults during airway management. Anticipation and management of these risks can prevent undesirable worsening of the existing medical condition. Airways that are at higher risk for failure or complication generally fall into three categories: the difficult airway, the failed airway, and the airway of the physiologically compromised patient.

There are methods for rapidly identifying the potential for a difficult airway and planning accordingly. A growing number of airway devices can assist with the identification, management, and rescue of the difficult airway. Preparation and pretreatment strategies can mitigate the risks of airway management in some conditions. Once a difficult airway is anticipated, the clinician can choose a strategy and technique based on the underlying anatomic difficulty. The amount of time available, primarily based on the ability to maintain oxygenation, will also determine the optimal management strategy.[1]

Assessment of the Difficult Airway

The difficult airway can be defined by anatomic characteristics that predict, through preintubation assessment, the potential for difficulty with bag-valve-mask (BVM) ventilation, laryngoscopy and intubation, cricothyrotomy, or placement of a rescue airway. A difficult airway has been defined by the American Society of Anesthesiologists (ASA) as one requiring more than two attempts at intubation with the same laryngoscope blade, a change in blade or use of an intubation stylet, or an alternative intubation technique or rescue.[2] Difficulty in visualization of the cords, described as a Cormack-Lehane grade 3 view (visualization of the glottis only) or grade 4 view (no visualization of the glottis), is associated with difficult laryngoscopy and failure to intubate successfully.[3] "Difficult BVM ventilation" is defined as the inability to maintain oxygen saturation above 90% despite optimal positioning and airway adjuncts.

KEY POINT

The difficult airway can be defined by anatomic characteristics that predict, through preintubation assessment, the potential for difficult BVM ventilation, difficult laryngoscopy and intubation, or difficult placement of a rescue airway.

The incidence of difficult airways in the emergent or critical care setting is less clearly defined than in the operating room.[4] The failure rate of the first laryngoscopic attempt during emergent rapid sequence intubation (RSI) is 10% to 23% and varies with the experience of the operator.[5-7] More than two attempts are needed in 3% of patients, and 99% of patients are intubated successfully by the third attempt.[8,9] The need for more than three attempts at intubation by an experienced operator is rarely met with success, and persistent attempts beyond this are associated with increased mortality and morbidity.[10]

PEARL

The need for more than three attempts at intubation by an experienced operator is rarely met with success. Persistent attempts beyond this are associated with increased mortality and morbidity.

Prior to any attempt at airway management, potential difficulties with BVM ventilation, laryngoscopy and intubation, and rescue must be assessed. The presence of a potentially difficult airway is not an absolute contraindication to RSI; however, early identification allows the clinician to plan appropriately and determine a rescue strategy. In some instances, the anticipated difficulty may present too great a risk for administration of paralytics, requiring an awake look or fiberoptic intubation to avoid the dangerous scenario of "cannot intubate/cannot ventilate" in a paralyzed patient.[11] If a difficult airway is predicted, optimal management can be determined based on airway difficulty and anatomy, the operator's experience, and the availability of alternative devices. How much time is available will also influence the strategy and is determined primarily by two factors: 1) the rate of progression of airway obstruction and 2) the ability to maintain oxygenation.[1]

PEARL

Plan for any anticipated difficulty or the failed airway. If special equipment may be needed, be sure it is immediately available and working.

Predicting Difficult Bag-Valve-Mask Ventilation

It is important to consider potential impediments of BVM ventilation before initiating RSI. In most circumstances, BVM ventilation should be the primary rescue following a failed attempt; therefore, it is critical for emergency physicians to master this skill. The physician must anticipate potential difficulties and use techniques to overcome any that are encountered. The presence of any two of the following five factors predicts difficult BVM ventilation: facial hair, obesity, edentulous patient, advanced age, and snoring.[12]

An inability to adequately ventilate with a BVM is often solved by better positioning, usually by alignment of the oral and tracheal axes through the "sniff position" and placing a pad under the occiput, if needed.[13] A jaw thrust and the use of oral and nasal airways can reduce obstruction caused by the tongue falling back into the posterior airway. A tighter seal can be obtained with two-person bagging and applying a lubricant to a man's facial hair.

PEARL

If dentures are present, they should be left in place to facilitate BVM ventilation.

KEY POINT

The presence of any two of the following five factors predicts difficult BVM ventilation: facial hair, obesity, edentulous patient, advanced age, and snoring.

Predicting Difficult Laryngoscopy and Tracheal Intubation

In some patients, such as those with anatomic disruption from trauma or certain congenital syndromes, the difficulty is obvious. Several readily visible external features are associated with difficult laryngoscopy and intubation: facial hair, obesity, short neck, small or large chin, buckteeth, high arched palate, and any airway deformity related to trauma, tumor, or inflammation.[1] However, identifying the more common subtle predictors of intubation difficulty before the initiation of neuromuscular blockade requires a systematic and focused clinical examination of the airway anatomy. In the critically ill patient, any practical approach must be rapid and able to be performed on a potentially uncooperative or unresponsive patient. The results of this evaluation should guide the development of an airway management plan.

The LEMON Airway Assessment

The LEMON mnemonic represents a practical, systematic assessment that can be performed rapidly on any critically ill patient. Based on known independent predictors, this approach was introduced by Murphy and Walls as a tool for the identification of difficult laryngoscopy and intubation.[14] A recent study demonstrated predictive value in the emergent setting,[15] and the most recent Advanced Trauma Life Support (ATLS) guidelines recommend the mnemonic as a method of evaluating airway difficulty.[16] This mnemonic refers to the assessment of five predictors: looking at external features, evaluating the geometry of the airway, the Mallampati score, obstruction, and neck mobility (Table 2-1).

Looking at external features is an assessment of potential airway difficulty based on obvious anatomic distortion or external features associated with difficulty such as obesity; facial hair; a short, thick neck; or a receding mandible. With experience, the physician can usually predict difficulty through simple observation; however, this will not occur unless a conscious effort is made to do so.

Evaluate the airway geometry using the 3-3-2 rule to predict the ability to align the oral, pharyngeal, and tracheal axes. The mandibular opening in an adult should be at least 4 cm (approximately three fingerbreadths). If it is less than this, visualization is reduced. A restricted oral opening may dictate the size of the device that can be employed. The distance between the mentum and the hyoid bone, which should be three to four fingerbreadths, assesses the ability of the mandible to accommodate the tongue during laryngoscopy. In a smaller mandible, the tongue is more likely to fill the oral cavity and obstruct visualization, and an unusually large mandible can elongate the oral axis, making visual alignment more challenging. The anterior larynx may be high if the space between the mandible and the top of the thyroid cartilage is less than two fingerbreadths, increasing the likelihood of a Cormack-Lehane grade 3 or 4 view.

The Mallampati score is used to assess the degree to which the tongue obstructs the visualization of the posterior pharynx. It is loosely associated with the ability to visualize the glottis.[17] Four views are described:

Class I: Faucial pillars, soft palate, and uvula can be visualized

Class II: Faucial pillars and soft palate can be visualized, but the uvula is masked by the base of the tongue

Class III: Only the base of the uvula can be visualized

Class IV: None of the three structures can be visualized

Simply put, the less posterior pharynx seen, the less likely the cords are to be seen. Class III is associated with a 5% failure rate and class IV with up to 20% failure.

Obstruction presents a uniquely challenging airway that is usually readily apparent. The development of a management plan for airway obstruction requires consideration of three aspects: 1) the location of the obstruction, 2) whether it is fixed (eg, tumor) or mobile (eg, epiglottis), and 3) how rapidly it is progressing. The location can determine which approach or rescue device should be used. For example, oral airway obstruction from angioedema of the tongue can limit the options to nasal techniques or surgical airways through the cricothyroid membrane. BVM ventilation is more likely to be successful in patients with mobile, inflammatory obstructions such as croup than in those with the fixed obstruction of a hard foreign body. The speed of progression determines whether management can await patient transport to another facility or to the operating room or whether it must occur immediately at the bedside.

Neck mobility can interfere with the ability to align the visual axes by preventing the desired "sniffing position." Most commonly, neck immobility is imposed by a cervical collar.

It is important to remove the anterior portion of the cervical collar, while maintaining cervical immobilization, to increase the chance of success during laryngoscopy. If there is no suspicion of cervical injury, atlanto-occipital extension should be assessed, even in the unconscious patient.

Predicting Difficult Airway Rescue

Alternative airway devices play an important role in airway management, either as a rescue from failed laryngoscopy or as a primary alternative when laryngoscopy is predicted to be difficult. In rare circumstances, such as the "cannot intubate/cannot ventilate" scenario, surgical cricothyrotomy is the only airway option remaining. It is therefore important to anticipate difficulties with rescue devices or the ability to surgically create an airway.

Extraglottic airway devices, such as the laryngeal mask airway (LMA) and the Combitube (Tyco-Kendall, Mansfield, MA), are commonly employed for rescue from failed intubation and can be a primary technique in selected circumstances.[18] As for the more commonly used techniques, patient characteristics may suggest difficulty and potential failure with an extraglottic device.[4] Adequate oral access and infraglottic patency are necessary for ventilation to occur; therefore, these devices will not succeed in the presence of oral, laryngeal, or infraglottic obstruction. The seal above the glottis, necessary for ventilation, may not be achievable if there is significant disruption or abnormal anatomy of the upper airway. Ventilation can also be difficult in patients with high airway resistance, such as those with asthma, and can fail at airway pressures exceeding 25 cm H_2O.

Flexible fiberoptic scopes are excellent tools for airway evaluation and facilitation of intubation; however, their use requires adequate time to prepare the equipment and the patient—time not always present in emergency departments. Visibility through any fiberoptic device can be obscured by excessive secretions or blood in the airway.[19] Compared with other rescue devices, flexible fiberoptic scopes require significant operator skill.

TABLE 2-1.	
The LEMON mnemonic. Adapted with permission from: "The Difficult Airway Course: Emergency," Airway Management Education Center, www.theairwaysite.com, and from: Murphy MF, Walls RM. Identification of the difficult and failed airway. In: Walls RM, Murphy MF, eds. *Manual of Emergency Airway Management.* 3rd ed. Philadelphia, PA: Lippincott Williams & Wilkins; 2008:81-93.	
Look externally	Look for external features predictive of airway difficulty.
Evaluate 3-3-2 (airway geometry)	The oral opening, the mentum to hyoid distance, and the mandible to thyroid cartilage distance are measured in fingerbreadths. Reduced distance may suggest difficulty aligning the oral, pharyngeal, and laryngeal axes.
Mallampati score	The degree of posterior pharynx visualized is associated with visualization of the vocal cords during laryngoscopy.
Obstruction and obesity	Identification of where the obstruction is and how quickly it is progressing will guide the management.
Neck mobility	Inability to flex or extend the neck could restrict visualization and the ability to reposition during BVM ventilation or laryngoscopy.

A surgical airway is a potential rescue strategy when all other alternatives are predicted to be difficult. The biggest challenge to a surgical airway is the decision to proceed. Some anatomic variables make surgical cricothyrotomy more difficult. Obesity or a very short "bull" neck can present a challenge to identification of landmarks. Overlying hematoma, abscess, or tumor and scarring from previous surgery, radiation, or burns can cause technical difficulties.[20]

The Failed Airway

The failed airway in emergency management has been defined as 1) inability to maintain adequate oxygenation following a failed intubation attempt or 2) three failed attempts at intubation by an experienced provider, even if oxygenation can be maintained.[4] The rate of failed airways in emergent patients undergoing RSI is approximately 1%.[7,8] Despite thorough assessment of airway difficulty and appropriate patient selection for RSI, failed airways can still be expected, particularly in the emergent setting. Therefore, any clinician providing emergent airway management to critically ill patients must have facility with rescue devices and surgical airways. It is essential to have a plan to address the failed airway before initiating paralytics, so that the anticipated necessary equipment can be gathered. Ideally, this plan should be shared with the team managing the patient (Table 2-2).

KEY POINT

The failed airway is defined as 1) the inability to maintain adequate oxygenation following a failed intubation attempt or 2) three failed attempts at intubation by an experienced provider.

Management of the Difficult Airway

The most important aspect of airway management is thoughtful preparation, and this is particularly true for the emergent, critically ill patient. Some planning is essential long before the patient arrives in the emergency department; ongoing physician education is necessary to maintain rarely performed airway and cricothyrotomy skills, and a well-stocked difficult-airway cart must be immediately available (Table 2-3). Steps such as pre-

oxygenation and premedication should be taken to prepare the patient for RSI and mitigate the potential harm that intubation can cause. Despite the urgency associated with emergent airway management, it is essential that the clinician take the time to assess airway difficulty, optimize the physiologic state of the patient, and develop a management plan.

Physiologic Challenges in Airway Management

For some patients, because of an underlying chronic or acute medical condition, airway management poses an increased risk of hypoxia or hypotension or exacerbation of an underlying disease state. Critically ill patients who have respiratory or hemodynamic compromise prior to the procedure are at particular risk. Certain conditions can be exacerbated by the drugs used to facilitate RSI or the physiologic effects from the procedure itself.[21] Many of these undesirable effects could be prevented or mitigated through recognition of the risk, adequate resuscitation, and attention to drug selection.

Preoxygenation

Preoxygenation should begin as soon as intubation is anticipated, regardless of the patient's oxygen saturation.[22] Preoxygenation displaces nitrogen with oxygen in the alveolar space, creating a reservoir of oxygen that can prevent hypoxia for several minutes of apnea. Hypoxia develops more quickly in children, pregnant women, obese patients, and physiologically compromised patients. The patient should be preoxygenated for at least 3 minutes using a nonrebreathing mask supplied with 15 L/min of oxygen. Nasal cannulas do not provide optimal preoxygenation. Patients with decreased respiratory rate or hypoxia despite use of a nonrebreathing mask could require preoxygenation with BVM ventilation, which can deliver 90% to 97% oxygen.

TABLE 2-3.

Contents of the difficult-airway cart

A surgical airway kit (open surgical, Seldinger wire-guided kit, or both)
A gum-elastic bougie (intubating stylet)
One of the blind insertion devices (eg, intubating LMA, Combitube [Tyco-Kendall, Mansfield, MA], King-LT [King Systems, Noblesville, IN])
One of the optical intubating stylets (eg, Shikani [Carus Medical, Minneapolis, MN], Levitan [Clarius Medical, Minneapolis, MN], RIFL [AI Medical Devices, Inc, Williamstown, MI])
One of the hand-held videolaryngoscopes (eg, GlideScope [Verathon, Bothell, WA], McGrath [LMA North American, San Diego, CA], Storz [Storz, Tallinn, Estonia], Pentax [Pentax, Tokyo, Japan])
Flexible fiberoptic scopes (nasopharyngoscope, intubating scope) (optional)
Medications to facilitate awake laryngoscopy

TABLE 2-2.

Verbal checklist prior to initiating RSI

Is this a difficult airway? What is the plan?
Is the patient ready? Preoxygenation, premedication, and blood pressure optimized?
Is the support equipment ready? IV, suction, and bag-mask?
Is the correct equipment ready? Correct endotracheal tube, stylet, and laryngoscope? Rescue devices?
Are the right drugs in the right doses ready?
Is the team ready? Does everyone understand the plan if intubation fails?

Pretreatment Agents in the Critically Ill Patient

Critically ill patients with elevated intracranial pressure (ICP), reactive airway disease, and cardiovascular disease can experience an exacerbation of their condition from the direct physiologic effects of laryngoscopy. Theoretically, pretreatment agents (Table 2-4) attenuate adverse physiologic responses to laryngoscopy and intubation; however, evidence-based studies demonstrating improved outcome using pretreatment in the emergent setting are lacking.[23–30] Laryngoscopy can cause increases in heart rate and blood pressure secondary to a reflex sympathetic response, which may be harmful in patients with elevated ICP, myocardial ischemia, and aortic dissection. Patients who have lost cerebral autoregulation can also experience a centrally mediated increase in ICP. In children, the increased vagal response can result in significant bradycardia, particularly in the presence of succinylcholine. Laryngeal stimulation can have adverse respiratory effects (eg, laryngospasm, cough, and bronchospasm). When pretreatment agents are used, they should be administered 3 to 5 minutes before initiation of RSI.

Lidocaine has been recommended as a pretreatment agent in patients with possible elevated ICP and in those with bronchospasm. There is suggestive evidence that lidocaine mitigates the ICP response to laryngeal manipulation; however, studies demonstrating a favorable effect on outcomes are lacking.[25,26] Studies of lidocaine as a pretreatment agent in patients with severe asthma are also inconclusive.[27] Clinicians must balance the potential benefit of a relatively benign medication in a critically ill patient against the lack of clear outcome data.

Fentanyl is an opioid that is known to attenuate the reflex sympathetic response to airway manipulation.[23,28,29] It may be used as a pretreatment when an increase in blood pressure and heart rate could be detrimental, as in patients with elevated ICP and certain cardiovascular diseases (eg, aortic dissection and ischemic heart disease). Although fentanyl is less likely than other opioids to produce hypotension in the suggested doses, it should not be given to patients who are dependent on their sympathetic drive such as those in compensated shock. Adverse reactions such as respiratory depression and chest rigidity can occur but are minimized when fentanyl is given slowly.

Pretreatment with atropine does not consistently prevent bradycardia in children and is no longer recommended for all children undergoing emergent intubation; however, it should be available at the bedside for administration if symptomatic bradycardia occurs.[30] Pretreatment of head-injured patients with a small dose of a nondepolarizing neuromuscular blocking agent is no longer recommended.[26]

Selecting an Induction Agent in the Critically Ill Patient

Etomidate, a nonbarbiturate hypnotic, is a commonly used induction agent for RSI (Table 2-4). Its advantages in critically ill patients include relative protection from myocardial and cerebral ischemia, minimal histamine release, a stable hemodynamic profile, and a short duration of action. There is no conclusive evidence that a single dose of etomidate given for RSI affects patient outcome through cortisol inhibition, even in septic shock.[31]

PEARL

Despite being regarded as having a stable hemodynamic profile, etomidate can cause some myocardial suppression; therefore, reduced doses (0.1–0.2 mg/kg) should be used in hypotensive patients and in those with significant left ventricular dysfunction.

Propofol is another effective induction agent for emergent RSI. Compared with etomidate, it has a more rapid onset of action and a shorter duration of action. Some of the pharmacologic advantages include its anticonvulsant properties and its ability to lower intracranial pressure. It does not cause his-

TABLE 2-4.

RSI drugs for the critically ill patient

	Drugs	Dose	Indication	Dose in Shock States
Pretreatment agents	Lidocaine	1.5 mg/kg IV	Increased ICP Bronchospasm	Not indicated
	Fentanyl	3 mcg/kg IV	Increased ICP Cardiac ischemia Aortic dissection	Not indicated
	Atropine	0.02 mg/kg IV	Bradycardia from laryngoscopy or succinylcholine	0.02 mg/kg IV
Induction agents	Etomidate	0.3 mg/kg IV	RSI	0.1 mg/kg IV
	Propofol	0.5–1.5 mg/kg IV	RSI in hemodynamically stable patients	Not indicated
	Ketamine	1–2 mg/kg IV	Hypotension Status asthmaticus	0.5 mg/kg IV

tamine release but can cause hypotension through myocardial suppression and vasodilation. Because of its potential to cause hypotension, propofol should be avoided in patients with potential hemodynamic compromise.

Ketamine is a dissociative induction agent that also provides analgesia and amnesia. In many ways, it is an ideal agent to consider in critically ill patients. It causes increases in blood pressure and heart rate through catecholamine release and is therefore useful in hypotensive patients. Ketamine causes direct smooth muscle relaxation and bronchodilation and is the induction agent of choice for patients with refractory status asthmaticus. Its ability to preserve the respiratory drive makes it an ideal agent for sedation during awake intubation and when using flexible fiberoptics. Despite its potential to increase heart rate and blood pressure, ketamine does not appear to cause an increase in ICP. Some studies suggest that it has possible cerebroprotective effects.[32] Because of its inotropic and chronotropic cardiac effects, ketamine is not preferred in the elderly or in patients with a potential for cardiac ischemia. When being used with fiberoptics in awake patients, pretreatment with atropine can attenuate the increased secretion production that ketamine can cause (Table 2-4).

Paralytics in the Critically Ill Patient

The most commonly used neuromuscular blocking agents during RSI are succinylcholine, rocuronium, and vecuronium. Succinylcholine has the most rapid onset and, compared with other agents, appears to provide the best intubating conditions at 60 seconds.[33,34] Its duration of action (8–10 minutes) is also much shorter, which is an advantage should difficulty with intubation occur. It is rapidly hydrolyzed by cholinesterase; therefore, its clearance is independent of hepatic or renal function. Succinylcholine is a depolarizing agent and will cause a transient increase in serum potassium of about 0.5 mEq/L; however, in patients with receptor up-regulation, a significant life-threatening hyperkalemic response can occur. Critically ill patients who sustained a significant burn, crush injury, or denervation injury more than 5 days earlier are at risk, as well as patients with preexisting myopathies (Table 2-5).

Rocuronium is an intermediate-duration, nondepolarizing agent that is another option for RSI if there is a potential contraindication to succinylcholine. Some clinicians prefer rocuronium as the primary neuromuscular blocking agent for RSI.[33] By increasing the dose of rocuronium to 1 mg/kg, the onset of action approximates that of succinylcholine, but its duration of action is prolonged to approximately 45 minutes. Vecuronium can also be used in a higher dose (0.2 mg/kg) to achieve a more rapid onset (between 1 and 2 minutes); however, the duration of paralysis can be 60 to 120 minutes.

A new class of reversal agents, called selective relaxant binding agents, can reverse a long-acting nondepolarizing neuromuscular blocker prior to spontaneous recovery. Sugammadex, a selective relaxant binding agent, reverses blockade within a few minutes. However, studies have raised concerns over hypersensitivity reactions.[35] As of early 2010, sugammadex has been approved for use in Europe but not the United States.

Patients in Shock

Critically ill patients who present in shock are, by definition, hemodynamically compromised and could have limited pulmonary reserve. Any procedure that exacerbates the underlying cardiopulmonary deficit could lead to significant morbidity or death. The clinician must weigh the potential detrimental effects of intubation and the time it could take to mitigate them against the urgency of airway protection, oxygenation, and ventilation.

Preoxygenation is critical in the patient with compromised tissue perfusion. In the absence of significant airway difficulty, RSI remains the preferred method of intubation; however, appropriate drug selection is important. In patients in shock, pretreatment agents are not indicated and, in some cases, could exacerbate hypotension. Induction agents must be selected carefully to avoid further deterioration of cardiac output and perfusion. Rarely, some situations preclude any induction agent; however, a reduced dose of etomidate or ketamine, or possibly an amnestic (non-induction) dose of midazolam, should be considered. Propofol should not be used as an induction agent in patients with cardiogenic or septic shock because of its propensity to cause hypotension through myocardial suppression and venous dilatation. There is also a possible association with cardiac failure and acidosis when propofol is used in critically ill patients, referred to as the propofol infusion syndrome. This is usually described in the context of prolonged infusions or very high doses.[36,37]

Once the patient is intubated, positive-pressure ventilation can impair venous return and cardiac filling, reducing cardiac output and potentially exacerbating hypotension. If time allows, hypotension responsive to intravenous fluids should be managed aggressively prior to intubation. Rapid boluses of crystalloid should be considered as possible pretreatment in all anticipated intubations in critically ill patients. Because these patients might also have an associated metabolic acidosis, some consideration might be given to increased minute ventilation if cardiac output is not compromised. Even transiently impaired ventilation during an otherwise rapid and effective intubation will significantly worsen an acidosis and cause further cardiovascular compromise. This can also occur in patients with severe metabolic acidosis secondary to causes other than shock (eg, acute aspirin overdose).

TABLE 2-5.

Conditions associated with succinylcholine-induced hyperkalemia

More than 5 days after the following:
Burns
Denervation injury
Significant crush injuries
Severe infection
Preexisting myopathies
Preexisting hyperkalemia

KEY POINT

Rapid boluses of crystalloid should be considered as possible pretreatment in all anticipated intubations in critically ill patients.

Techniques to Improve Laryngoscopy

The intubation success rate using RSI approaches 99% for both emergency physicians and anesthesiologists. Success varies with level of training and experience; therefore, one response to a failed intubation should be an immediate intubation attempt by a more experienced clinician, if one is available.[8,9]

The most common reasons for intubation failures are inadequate equipment preparation and poor patient positioning. Before proceeding with RSI, it is critical that the clinician pause to run through a short checklist with the team, ensuring that all the equipment is working and at the bedside (Table 2-2). Following a failed intubation attempt, simple maneuvers to optimize the patient's position should be the first step. Proper bed height, positioning the head of the patient at the end of the stretcher, and, in the absence of cervical spine precautions, extension at the atlanto-occipital joint can improve visualization. Elevation of the head with a pad under the occiput can help align the pharyngeal and tracheal visual axes, particularly in obese patients. Ideally, the ear canal should lie in a horizontal plane with the anterior shoulder. A laryngoscopic technique that involves the application of backward-upward-rightward pressure (BURP) on the thyroid cartilage (not the cricoid ring) can enhance visualization of an anterior glottis.[38,39] In a modification of this maneuver, called bimanual laryngoscopy, the intubator manipulates the larynx with the right hand until ideal visualization is achieved and then an assistant maintains this position.[38] Direct cricoid pressure, the Sellick maneuver, has

TABLE 2-6.

Airway management tools. Adapted from: Vissers RJ, Gibbs M. The high risk airway. *Emerg Med Clin North Am.* 2010:28;203-217. Copyright 2010. Adapted with permission.

BVM ventilation

Direct laryngoscopy

Intubating stylets (the bougie)

Supraglottic rescue devices
  Blind insertion devices
    Double-balloon esophageal airways
    Laryngeal mask airways
  Direct visualization
    Video laryngoscopy
    Flexible fiberoptics
    Fiberoptic stylets

Subglottic rescue devices
    Open surgical cricothyrotomy
    Percutaneous cricothyrotomy
    Retrograde intubation
    Transtracheal jet ventilation

been recommended to prevent passive regurgitation of gastric contents during intubation of an unconscious or paralyzed patient. However, its effectiveness is in question, and it has been shown to impair the laryngoscopic view and insertion of the endotracheal tube.[40] In a difficult laryngoscopy, cricoid pressure should be released.

When an intubation attempt fails, the first priority is to oxygenate through BVM ventilation. Between attempts, it is critical that the technique, position, provider, or equipment is changed to improve the likelihood of success. Preparation for a possible rescue airway must be considered. Persistence without altering the technique and attempts at blind passage are usually met with failure and anoxia and are therefore discouraged. It is important to recognize when further attempts at laryngoscopy are unlikely to succeed.

KEY POINT

Persistence in laryngoscopy beyond three attempts has been associated with low success and increased morbidity and mortality and should be abandoned in favor of an alternative management strategy.[41]

Rescue Devices

The number of airway rescue devices available to the clinician managing the critically ill patient in the emergent setting has increased dramatically. In some cases, this represents an enhancement or adoption of devices with a long history of use and success within the specialty of anesthesia, making them effective or affordable in the emergency setting. The recent introduction and proliferation of the use of video laryngoscopy are changing the approach to high-risk airway management in critically ill patients. The drive toward lower-cost and durable or disposable items, combined with rapid technological advances, suggests the number of airway options will continue to grow, and one of them may indeed replace traditional laryngoscopy as the primary airway management technique.

Although the variety of choices is exciting, it can be intimidating as well. The relative infrequency of emergent, difficult airway management suggests that it is not possible for emergency physicians to be proficient with all techniques, and having all the devices available would be cost prohibitive. Fortunately, most of these rescue devices fall into a few discrete categories, based on their anatomic approach (supraglottic versus subglottic) and whether they provide direct glottic visualization or not (blind insertion) (Table 2-6).

The first "rescue" from failed intubation or BVM ventilation should be better laryngoscopic and BVM ventilation techniques. Following that, the emergency physician should be comfortable using an intubating stylet and have at least one supraglottic rescue device and one subglottic surgical airway technique in the armamentarium. Facility with a fiberoptic or video laryngoscopic device is becoming increasingly desirable and achievable.

A mobile difficult-airway cart containing an appropriate variety of rescue devices should be available in all acute care settings (Table 2-3). The clinician should be familiar with the contents of this cart and be proficient with the available devices.

Management of a difficult airway in a critically ill patient is needed relatively infrequently; an emergency is not the time to learn a new technique. Expertise can be obtained in a number of ways outside the acute care setting. The controlled environment of the operating room has been used as a learning environment. High-fidelity simulation labs are increasingly available as optimal learning environments for development of skills and management approaches for the difficult airway in critically ill patients. A number of national courses are designed specifically to teach airway skills. Devices such as intubating stylets and video laryngoscopes can be used safely as the primary technique in routine, nondifficult airways.

Choosing a Rescue Strategy

Regardless of the rescue devices available, the clinician must integrate these techniques into a well-thought-out plan for managing the difficult or failed airway. Developing a thoughtful strategy, based on patient characteristics, that incorporates appropriate preparation and employs the optimal technique is always more important than the tools themselves. Because these are low-frequency events that can evolve rapidly, decision-making tools should be used to help frame a management strategy. Several algorithms have been proposed, such as the American Society of Anesthesiologists' difficult airway algorithm, which works well in the controlled operating room setting but is difficult to apply in the emergency department or critical care setting.[2] Other algorithms designed specifically for the emergency setting provide a logical framework for dealing with difficult and failed airways in critically ill patients.[42]

Whatever algorithm is chosen, elements common to all strategies are critical to successful airway management. Appropriate preparation of the patient and the equipment is essential. All patients should be preoxygenated and any physiologic chal-

FIGURE 2-2.

Difficult airway grid. From: Vissers RJ, Gibbs M. The high-risk airway. *Emerg Med Clin North Am.* 2010:28;203-217. Copyright 2010. Used with permission.

	Is anatomy normal or abnormal?	
	Normal anatomy Adequate oxygenation	Abnormal anatomy Adequate oxygenation
	Normal anatomy Inadequate oxygenation	Abnormal anatomy Inadequate oxygenation

(Row label, left side: Is oxygenation adequate?)

TABLE 2-7.

Principles and solutions for clinical scenarios in Figure 2-2. Based on: Vissers RJ, Gibbs M. The high-risk airway. *Emerg Med Clin North Am.* 2010:28;203-217. Copyright 2010. Used with permission.

Principles	Solutions
Normal Anatomy + Adequate Oxygenation	
You have time.	Hand-held fiberoptics are available.
No need for a surgical airway	Any of these should work.
Blind-insertion devices (BID) are appropriate.	Hand-held fiberoptics are not available.
Hand-held fiberoptics are ideal.	First choice: I-LMA
Cuffed tube is the goal.	Second choice: intubating stylet
Normal Anatomy + Inadequate Oxygenation	
No time	Hand-held fiberoptics are available.
Multiple BID attempts are inappropriate.	Limited attempts with these, then surgical airway
Use what you know best.	Hand-held fiberoptics are not available.
Surgical airway if first rescue plan fails	Limited attempts with I-LMA, then surgical airway
Abnormal Anatomy + Adequate Oxygenation	
BID is risky.	Hand-held fiberoptics are available.
Direct airway visualization is preferred.	Limited attempts with fiberoptic
Fiberoptic okay if view not obscured by blood	Surgical airway if unsuccessful
Surgical airway backup	Hand-held fiberoptics are not available.
	Surgical airway
Abnormal Anatomy + Inadequate Oxygenation	
No time	Hand-held fiberoptics are available.
BIDs are contraindicated.	One attempt with fiberoptic
Fiberoptic okay if view not obscured by blood	Surgical airway if unsuccessful
Surgical is often the best first choice.	Hand-held fiberoptics are not available.
	Surgical airway

lenges should be addressed to mitigate the undesirable effects of emergent intubation. The use of an "awake look" is an important technique in emergent difficult airway assessment and is becoming easier to perform with the increased availability of video-assisted airway devices. Recognizing the need for help from other consultants or colleagues is the key to success in some circumstances. Finally, the subglottic surgical airway is the "last resort" strategy in most difficult airway management situations.

Selecting the airway device most appropriate for the particular airway scenario can be challenging. Which tool to use may be limited by what is available and the skill set of the clinician. Because of the variety of devices and the variability of what is available in different settings, it may be best to consider rescue devices by their category. One approach uses a four-box grid based on the responses to two basic questions to help develop an appropriate plan and a rescue strategy (Figure 2-2, Table 2-7).[1] In the context of this framework, an "abnormal anatomy" implies disrupted or altered anatomy, not just anticipated difficulty in visualizing the glottis. Examples of a difficult airway with "abnormal anatomy" include trauma, burn, hematoma, cancer, abscess, foreign body, and angioedema. Examples of a difficult airway with "normal anatomy" include obesity, a small mouth, and a high anterior larynx.

Conclusion

Airway management is essential to the practice of emergency medicine. Critically ill patients will require emergent airway management for a myriad of reasons. It is crucial that emergency physicians be able to assess critically ill patients for the presence of a difficult airway, predict difficulty with BVM ventilation and intubation, and select appropriate rescue devices should direct laryngoscopy fail. Equally important in managing the difficult airway is the selection of appropriate pretreatment, induction, and paralytic medications for patients who are hemodynamically unstable.

References

1. Vissers RJ, Gibbs M. The high-risk airway. *Emerg Med Clin North Am.* 2010;28;203-217.
2. Practice Guidelines for Management of the Difficult Airway: an updated report by the American Society of Anesthesiologists Task Force on Management of the Difficult Airway. *Anesthesiology.* 2003;98:1269-1277.
3. Cormack RS, Lehane J. Difficult trachea intubation in obstetrics. *Anaesthesia.* 1984;39:1105-1111.
4. Murphy MF, Walls RM. Identification of the difficult and failed airway. In: Walls RM, Murphy MF, eds. *Manual of Emergency Airway Management.* 3rd ed. Philadelphia, PA: Lippincott Williams & Wilkins; 2008:81-93.
5. Sagarin MJ, Barton ED, Chang YM, et al. Airway management by U.S. and Canadian emergency medicine residents: a multicenter analysis of more than 6,000 endotracheal intubation attempts. *Ann Emerg Med.* 2005;46:328-336.
6. Levitan RM, Rosenblatt B, Meiner EM, et al. Alternating day emergency medicine and anesthesia resident responsibility for management of the trauma airway: a study of laryngoscopy performance and intubation success. *Ann Emerg Med.* 2004;43:48-53.
7. Sackles JC, Laurin EG, Rantapaa AA, et al. Airway management in the emergency department: a one-year study of 610 tracheal intubations. *Ann Emerg Med.* 1998;31:325-332.
8. Bair AE, Filbin MR, Kulkami R, et al. Failed intubation in the emergency department: analysis of prevalence, rescue techniques, and personnel. *J Emerg Med.* 2002;23:131-140.
9. Tayal VS, Riggs RW, Marx JA, et al. Rapid-sequence intubation at an emergency medicine residency: success rate and adverse events during a two-year period. *Acad Emerg Med.* 1999;6:31-37.
10. Peterson GN. Management of the difficult airway: a closed claims analysis. *Anesthesiology.* 2005;103:33-39.
11. Murphy M, Hung O, Launcelott G, et al. Predicting the difficult laryngoscopic intubation: are we on the right track? *Can J Anaesth.* 2005;52:231-235.
12. Langeron O, Masso E, Huraux C, et al. Prediction of difficult mask ventilation. *Anesthesiology.* 2000;92:1229-1236.
13. Kheterpal S, Han R, Tremper KK, et al. Incidence and predictors of difficult and impossible mask ventilation. *Anesthesiology.* 2006;105:885-891.
14. Murphy MF, Walls RM. The difficult and failed airway. In: Walls RM, Luten RC, Murphy MF, et al, eds. *Manual of Emergency Airway Management.* Philadelphia, PA: Lippincott Williams & Wilkins; 2000:31-39.
15. Reed MJ, Dunn MJ, McKeown DW. Can an airway assessment score predict difficulty at intubation in the emergency department? *Emerg Med J.* 2005;22:99-102.
16. Kortbeck JB, Al Turki SA, Ali J, et al. Advanced trauma life support, 8th edition, the evidence for change. *J Trauma.* 2008;64:1638-1650.
17. Lee A, Fan LT, Gin T, et al. A systematic review (meta-analysis) of the accuracy of the Mallampati tests to predict the difficult airway. *Anesth Analg.* 2006;102:1867-1878.
18. Parmet JL, Colonna-Romano P, Horrow JC, et al. The laryngeal mask airway reliably provides rescue ventilation in cases of unanticipated difficult tracheal intubation along with difficult mask ventilation. *Anesth Analg.* 1998;87:661-665.
19. Kovacs G, Law JA, Petrie D. Awake fiberoptic intubation using an optical stylet in an anticipated difficult airway. *Ann Emerg Med.* 2007;49:81-83.
20. Vissers RJ, Bair AE. Surgical airway techniques. In: Walls RM, Murphy MF, eds. *Manual of Emergency Airway Management.* 3rd ed. Philadelphia, PA: Lippincott Williams & Wilkins; 2008:193-220.
21. Fox EJ, Sklar GS, Hill CH, et al. Complications related to the pressor response to endotracheal intubation. *Anaesthesiology.* 1977;47:524-525.
22. Benumof JL, Dagg R, Benumof R. Critical hemoglobin desaturation will occur before return to an unparalyzed state following 1 mg/kg of intravenous succinylcholine. *Anesthesiology.* 1997;87:979-982.
23. Caro DA, Bush S. Pretreatment agents. In: Walls RM, Murphy MF, eds. *Manual of Emergency Airway Management.* 3rd ed. Philadelphia, PA: Lippincott Williams & Wilkins; 2008:222-233.
24. Bozeman WP, Idris AH. Intracranial pressure changes during rapid sequence intubation: a swine model. *J Trauma.* 2005;58:278-283.
25. Robinson N, Clancy M. In patients with head injury undergoing rapid sequence intubation, does pretreatment with intravenous lignocaine/lidocaine lead to an improved neurological outcome? A review of the literature. *Emerg Med J.* 2001;18:453-457.
26. Butler J, Jackson R. Towards evidence based emergency medicine: best BETS from Manchester Royal Infirmary. Lignocaine premedication before rapid sequence induction in head injuries. *Emerg Med J.* 2002;19:554.
27. Maslow A, Regan M, Israel E, et al. Inhaled albuterol, but not intravenous lidocaine, protects against intubation-induced bronchoconstriction in asthma. *Anesthesiology.* 2000;93:1198-1204.
28. Reynolds SF, Heffner J. Airway management of the critically ill patient: rapid sequence intubation. *Chest.* 2005;127:1397-1412.
29. Weiss-Bloom L, Reich D. Haemodynamic responses to tracheal intubation following etomidate and fentanyl for anaesthetic induction. *Can J Anaesth.* 1992;39:780-785.
30. Fleming B, McCollough M, Henderson SO. Myth: atropine should be administered before succinylcholine for neonatal and pediatric intubation. *Can J Emerg Med.* 2005;7:114-117.
31. Walls RM, Murphy MF. Clinical controversies: etomidate as an induction agent for endotracheal intubation in patients with sepsis: continue to use etomidate for intubation of patients with septic shock. *Ann Emerg Med.* 2008;52:13-14.
32. Sehdev RS, Symmons DA, Kindl K. Ketamine for rapid sequence induction in patients with head injury in the emergency department. *Emerg Med Australas.* 2006;18:37-44.
33. Mallon WK, Keim SM, Schoenberg JM, et al. Rocuronium vs succinylcholine in the emergency department: a critical appraisal. *J Emerg Med.* 2009;37:183-188.
34. Naguib M, Samarkandi AH, El-Din ME, et al. The dose of succinylcholine required for excellent endotracheal intubating conditions. *Anesth Analg.* 2006;102:151-155.
35. Sparr HJ, Vermeyen KM, Beaufort AM, et al. Early reversal of profound rocuronium-induced neuromuscular blockade by sugammadex in a randomized multicenter study: efficacy, safety, and pharmacokinetics. *Anesthesiology.* 2007;106:935-943.
36. Vernooy K, Delhaas T, Cremer O, et al. Electrocardiographic changes predicting sudden death in propofol-related infusion syndrome. *Heart Rhythm.* 2004;3;131-137.
37. Perrier ND, Baerga-Varela Y, Murray MJ. Death related to propofol use in an adult patient. *Crit Care Med.* 2000;28:3071-3074.
38. Levitan RM, Kinkle WC, Levin WJ, Everett WW. Laryngeal view during laryngoscopy: a randomized trial comparing cricoid pressure, backward-upward-rightward pressure, and bimanual laryngoscopy. *Ann Emerg Med.* 2006;47:548-555.
39. Knill RL. Difficult laryngoscopy made easy with a "BURP." *Can J Anaesth.* 1993;84:419-421.
40. Hartsilver EL, Vanner RG. Airway obstruction with cricoid pressure. *Anaesthesia.* 2000;55:208-211.

41. Mort TC. Emergency tracheal intubation: complications associated with repeated laryngoscopic attempts. *Anesth Analg.* 2004;99:607-613.

42. Walls RM. The emergency airway algorithms. In: Walls RM, Murphy MF, eds. *Manual of Emergency Airway Management.* 3rd ed. Philadelphia, PA: Lippincott Williams & Wilkins; 2008:9-22.

CHAPTER 3

The Crashing Ventilated Patient

Jairo I. Santanilla

IN THIS CHAPTER

Evaluation of hemodynamically unstable ventilated patients in distress

Management of hemodynamically unstable ventilated patients

Special scenarios: pediatric patients and patients with a tracheostomy

Introduction

Critically ill patients present to the emergency department every day. Some of them required intubation in the prehospital setting; others are intubated on arrival or during emergency department evaluation. After their airways have been secured and their conditions stabilized, patients can remain in the emergency department because of a lack of critical care beds. In some hospitals, a dedicated intensivist will take charge of these patients, but in others this type of coverage is not available at all or not around the clock. Thus, acute complications or deteriorations must be handled by emergency physicians.

This chapter provides a framework for managing the crashing mechanically ventilated patient. The information provided will assist the practitioner in determining if the patient's condition is related to the underlying pathology that necessitated mechanical ventilation or if it is being caused by mechanical ventilation itself. This chapter does not fully address basic ventilator management, noninvasive positive-pressure ventilation, advanced trauma life support, or advanced cardiovascular life support (ACLS).

Determine Hemodynamic Stability

The initial step in managing the crashing ventilated patient is to determine the patient's hemodynamic stability. The ventilated patient is, by definition, critically ill. However, he or she can fall anywhere on the spectrum from being ventilated for airway protection, with normal vital signs, blood pressure, and oxygen saturation, to being ventilated and in cardiac arrest. Determining where the patient is on this spectrum, including assessing for hypotension and hypoxia, will dictate how much time the practitioner has to implement rescue strategies. In addition, it is important to anticipate the patient's clinical course. The approach to a patient who is intubated for hypoxia stemming from pneumonia and whose blood pressure and oxygenation gradually trend down over hours or days is different from the approach to a patient who is declining over a span of minutes (Figure 3-1).

As a general rule, the following evaluation should be performed within 1 hour on patients with new unexplained hypotension (systolic blood pressure [SBP] <90 mm Hg), new unexplained hypoxia (SaO_2 <90%), or a new marked change in vital signs (a drop in SBP by more than 20 points or a drop in SaO_2 by more than 10%). Patients with *stable* SBP between 80 and 90 mm Hg and SaO_2 between 80% and 90% should be evaluated expeditiously, with the hope of halting the decline. Those with SBP <80 mm Hg or an SaO_2 <80% and those who continue to decline rapidly should be evaluated quickly, with consideration given to entering the cardiac arrest/near arrest algorithm. These

FIGURE 3-1.

The crashing ventilated patient algorithm. The steps are discussed in more detail in the main text. For the differential diagnosis in difficult-to-ventilate patients, see Table 3-2.

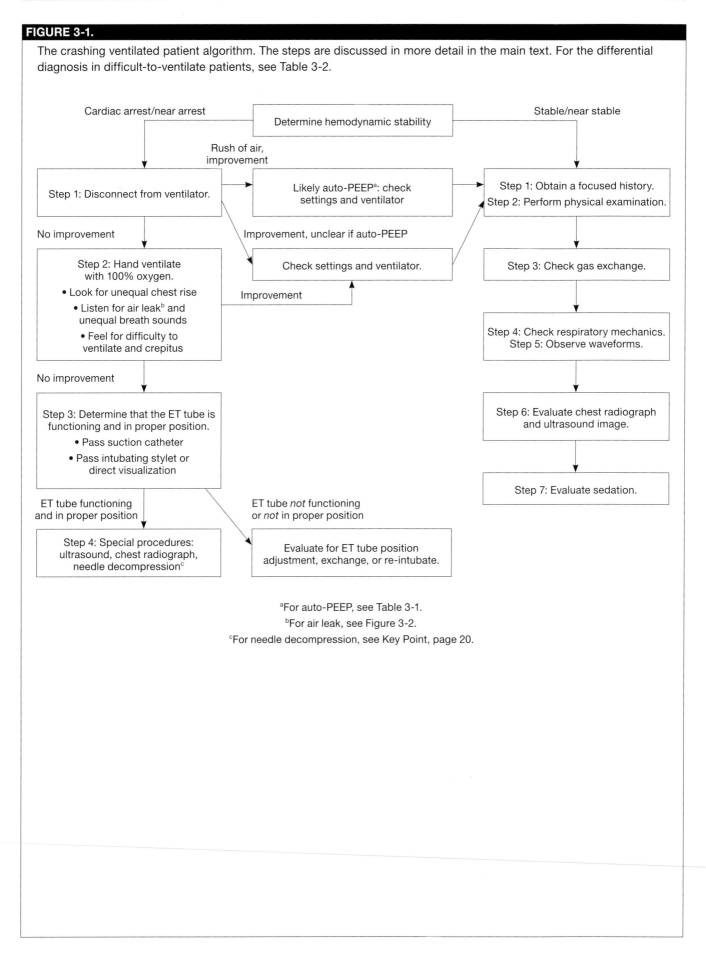

[a]For auto-PEEP, see Table 3-1.
[b]For air leak, see Figure 3-2.
[c]For needle decompression, see Key Point, page 20.

FIGURE 3-2.

Approach to the ventilated patient with an air leak

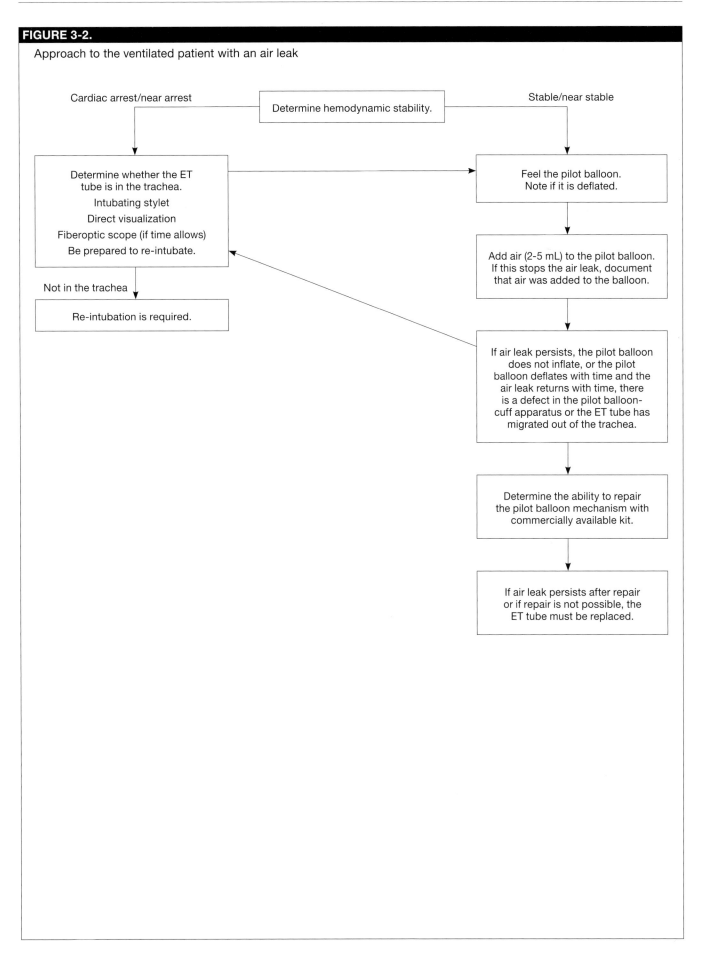

values are arbitrary demarcation points and do not take precedence over clinical judgment.

PEARL

The initial step in managing the crashing ventilated patient is to determine the patient's hemodynamic stability.

KEY POINT

Important questions to ask:

- How stable is the patient?
- How rapidly is the patient deteriorating?
- How much time is there to determine the cause of the instability and address the problems?

The Cardiac Arrest/Near Arrest Patient

Time is of the essence in the patient with cardiac arrest or near arrest. ACLS algorithms should be implemented quickly. Additionally, there are some key points to remember in the ventilated patient who has a cardiac arrest or becomes acutely hemodynamically unstable. The emergency department practitioner should develop a step-wise approach in this situation. During each step, the practitioner should "look, listen, and feel" to run through the differential diagnosis.

During the stabilization of these patients, it is important to keep in mind the original pathology that necessitated intubation. The crashing ventilated patient could simply be growing worse from the primary pathology. The multitrauma patient could have an intrathoracic or intraabdominal catastrophe, and the septic patient could be deteriorating clinically from lack of source control.

However, it is also important to determine and address special circumstances that the ventilator can precipitate. The most significant of these are tension pneumothorax and severe auto-positive end-expiratory pressure (auto-PEEP). Tension pneumothorax can lead to marked hypotension because of decreased cardiac output and marked hypoxia from ventilation perfusion mismatch.[1] Auto-PEEP (also referred to as intrinsic PEEP, breath stacking, or dynamic hyperinflation) is caused by trapped volume in the pulmonary system. If severe enough, it will eventually lead to increased intrathoracic pressure. This can cause hypotension and decreased cardiac output from decreased venous return as well as marked hypoxia from ventilation perfusion mismatch.[2]

KEY POINT

Patients on volume-targeted modes with obstructive or reactive airway disease, those on volume-targeted modes receiving a high minute ventilation, and those receiving inverse-ratio ventilation are at risk for auto-PEEP (breath stacking).

PEARL

Tension pneumothorax and severe auto-PEEP are important causes of ventilator-induced hemodynamic instability.

In critically ill ventilated patients who develop respiratory distress and are hemodynamically unstable, the following steps will assist the emergency physician in determining the cause of decompensation (Figure 3-1).

Step 1: Disconnect the patient from the ventilator.

This is perhaps the easiest step to perform. It can be both diagnostic and therapeutic in the crashing ventilated patient. A quick rush of air or a prolonged expiration of trapped air from the endotracheal (ET) tube can be diagnostic of ventilator-induced auto-PEEP (Table 3-1). A few seconds of observation can determine if this is the case. Return of hemodynamic stability implies that the maneuver was successful.

Patients undergoing cardiopulmonary resuscitation (CPR) should not be connected to a ventilator. The intrathoracic pressure variations caused by CPR will trigger ventilator breaths at high rates if the ventilator is set on assist-control. Patients on inhaled nitric oxide should not be removed from the nitric oxide abruptly, and efforts should be made to quickly reestablish the supply through the bag-valve-mask system. In addition, care should be taken when disconnecting patients who are on high PEEP such as those with acute respiratory distress syndrome (ARDS). Although it is important to disconnect the patient from the ventilator to address causes of auto-PEEP, derecruitment could occur and hypoxia could be worsened. Once auto-PEEP has been ruled out, PEEP valves may be used to maintain the extrinsic PEEP levels and thus avoid derecruitment. PEEP valves can be problematic in the markedly hypotensive patient, as they could increase intrathoracic pressures and thereby decrease venous return.

PEARL

Inhaled nitric oxide should not be discontinued abruptly because this could cause rebound pulmonary hypertension. Administration should be reestablished quickly through the bag-valve-mask system.

TABLE 3-1.
Managing auto-PEEP

Determine what caused the auto-PEEP   • High set respiratory rate, high patient respiratory rate, obstructive airway disease
Consider decreasing the tidal volume in patients with obstructive or reactive airway disease
Consider decreasing the set respiratory rate   • Will be ineffective in assist-control mode with a high intrinsic rate
Optimize sedation   • Use opiates to control respiratory rate
Monitor ventilator flow-time waveform
Consider changing to synchronized intermittent ventilation
Consider chemical paralysis

Step 2: Breathing—Hand ventilate with 100% oxygen.

Ensure that 100% oxygen is being delivered and limit the respiratory rate to 8 to 10 breaths per minute. Particular attention should be given to the delivery of hand ventilation. Inadvertent rates as high as 40 breaths per minute are often used in codes.[3,4] Excessive rates will increase intrathoracic pressures, leading to a decrease in venous return and cardiac output.[5] Look at both sides of the chest to determine if there is equal chest rise. Unequal chest rise can signify a main-stem intubation, pneumothorax, or mucus plug. Listen for air escaping from the mouth or nose (a sign of an air leak). Listen over the epigastric area and in both axilla. Decreased breath sounds could indicate main-stem intubation, pneumothorax, or atelectatic lung. Feel for subcutaneous crepitus (a sign of pneumothorax) and assess for difficulty in hand ventilating (a sign of low dynamic or static respiratory system compliance [Table 3-2]).

Step 3: Airway—Determine that the endotracheal tube is functioning and in the proper position.

The ET tube functions by providing a conduit to the lower trachea. Its cuff attempts to create a seal between it and the inner wall of the trachea. To determine if it is functioning properly, pass the suction catheter and listen for an air leak (Figure 3-2). Easy passage of the suction catheter does not guarantee that the ET tube is in the trachea because the catheter could be passing down the esophagus; however, if it is difficult or impossible to pass the suction catheter, the tube is either dislodged,

TABLE 3-2.
Causes of decreased respiratory system compliance

Causes of high peak pressures (increased airflow resistance, decreased dynamic compliance)
Airway
- Biting on the ET tube
- Bronchospasm
- Obstruction of the ET tube by secretions, mucus, blood
- Twisted ET tube

Pulmonary
- Partial mucus plugging

Causes of high plateau pressures (low respiratory system compliance, decreased static compliance)
Pulmonary
- ARDS/acute lung injury (ALI)
- Atelectasis
- Auto-PEEP
- Mucus plugging
- Pneumonia
- Pneumothorax
- Pulmonary edema
- Unilateral intubation

Chest wall
- Chest wall rigidity
- Circumferential chest wall burn
- Obesity

Other
- Abdominal distention/pressure

obstructed, or twisted or the patient is biting the tube. Attempt to correct a twisted or bent ET tube by repositioning the patient's head; if the patient is biting on the tube, insert a bite block. Dislodged or obstructed ET tubes require re-intubation. Patients with dislodged tubes should be treated as difficult intubations because unplanned extubations are notorious for causing trauma to the glottis, leading to vocal cord edema.[6]

In the cardiac arrest or near arrest patient, the best choice for determining that the ET tube is in the proper position is direct visualization of the tube passing through the cords. This step is often omitted in the crashing ventilated patient because of the belief that the tube has not migrated. Unfortunately, unrecognized ET tube migration can occur during routine care of the critically ill patient. Patients are frequently moved in and out of EMS vehicles, transferred to and from stretchers for imaging studies, and turned for procedures or bathing, all of which can dislodge the tube. This visualization step can be performed while providing hand ventilation.

Other simple techniques may be used to confirm that the ET tube is in the trachea. Direct visualization of the carina with a fiberoptic scope is an option, but this device is typically not readily available in an emergency department. Another quick and readily available technique is to pass an intubating stylet (gum elastic bougie or Eschmann introducer) gently through the ET tube.[7] If resistance is met at 30 cm, the ET tube is in the trachea. If however, the stylet passes beyond 35 cm without resistance, the tube is likely in the esophagus. If resistance is met too soon, the intubating stylet may be catching on the tube.

At least one of these techniques to determine proper positioning should be employed early enough in the code to correct any airway issues. In addition, improper positioning should be confirmed before simply removing the tube and re-intubating the patient, particularly if the patient is thought to have a difficult airway (unless it is glaringly evident that the patient is extubated).

PEARL
If it is difficult or impossible to pass the suction catheter, the ET tube is either dislodged, obstructed, or twisted or the patient is biting the tube.

KEY POINT
Passage of an intubating stylet (gum elastic bougie or Eschmann introducer) is a quick, simple, and readily available technique for confirming that the ET tube is in the trachea.

- Gently pass the intubating stylet through the ET tube—do not force it.
- Resistance should be encountered at approximately 30 cm.
- Passage of the stylet beyond 35 cm without resistance implies that the ET tube is in the esophagus.

Step 4: Special Procedures

If the patient is still in cardiac arrest or near arrest after being disconnected from the ventilator, ensuring proper placement of the ET tube, and hand ventilating with 100% oxygen, a clinical decision will be required regarding needle decompression of the chest. If time permits, a focused history from the bedside nurse, respiratory therapist, or paramedic and a focused physical examination will indicate which side of the chest to decompress. In addition, depending on the urgency of the situation, bedside ultrasonography and chest radiography may be employed. The presence of a "lung-slide" artifact on bedside ultrasonography excludes pneumothorax. The lung slide artifact appears in M-mode as the "seashore sign" (Figure 3-3); its absence appears as the "stratosphere sign/bar-code sign" (Figure 3-4).[8-10]

At times, the clinical situation does not allow for imaging studies, and the focused history and physical examination may not be helpful. In these cases, needle decompression of both sides of the chest should be considered if other more likely causes of acute decompensation are not found. It is important to remember that chest tube placement is required in patients after needle decompression.[11-13]

PEARL

Use ultrasonography to quickly evaluate for pneumothorax.

KEY POINT

Needle Decompression

- Determine which side to decompress first.
- Identify the second intercostal space, in the midclavicular line.
- Prepare the area with chlorhexidine if time permits.
- Anesthetize the area if the patient is conscious and time permits.
- Insert an over-the-needle catheter over the rib.
  - A 14-gauge catheter, at least 5 cm is preferred
  - May need a different size needle depending on the size of the patient
- Puncture the parietal pleura while listening for a sudden escape of air.
- Remove the needle while leaving the catheter in place.
- Secure the catheter with a bandage or small dressing.
- Prepare for chest tube thoracostomy.

The Stable/Near Stable Patient

If the patient is deemed stable or near stable or quickly regains stability after disconnection from the ventilator and hand ventilation, the event should be approached in a systematic manner (Figure 3-1). The patient should be placed on 100% oxygen during this evaluation.

Step 1: Obtain a focused history.

A focused history should be obtained from the practitioners most involved with the patient's care (bedside nurse, respiratory therapist, resident, and paramedic). Valuable information includes the indication for intubation, the difficulty of the intubation, the depth of the ET tube, the ventilator settings, and recent procedures or moves (central line insertion; chest tube placement; removal or transition to water seal; thoracentesis;

endotracheal tube manipulation; transport off stretcher; rotation for cleaning, a procedure, or chest radiograph).

Step 2: Perform a focused physical examination.

Take a general survey of the patient. Observe for agitation, attempts to pull at the ET tube and lines, gasping for breath (the patient will have the mouth open and appear dyspneic), and tearing of the eyes.

Airway. Look at the ET tube, and determine if it has migrated from its previous position. It is possible that it has migrated out of the trachea or into a main bronchus. Adjust if necessary. Listen for escaping air (an air leak) from the mouth or nose (Figure 3-2). This typically signifies that the tube has lost its seal with the trachea and occurs in extubation or cuff failure. Feel the pilot balloon; if it is deflated, the cuff is deflated. Add air to the pilot balloon. If this stops the air leak, make a note that air was added to the balloon. If the pilot balloon does not inflate or deflates with time, there is a defect in the pilot balloon-cuff apparatus and the ET tube will likely need to be exchanged. Occasionally it may be possible to repair the pilot balloon mechanism with commercially available kits. This is a good option in patients who are difficult to intubate.

PEARL

If the pilot balloon does not inflate or deflates with time, there is a defect in the pilot balloon-cuff apparatus, and the ET tube will likely need to be exchanged.

Determine that the ET tube is functioning properly by passing the suction catheter. If it is difficult or not possible to pass the suction catheter, the endotracheal tube is either dislodged, obstructed, or twisted, or the patient is biting the tube. Attempt to correct a twisted or bent ET tube by repositioning the head; insert a bite block if the patient is biting on the tube. Dislodged or obstructed tubes require re-intubation.

If extubation is suspected at any point in the evaluation, determine that the ET tube is in proper position. Any of the techniques discussed in the previous section may be used.

TABLE 3-3.

Initial ventilator settings for ALI/ARDS

Volume-targeted, assist control
Tidal volume: 6–8 mL/kg ideal body weight • Can start at 8 mL/kg ideal body weight and work down to 6 within 4 hours
Respiratory rate: Set to approximate baseline minute ventilation (not to exceed 35 breaths/min)
PEEP: 5–8 cm H_2O • Titrate up based on protocol
F_{IO_2}: 100% • Titrate down based on protocol
Flow rate: 60 L/min
Keep plateau pressures <30 cm H_2O

KEY POINTS

- Is the ET tube in proper position?
  - Did it migrate out of the trachea?
  - Did it migrate down into the main bronchus?
- Is it functioning properly?

Breathing. Look at both sides of the chest to determine if there is equal chest rise. Unequal chest rise can signify a main-stem intubation, pneumothorax, or mucus plug. Look at the ventilator tubing and determine if there is an oscillating water collection. Listen for air escaping from the mouth or nose (a sign of an air leak). Listen over the epigastric area and in both axilla. Decreased breath sounds may provide clues regarding main-stem intubation, pneumothorax, or atelectatic lung. Feel for subcutaneous crepitus (a sign of pneumothorax).

KEY POINT

Dealing with whole-lung atelectasis:

- Use recruitment maneuvers
  - Disconnect from ventilator and provide hand ventilation at higher tidal volumes
- Provide frequent suctioning
- Rotate patient
- Perform chest percussion
- Administer bronchodilators
- Perform bronchoscopy

Circulation. Check for pulses, and cycle the blood pressure cuff frequently. If the patient has an arterial line, make sure the transducer is level. Determine the need for fluid bolus and/or vasopressors.

Step 3: Assess gas exchange.

Hypoxia can be diagnosed based on pulse oximetry if the waveform is reliable. The waveform should not be highly variable, and the frequency of the waveform should match the heart rate on the cardiac monitor. In a few instances, such as carbon monoxide poisoning, pulse oximetry is not reliable.[14] In these cases, or if the pulse oximeter is not picking up, an arterial blood gas (ABG) sample should be obtained. Patients with a Pao_2/Fio_2 ratio less than 200 should be evaluated for ARDS. Those with a ratio between 200 and 300 should be evaluated for acute lung injury (ALI).[15] A lung-protective strategy should be implemented in those found to have ALI or ARDS (Table 3-3).[16] Hypoventilation cannot be identified based on pulse oximetry; ABG measurement is beneficial in this event.

PEARL

Hypoventilation cannot be identified based on pulse oximetry; ABG measurement is beneficial in this event.

Step 4: Check respiratory mechanics.

Determine if the peak pressures and plateau pressures have changed from their previous values. These values should be obtained on volume-targeted modes. Airway pressures are a function of volume and respiratory system compliance. The respiratory system incorporates the ventilator circuit, ET tube, trachea, bronchi, pulmonary parenchyma, and chest wall. A set volume with a set system compliance results in a specific pressure. Peak pressures are a function of the volume, resistance to airflow, and respiratory system compliance. The plateau pressure is obtained during an inspiratory pause, thus eliminating airflow, and therefore reflects only the respiratory system compliance. An isolated increase in the peak pressure is indicative of increased resistance to airflow; an isolated increase in the

FIGURE 3-3.

Seashore sign. The lung-slide artifact appears in ultrasound M-mode as the seashore sign. This excludes pneumothorax. Image courtesy of Dr. Christine Butts and Dr. Matthew Bernard, Louisiana State University Health Sciences Center.

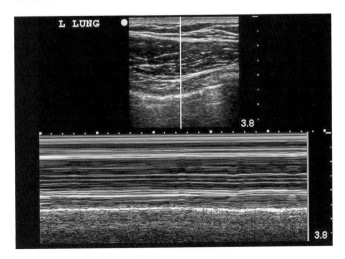

FIGURE 3-4.

Stratosphere/barcode sign. Absence of the lung-slide artifact is identified in ultrasound M-mode as the stratosphere/barcode sign. Pneumothorax cannot be excluded. Image courtesy of Dr. Christine Butts and Dr. Matthew Bernard, Louisiana State University Health Sciences Center.

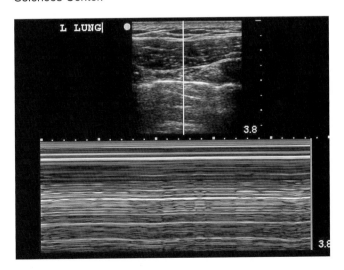

plateau pressure is indicative of a decrease in respiratory system compliance (Table 3-2). Note that the plateau pressure can never be higher than the peak pressure and that if the plateau pressure rises, so will the peak pressure. It is important to keep in mind the relationship of the Δ (peak pressure – plateau pressure). Also note that these measurements assume a comfortable patient. Peak pressures and plateau pressures are not reliable in the "bucking" patient.[17,18]

PEARL

Peak pressures and plateau pressures can be obtained only in volume-targeted modes.

Step 5: Observe ventilator waveforms.

The two most helpful ventilator waveforms are the flow-time curve and the pressure-time curve. The flow-time curve can be used to detect air trapping. The pressure-time curve can be used to determine plateau pressures with an inspiratory hold (Figure 3-5).

A notching in the pressure-time curve during inspiration can signify air hunger. In this situation, the patient desires a higher flow rate than the ventilator is delivering (Figure 3-6). It is commonly seen in volume-targeted modes. Increasing the flow rate will often alleviate this phenomenon. Another solution is to change to a pressure-targeted mode.

Double triggering can also be seen on ventilator waveforms. This occurs when the patient desires a higher tidal volume than the ventilator is set to deliver. The patient is still inspiring when the first breath has finished cycling and the ventilator immediately gives a second mechanical breath (Figure 3-7). This is frequently seen in low-tidal-volume ventilation, as used for patients with ARDS and status asthmaticus. It is important to recognize because the actual tidal volume being provided is essentially twice the set tidal volume. This has important ramifications for patients with ARDS and obstructive processes such as asthma and chronic obstructive pulmonary disease in which the goal is lower tidal volumes. Typically, improved sedation with emphasis on blunting the respiratory drive with opiates alleviates double triggering. Other adjustments that could help are increasing the flow, increasing the tidal volume by 1 mL/kg predicted body weight up to 8 mL/kg, or changing from a volume-targeted mode to a pressure-targeted mode.

Step 6: Imaging Studies—Chest Radiograph and Bedside Ultrasonography

Evaluate the chest radiograph for ET tube position, mainstem intubation, lung atelectasis, pneumothorax, and worsening parenchymal process. Bedside ultrasonography, if available, is typically quicker in evaluating for pneumothorax; however, it will not provide information on the location of the ET tube, lung atelectasis, or parenchymal processes (Figures 3-3 and 3-4).

Step 7: Evaluate sedation.

Some patients, such as those with drug overdoses or traumatic head injuries, may not require any sedation. Others may tolerate intubation quite well while almost fully awake. However, most patients require some form of sedation or analgesia to make the ET tube and ventilation tolerable.

Agents should be chosen based on the desired effect. If a patient appears agitated, sedative-hypnotics such as benzodiazepines, propofol, and dexmedetomidine should be used; however, it is important to note that these agents do not provide an analgesic component. If a patient is being given adequate sedative doses and still appears agitated, consider pain as a cause. For example, the agitated patient with a femur fracture and receiving high-dose benzodiazepines may simply need an opiate for pain control. Opiates that can usually be used are fentanyl, hydromorphone, and morphine. The goal of sedation and anesthesia in ventilated patients who are not being evaluated for extubation is to achieve a state in which the patient will arouse to gentle stimulation but will return to a sedated state when left alone. Patients who are being sedated and require deep stimulation to get a response are oversedated.

Patients who display air hunger and a high respiratory rate can be given a trial of opiates to relieve symptoms. Proper sedation and analgesia are paramount in patients being treated with a strategy that allows or induces hypercapnia such as those with status asthmaticus and ARDS. Hypercapnia is a powerful stimulus to the respiratory drive, and opiates are often required to control respiratory rates. Patients who tend to be difficult to control (besides those with status asthmaticus and ARDS) include those with hepatic encephalopathy or intracranial processes such as mass effect and hemorrhage. Chemical weakening with intermittently dosed paralytics can be required if patients have had a good trial of sedation, analgesia, and ventilator changes and are still markedly tachypneic. Careful consideration should be given prior to this step, as prolonged paralysis

FIGURE 3-5.

Pressure-time curve indicating inspiratory hold and plateau pressure

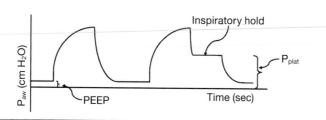

FIGURE 3-6.

Air hunger on ventilator waveform

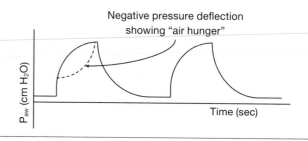

has been implicated in critical illness polyneuropathy.[19,20] In addition, expert consultation should be obtained prior to prolonged paralysis of neurosurgical patients. The goal of chemical paralysis in these patients is to weaken them enough to control their interaction with the ventilator. Usually, this does not require a full dose of the paralytic.

Hemodynamic instability in mechanically ventilated and sedated patients can be a result of medication; sedatives and analgesics can precipitate or worsen hypotension. As a general rule, continuous infusions should be held in these cases. Patients who are hypoxic and agitated, but not hypotensive, could benefit from improved sedation. It is possible that their pulmonary status is so tenuous that they are agitated from the hypoxia and their condition is worsened by the oxygen consumption caused by their agitation. Patients who are agitated and hypotensive may respond well to a low-dose benzodiazepine and opiate if the agitation is a precipitant of hypotension. In all these cases, it is imperative to determine if sedation is a factor in the decompensation. Chemical paralysis should be reserved as a final option.

PEARL

Hemodynamic instability in mechanically ventilated and sedated patients could be a result of medication.

KEY POINT

The goal of sedation is a patient who arouses to gentle stimulation but returns to a sedated state when left alone. If deep stimulation is required to get a response, the patient is oversedated.

FIGURE 3-7.

Double-triggering ventilator waveform

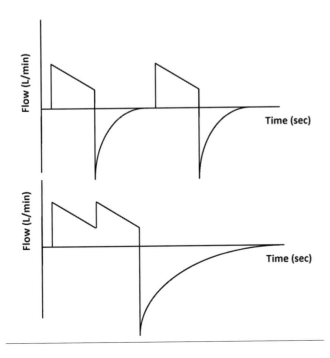

Special Scenarios

Two special scenarios should be mentioned. One is the crashing intubated pediatric patient, and the second is the patient with a tracheostomy (Table 3-4). The previously described approach can be used in pediatric patients; however, there are a few caveats that can improve the approach. The first is to recognize that ET tube migration is common with small movements of the head and neck. A simple solution is to use a cervical collar for immobilization. Second, small ET tubes are often uncuffed and do not have a pilot balloon. Air leaks in this scenario should prompt the clinician to consider that the tube is either dislodged or too small. Finally, specialized equipment such as intubating stylets and fiberoptic scopes are typically not available for pediatric sizes.

Important questions that have ramifications for the care of the crashing ventilated patient with a tracheostomy are these: 1) Does the patient have a laryngectomy? 2) Why does the patient have a tracheostomy? and 3) How old is the tracheostomy? These are important questions because patients with a laryngectomy cannot be intubated orally, patients with a tracheostomy secondary to anatomic considerations or difficult/failed airway can be difficult to intubate orally, and the track in a patient with a recent tracheostomy (less than 1 week) may not have matured enough to safely reintroduce a tracheostomy tube.

TABLE 3-4.

Special scenarios

Children
- Commonly, ET tubes migrate in and out of position with small manipulations of head position.
- Place a cervical collar to help stabilize head position.
- Document that the purpose is not for cervical spine protection.
- Small ET tubes are uncuffed.
- Most readily available intubating stylets and fiberoptic scopes are too large for pediatric ET tubes.

The Tracheostomy Patient – Unintentional Extubation
- Determine if patient had a laryngectomy.
  - Oral intubation is an option if the patient did not have a laryngectomy.
- Determine reason for tracheostomy.
  - Anatomic reason, difficult or failed airway – oral intubation may not be an option
  - Traumatic brain injury, chronic respiratory failure – oral intubation may be an option
- Determine age of tracheostomy.
  - <1 week – site may not be mature enough for manipulation; high risk of creating false tract
- Gently place a 6.0 ET tube in the stoma.
  - May confirm with fiberoptic visualization.
  - Stop if there is any resistance.

The Tracheostomy Patient – Obstruction
- Remove inner cannula and replace with same-sized cannula.

Conclusion

Mechanically ventilated patients are typically the most critically ill patients that the emergency department practitioner will manage. The underlying disease process that required intubation is typically life threatening. When patients become unstable, the physician should take a step-wise approach toward determining if the patient is deteriorating because of the underlying disease process or because of interaction with the ventilator. It is hoped that the approach presented here will assist practitioners with a framework to evaluate and stabilize the crashing ventilated patient.

References

1. Chen KY, Jerng JS, Liao WY, et al. Pneumothorax in the ICU: patient outcomes and prognostic factors. *Chest.* 2002;122:678-683.

2. Pepe PE, Marini JJ. Occult positive end-expiratory pressure in mechanically ventilated patients with airflow obstruction: the auto-PEEP effect. *Am Rev Respir Dis.* 1982;126:166-170.

3. O'Neill JF, Deakin CD. Do we hyperventilate cardiac arrest patients? *Resuscitation.* 2007;73:82-85.

4. Abella BS, Alvarado JP, Myklebust H, et al. Quality of cardiopulmonary resuscitation during in-hospital cardiac arrest. *JAMA.* 2005;293:305-310.

5. Aufderheide TP, Sigurdsson G, Pirrallo RG, et al. Hyperventilation-induced hypotension during cardiopulmonary resuscitation. *Circulation.* 2004;109:1960-1965.

6. Christie JM, Dethlefsen M, Cane RD. Unplanned endotracheal extubation in the intensive care unit. *J Clin Anesth.* 1996;8:289-293.

7. Bair AE, Laurin EG, Schmitt BJ. An assessment of a tracheal tube introducer as an endotracheal tube placement confirmation device. *Am J Emerg Med.* 2005;23:754-758.

8. Lichtenstein DA, Meziere G, Lascols N, et al. Ultrasound diagnosis of occult pneumothorax. *Crit Care Med.* 2005;33:1231-1238.

9. Blaivas M, Lyon M, Duggal S. A prospective comparison of supine chest radiography and bedside ultrasound for the diagnosis of traumatic pneumothorax. *Acad Emerg Med.* 2005;12:844-849.

10. Wilkerson RG, Stone MB. Sensitivity of bedside ultrasound and supine anteroposterior chest radiographs for the identification of pneumothorax after blunt trauma. *Acad Emerg Med.* 2010;17:11-17.

11. Harcke HT, Pearse LA, Levy AD, et al. Chest wall thickness in military personnel: implications for needle thoracentesis in tension pneumothorax. *Mil Med.* 2007;172:1260-1263.

12. Givens ML, Ayotte K, Manifold C. Needle thoracostomy: implications of computed tomography chest wall thickness. *Acad Emerg Med.* 2004;11:211-213.

13. Zengerink I, Brink PR, Laupland KB, et al. Needle thoracostomy in the treatment of a tension pneumothorax in trauma patients: what size needle? *J Trauma.* 2008;64:111-114.

14. Lee WW, Mayberry K, Crapo R, Jensen RL. The accuracy of pulse oximetry in the emergency department. *Am J Emerg Med.* 2000;18:427-431.

15. Bernard GR, Artigas A, Brigham KL, et al. The American-European Consensus Conference on ARDS. Definitions, mechanisms, relevant outcomes, and clinical trial coordination. *Am J Respir Crit Care Med.* 1994;149(3 Pt 1):818-824.

16. Ventilation with lower tidal volumes as compared with traditional tidal volumes for acute lung injury and the acute respiratory distress syndrome. The Acute Respiratory Distress Syndrome Network. *N Engl J Med.* 2000;342:1301-1308.

17. Tobin MJ. Advances in mechanical ventilation. *N Engl J Med.* 2001;344:1986-1996.

18. Tobin MJ. Respiratory monitoring. *JAMA.* 1990;264:244-251.

19. Douglass JA, Tuxen DV, Horne M, et al. Myopathy in severe asthma. *Am Rev Respir Dis.* 1992;146:517-519.

20. Kupfer Y, Namba T, Kaldawi E, Tessler S. Prolonged weakness after long-term infusion of vecuronium bromide. *Ann Intern Med.* 1992;117:484-486.

Fluid Management in the Critically Ill Patient

Alan C. Heffner and Matthew T. Robinson

IN THIS CHAPTER

Fluid distribution

Signs of hypovolemia

Volume responsiveness

Fluid selection

Special circumstances
Minimal volume resuscitation in hemorrhagic shock
Burn resuscitation
Maintenance fluid therapy

Introduction

Fluid therapy is a cornerstone in the management of acute critical illness. Relative and absolute hypovolemia complicate many clinical conditions. In practice, the clinician is routinely challenged with the complex tasks of assessing volume status and the need for fluid therapy and determining the best choice and dose of fluid for an individual patient and situation. Timely and appropriate fluid administration maintains macrocirculatory and microcirculatory support and reduces the mortality rate.[1] In contrast, both under- and over-administration of fluids adversely affect outcome. Inadequate resuscitation risks organ malperfusion resulting from persistent shock. Overly aggressive fluid administration results in volume overload without improving oxygen delivery and is associated with worse clinical outcomes.[2] A thorough understanding of the appropriate selection, timing, and goals of fluid therapy is vital to optimize patient care.

General Principles

Fluid Distribution and Movement

Water is the most abundant constituent of the body, accounting for 50% to 70% of total body weight. Variations in total body water depend primarily on lean body mass, since fat and other tissue contain very little water (Table 4-1). Water is distributed within intracellular and extracellular fluid compartments. The distribution of water in an average adult male is shown in Table 4-2. The intracellular space contains two thirds of the total body water, with the remainder distributed to the extracellular space, which is further divided into interstitial and intravascular spaces in a 4:1 ratio. These fluid compartments are not contiguous, but they may be treated as such because of their similar composition and behavior.

Water freely crosses cell membranes. Osmotic forces within fluid compartments determine water distribution within the body. Intracellular and extracellular fluid environments are iso-osmolar but are physiochemically distinct because of tight regulation of dissolved solutes and proteins. Membrane-bound sodium-potassium ATP-ase pumps compartmentalize sodium and potassium to the extracellular and intracellular spaces, respectively. Active restriction of sodium to the extracellular space is the foundation for isotonic sodium-based resuscitation solutions.

KEY POINT

Isotonic solutions maximize extracellular (including vascular) fluid retention and are indicated for resuscitation, regardless of accompanying electrolyte and water deficits.

The intravascular fluid, or plasma, differs from all other fluid compartments in that it exists as a single continuous fluid collection and contains trapped protein moieties in a higher concentration than is in the surrounding interstitial fluid. These trapped proteins produce the colloid oncotic pressure (COP) that favors fluid retention in the vascular space. Fluid flux across vascular endothelial membranes is governed by Starling forces (Table 4-3). In a healthy person, transcapillary hydrostatic force is nearly opposed by COP. Small net losses from the vascular space are returned to the systemic circulation via the lymphatic system. Albumin typically accounts for 80% of COP, while large cellular moieties such as red cells and platelets contribute less oncotic pressure effect. Positive hydrostatic pressure, hypoalbuminemia, and pathologic endothelial permeability are common clinical conditions that enhance fluid extravasation from the vascular compartment. The clinical consequence of ongoing fluid administration for cardiovascular support is the simultaneous evolution of pulmonary and tissue edema. Alteration of COP with enhanced retention of intravascular volume is one of the theoretic advantages of colloid-based fluids.

Effective Circulating Volume

Effective circulating volume (ECV) refers to the portion of intravascular volume contributing to organ perfusion. ECV falls with hypovolemia but does not necessarily correlate with volume status, as organ perfusion is also dependent on cardiac output, arterial tone, and circulatory distribution. For example, ECV may be compromised by limited cardiac output despite optimized volume status.

Pathophysiology

The immediate consequence of hypovolemia is impaired oxygen delivery, which triggers a swift compensatory response. Cardiac output is the most important determinant of oxygen delivery, with the flexibility to compensate for reduced oxygen-carrying capacity and/or increased metabolic demands (Figure 4-1). In the setting of hypovolemia, the body acts to defend itself through compensatory adjustments aimed at maintaining perfusion pressure and oxygen delivery.

At the macrocirculatory level, volume loss leads to decreased venous return and decreased cardiac output. Reduced stretch sensed by aortic and carotid baroreceptors leads to swift sympathetic catecholamine release, resulting in peripheral vasoconstriction, tachycardia, and enhanced cardiac contractility. These compensatory measures attempt to maintain cardiac output in the face of a falling stroke volume. Venoconstriction shunts blood from capacitance vessels and maintains intrathoracic blood volume and cardiac preload. Organ blood flow is directly proportional to perfusion pressure in most vascular beds, and peripheral arterial vasoconstriction maintains critical perfusion pressure. Preferential perfusion shunts limited cardiac output to vital organs at the expense of reduced blood flow to noncritical (hepatosplanchnic, renal, cutaneous) circulations. Therefore, mean arterial pressure (MAP) can be maintained despite hypovolemia and organ hypoperfusion.

Clinical Signs of Hypovolemia

Hypovolemia primarily manifests as circulatory insufficiency. Signs and symptoms reflect organ dysfunction and the counter-regulatory response set in motion to offset the hypovolemic state. Classically, hypovolemia is portrayed as following a stepwise progression of signs and symptoms based on the vol-

TABLE 4-1.

Total body water estimates

Adult male	60%
Adult female[a]	50%
Elderly[a]	50%
Obese[a]	50%
Infant	70%

Total body water represents 50% to 60% of lean body weight in adults.

[a]Lower total body water proportional to skeletal muscle mass.

TABLE 4-2.

Size and composition of body fluid compartments[a]

Compartment	% Body Weight	Volume (L)	H_2O (L)	Na (mmol/L)	K (mmol/L)	Cl (mmol/L)	HCO_3^- (mmol/L)
Total body	60	45	42				
Intracellular fluid	40	30	28 (60%)	16	150		10
Extracellular fluid	20	15	14 (40%)	140	4	103	26
Interstitial	16	12					
Plasma	4	3					
Blood	7	5					

[a]Values based on a 70-kg man.

ume deficit (Table 4-4). The clinical reality is that signs of hypovolemia are highly variable depending on the culprit disease, the speed of its evolution, and the individual's physiologic reserve for compensatory response. Compared with hemorrhage, sepsis presents a complicated hypovolemic state in which absolute fluid deficits are compounded by pathologic vasodilation and accelerated end-organ dysfunction. Children and healthy adults with vigorous compensatory mechanisms may tolerate large volume loss in the absence of severe clinical symptoms. In contrast, patients with limited cardiac reserve may poorly tolerate even minimal fluid loss.

Shock

Shock is defined as a state of inadequate tissue perfusion in which tissue oxygen delivery is inadequate to meet metabolic needs. Contrary to popular use, the term does not reflect perfusion pressure. Unfortunately, blood pressure is an unreliable indicator of adequate systemic oxygen delivery and perfusion. Shock can occur in patients with normal or elevated blood pressure. Many patients with significant blood or fluid loss demonstrate normotension, but this should not be seen as a sign of normal organ perfusion.[3] Inadequate perfusion in the setting of normal blood pressure is called *compensated shock*. The difficulty in identifying these patients spawned the terms *occult hypoperfusion* and *cryptic shock* to describe hemodynamically stable patients with microvascular insufficiency. Most critically ill patients present in compensated shock with normal or near-normal blood pressures.

Blood Pressure and Hypotension

Uncompensated shock is characterized by hypotension, which is a late sign of hypoperfusion that develops when physiologic attempts to maintain normal perfusion pressure are overwhelmed or exhausted. Hypotension should always be considered pathologic until proven otherwise. A MAP of less than 65 mm Hg, a systolic blood pressure (SBP) of less than 90 mm Hg, and/or a MAP of more than 20 mm Hg below baseline should raise clinical concern even in the absence of overt clinical hypoperfusion.

Brief self-limited hypotensive episodes represent progressive exhaustion of cardiovascular compensation and are the first sign of uncompensated shock. Transient hypotension is an important clue to recognize, as it is associated with adverse outcomes and often heralds further hemodynamic deterioration in the absence of intervention.

PEARL

Transient hypotension is an important clue to recognize, as it is associated with adverse outcomes and often heralds further hemodynamic deterioration in the absence of intervention.

It is important to understand the limitations of blood pressure measurements in critically ill patients. Automated blood pressure cuffs rely on the oscillometric method of blood pressure determination and may overestimate true arterial blood pressure in low-flow states.[4] Direct auscultation with reliance on Korotkoff sounds can underestimate actual SBP by as much as 30 mm Hg in low-flow states.[5] The potential for large measurement errors in hemodynamically unstable patients warrants consideration of invasive arterial monitoring in patients with severe cardiovascular deterioration.

The discriminative power of postural vital signs depends on appropriate testing and integration with specific clinical findings. Supine resting blood pressure and pulse rate should be

---

TABLE 4-3.

Starling law governing fluid flux across vascular endothelium

$$V = K_f \left[(P_{capillary} - P_{interstitium}) - \sigma(COP_{capillary} - COP_{interstitium}) \right]$$

P = Hydrostatic pressure
σ = Reflection coefficient that reflects membrane permeability; value range, 0–1. Inflammatory mediated endothelial permeability reduces σ.

FIGURE 4-1.

Determinants of systemic oxygen delivery

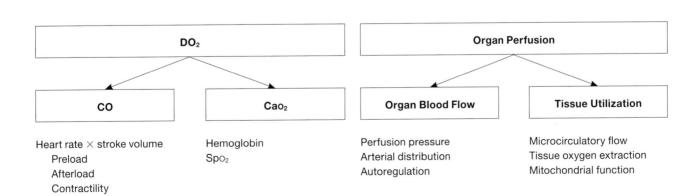

| Oxygen delivery (DO₂) = cardiac output (CO) × oxygen-carrying capacity (CaO₂) |

DO₂		**Organ Perfusion**	
CO	**CaO₂**	**Organ Blood Flow**	**Tissue Utilization**
Heart rate × stroke volume Preload Afterload Contractility	Hemoglobin SpO₂	Perfusion pressure Arterial distribution Autoregulation	Microcirculatory flow Tissue oxygen extraction Mitochondrial function

reassessed at least 2 minutes after standing because all patients have a brief orthostatic response after standing. Postural pulse change greater than 30 beats per minute is unusual in normovolemic patients.[5] Severe postural dizziness with intolerance of the upright position confirms hypovolemia in contrast to subjective symptoms that do not limit standing. Orthostatic hypotension, defined as an SBP decline of more than 20 mm Hg, is seen in 10% to 30% of normovolemic patients. The postural hemodynamic response may also be altered by aging and medications. Up to 30% of elderly patients demonstrate an orthostatic response in the absence of volume depletion.[6]

Heart Rate and Shock Index

Sinus tachycardia is nonspecific, but its presence should prompt careful clinical consideration of volume depletion, hemorrhage, and sepsis. Heart rate typically increases in the early stages of hypovolemia to maintain cardiac output in the face of falling stroke volume. However, the heart rate response to acute volume loss is highly variable. In normal patients, volume loss of up to 20% fails to induce a tachycardic response.[7] This compensatory response may be further blunted by comorbid disease and medications, especially β-blockers. Paradoxic and relative bradycardia are reported in up to 30% of patients with traumatic and nontraumatic hemoperitoneum.[8,9]

The shock index (SI) is the ratio of heart rate to systolic blood pressure. The index may predict uncompensated shock and must be interpreted relative to the individual patient. The normal range for SI is 0.5 to 0.7. An SI greater than 0.9 should raise suspicion of critical illness despite seemingly normal vital signs.[10] The SI has been shown to be a better correlate than either heart rate or SBP alone in identifying acute blood loss.[11] Unfortunately, elevated SI is not specific for hypovolemia and may be less accurate in clinical conditions involving fever-associated tachycardia.

Delayed capillary refill, dry axillae and mucous membranes, abnormal skin turgor, and sunken eyes are classic, but imperfect, hallmarks of hypovolemia. Symptoms of reduced cardiac output such as fatigue, dyspnea, postural dizziness, and near syncope are common but are neither specific nor sensitive. Nonfocal confusion, agitation, and lassitude are common manifestations of hypovolemia in elderly patients.[7] Organ dysfunction can be the heralding signal of hypovolemia and can occur in the absence of global hypoperfusion or hemodynamic instability. Oliguria, concentrated urine, and increased serum creatinine are exemplary signs of early renal dysfunction. Electrolyte and acid-base derangements associated with hypovolemia can also produce a constellation of associated symptoms.

Volume depletion describes the state of contracted extracellular fluid with clinical implications of compromised ECV, tissue perfusion, and function. It is distinguished from dehydration, which implies an intracellular water deficit characterized by plasma hypernatremia and hyperosmolarity.[7] Hypovolemia can occur as a consequence of blood loss, water and electrolyte loss, or primary water loss (Table 4-5).

TABLE 4-4.

Classes of acute hemorrhagic shock. Estimated blood loss[a] based on patient's initial presentation.[b] From: American College of Surgeons Committee on Trauma. *Advanced Trauma Life Support for Doctors.* 8th ed. Chicago, IL: American College of Surgeons; 2008. Used with permission.

	Class I	Class II	Class III	Class IV
Blood loss (mL)	Up to 750	750–1500	1500–2000	>2000
Blood loss (% blood volume)	Up to 15%	15%–30%	30%–40%	>40%
Pulse rate	<100	100–120	120–140	>140
Blood pressure	Normal	Normal	Decreased	Decreased
Pulse pressure	Normal or increased	Decreased	Decreased	Decreased
Respiratory rate	14–20	20–30	30–40	>35
Urine output (mL/hr)	>30	20–30	5–15	Negligible
CNS/mental status	Slightly anxious	Mildly anxious	Anxious, confused	Confused, lethargic
Fluid replacement	Crystalloid	Crystalloid	Crystalloid and blood	Crystalloid and blood

[a]Estimates based on a 70-kg man.

[b]The guidelines in this table are based on the 3-for-1 (3:1) rule, which derives from the empiric observation that most patients in hemorrhagic shock require as much as 300 mL of electrolyte solution for each 100 mL of blood loss. Applied blindly, these guidelines may result in excessive or inadequate fluid administration. For example, a patient with a crush injury to an extremity may have hypotension that is out of proportion to his or her blood loss and may require fluids in excess of the 3:1 guidelines. In contrast, a patient whose ongoing blood loss is being replaced by blood transfusion requires less than 3:1. The use of bolus therapy with careful monitoring of the patient's response may moderate these extremes.

Shock is defined by inadequate tissue perfusion, not systemic blood pressure.

Most emergency department patients requiring resuscitation present in compensated shock with normal blood pressure.

Early recognition of circulatory insufficiency must be coupled with timely resuscitation to improve patient outcome.

Fluid Resuscitation

Circulatory failure is the final common pathway of many diseases and carries a wide differential diagnosis (Table 4-6). Inadequate circulating volume is the most common primary cause of shock. Rapid restoration of the underlying fluid deficit is necessary to reverse hypoperfusion. Acute cardiac decompensation and pulmonary embolus are two exceptional situations in which limited volume resuscitation, giving priority to mechanical and catecholamine resuscitation, is recommended.

TABLE 4-5.

Anatomic sites of nonhemorrhagic fluid loss

Gastrointestinal	Vomiting
	Diarrhea
	Drainage (ostomy, fistula, nasogastric)
Renal	Diuresis (medication, osmotic)
	Salt wasting
	Diabetes insipidus
Skin	Burn
	Wound
	Exfoliative rash
	Sweat
Third-space sequestration	Intestinal obstruction
	Peritonitis
	Crush injury
	Pancreatitis
	Ascites
	Pleural effusion
	Capillary leak
Insensible loss	Respiratory
	Fever

Intravenous Access

Appropriate intravenous access is vital to resuscitation. The determinants of flow through a rigid tube are listed in Table 4-7. The rate of volume infusion is determined by the dimension of the vascular catheter, not by the size of the cannulated vein. Flow is directly proportional to the fourth power of the catheter radius and inversely proportional to the catheter length. Therefore, doubling the catheter size results in a 16-fold increase in flow, whereas doubling the cannula length decreases flow by half.

Central venous catheters (CVCs) allow hemodynamic monitoring and provide a reliable portal for volume therapy, vasoactive drug infusion, and serial blood sampling. Because of differences in length, infusion rates through adult CVCs are up to 75% less than through peripheral catheters of equal diameter. Many patients can be adequately resuscitated with peripheral venous access. In some circumstances, massive volume infusion may require the use of large-bore introducer catheters (8.5F–9.5F) that support flow rates approaching those of intravenous tubing at almost 1 L/min (Table 4-8).[12,13] Manual compression of the bag is an inefficient method of improving flow compared with use of an external pressure bag.[14]

End Points of Resuscitation

End points or targets of resuscitation are critical to guide therapy during acute critical illness. Rapid restoration of perfusion pressure is a priority. Restoration of MAP to 60 to 65 mm Hg supports vital organ autoregulation.[15] However, normalization of traditional markers of blood pressure, heart rate, and urine output does not guarantee adequate organ perfusion.[1,16,17] Resuscitation aimed at these markers risks leaving the patient in persistent compensated shock.

Resuscitation aims to stabilize oxygen delivery to meet

TABLE 4-6.

Differential diagnosis of undifferentiated shock and hypotension

Hypovolemia
  Blood loss
  Fluid loss
    Gastrointestinal
    Renal
    Insensible (skin, respiratory)
    Third space (interstitium, body cavity)

Vasodilatory
  Sepsis
  Anaphylaxis
  Adrenal crisis
  Neurogenic shock
  Toxin/medication induced

Obstructive/Central
  Cardiac dysfunction
  Cardiac tamponade
  Pulmonary embolus
  Tension pneumothorax

global and regional metabolic requirements. Central venous oxygen saturation ($ScvO_2$) and serum lactate concentration have emerged as rapid and reliable global perfusion markers. $ScvO_2$ reflects the systemic balance of oxygen delivery and utilization. Decreasing oxygen delivery is compensated by increased tissue oxygen extraction, which results in a fall in $ScvO_2$ below the normal 70%. $ScvO_2$ is a practical bedside measurement that is sampled from a catheter (CVC or percutaneously inserted central venous catheter) positioned in the superior vena cava. $ScvO_2$ response is rapid and dynamic, so monitoring provides immediate feedback on resuscitation efforts (or clinical deterioration).

Admission lactate concentration and base deficit predict morbidity and mortality independent of hemodynamics.[18] These markers of illness severity are also useful to corroborate response to therapy and as end points of resuscitation. Although initial base deficit correlates with lactate concentration, confounding by resuscitation fluid, other therapies, and evolving organ dysfunction decreases the utility of serial base deficit calculations as a resuscitation end point. However, rapid lactate clearance is associated with decreased mortality rates across a number of critical conditions.[19-21] Persistent hyperlactatemia is associated with higher rates of multiple organ failure and death.[22] As such, serial lactate levels provide an important gauge of resuscitation.

The optimal end point of resuscitation remains controversial. Novel markers such as measurements obtained with tissue capnometry, oximetry, and near-infrared spectroscopy hold promise, but their roles remain to be clarified. Most important, we cannot expect a single resuscitation end point to perform in all clinical circumstances. As such, a multimodal approach that seeks to normalize a combination of both global and regional perfusion markers is most prudent (Table 4-9).

KEY POINTS

Normalization of vital signs does not ensure adequate systemic perfusion or completion of resuscitation.

A combination of global and regional markers should be used to guide adequacy of therapy during resuscitation.

Central venous oxygen saturation and lactate clearance have emerged as reliable targets of acute resuscitation.

The Empiric Volume Challenge

The immediate goal of cardiovascular support is to restore and maintain systemic oxygen delivery and end-organ perfusion. Restoration of oxygen delivery through fluid resuscitation relies on optimizing preload to maximize stroke volume. The

TABLE 4-7.

Determinants of flow through a rigid tube

Hagen-Poiseuille equation: $Q = (P_{in} - P_{out}) \times (\pi r4/8\mu L)$

Q = Flow
$P_{in} - P_{out}$ = Pressure gradient
r = Radius
μ = Viscosity
L = Tube length

empiric volume challenge remains the standard means of initial fluid resuscitation. In the setting of acute undifferentiated shock or overt hypovolemia, volume expansion is achieved by infusing serial aliquots of isotonic fluid under direct observation. Crystalloid (10–20 mL/kg) or colloid (5–10 mL/kg) boluses should be infused quickly (over 15–20 minutes), with serial boluses titrated to the clinical end point objective while the patient is monitored for adverse effects such as pulmonary congestion. A positive clinical response to volume loading confirms volume responsiveness but does not predict further response to therapy. This can contribute to overly aggressive volume expansion and fluid excess.

PEARL

A positive clinical response to volume loading confirms volume responsiveness but does not predict further response to therapy.

Total volume requirements are difficult to predict at the onset of resuscitation and are most often underestimated. Classic hypovolemia, as occurs with acute hemorrhage or fluid loss, may stabilize rapidly with appropriate volume expansion. The 3:1 rule of hemorrhage resuscitation suggests that three volumetric units of crystalloid are required to replete the extracellular fluid deficit of 1 unit of blood loss.[23,24] However, experimental models confirm the experience in severely traumatized patients for whom fluid requirements exceed the 3:1 suggestion. Pathologic vasodilation and transcapillary leak contribute to the need for ongoing volume replacement. Crystalloid requirements average 40 to 60 mL/kg in the first hour of septic shock but can be as high as 200 mL/kg to normalize perfusion parameters.[16,25]

TABLE 4-8.

Intravenous fluid flow rate through peripheral and central venous catheters

Size of Cannula	Length (mm)	Internal Diameter (mm)	Flow Rate (mL/min)
20 gauge IV	32	0.7	54
18 gauge IV	32	0.9	104
18 gauge IV	45	0.9	90
16 gauge IV	32	1.2	220
16 gauge IV	45	1.2	186
14 gauge IV	32	1.6	302
14 gauge IV	45	1.6	288
9F sheath	100	2.5	838
IV tubing	3	3	1030

Volume Responsiveness

The effectiveness of fluid administration in improving stroke volume depends on a number of variables, including venous tone and ventricular function. Following initial fluid resuscitation, subsequent fluid administration often fails to achieve its desired effect. Fluid therapy does not affect macrocirculatory flow in 50% of critically ill patients.[26,27] Volume or preload responsiveness refers to the the potential for fluid administration to augment stroke volume. *In contrast to the empiric volume challenge, volume responsiveness should be gauged prior to fluid administration, and the information used to guide whether fluid administration is part of the solution to reverse clinical hypoperfusion.* Fluid loading in volume unresponsive patients should be avoided, as it delays appropriate therapy and contributes to fluid excess with organ dysfunction, including hypoxemic respiratory failure and abdominal compartment syndrome.[2] Recent trials highlight the importance of fluid balance on organ function and morbidity.[2] A more rational approach for patients who remain hypoperfused after initial management with empiric volume challenges incorporates selection and titration of subsequent therapy under the guidance of objective cardiovascular monitoring.

PEARL

Predicting volume responsiveness before fluid administration aims to identify patients unlikely to respond to fluid, thus preventing delays in appropriate therapy and fluid excess stemming from continued empiric fluid administration.

Predicting Volume Responsiveness

Invasive hemodynamic measurements are used frequently as surrogates of preload and predictors of volume responsiveness. Central venous pressure (CVP) monitoring is widely advocated. In the absence of conflicting data, a target CVP of 8 to 12 mm Hg is recommended to optimize preload prior to the institution of pressor and inotropic support.[26]

Unfortunately, cardiac pressure surrogates of preload (CVP and pulmonary artery occlusion pressure) reflect the net influences of intravascular volume, venous tone, cardiac function,

---

TABLE 4-9.

Prioritized end points of fluid therapy

Adequate intravenous access

MAP >65 mm Hg

Optimize oxygen delivery and organ perfusion
    Regional markers
        Cutaneous perfusion
        Urine output
        Mental status
    Systemic markers
        Scvo$_2$ >70%
        Serum lactate clearance and normalization

---

and intrathoracic pressure. These myriad influences confound their ability to reflect intravascular volume status or preload responsiveness in an individual patient. There is no consistent threshold CVP to reliably estimate response to fluid administration. Values that are considered low, normal, or high can be found in patients who respond positively to fluid.[27,28] Obstructive lung disease, positive-pressure ventilation, myocardial dysfunction, reflex venoconstriction, and erroneous measurements are examples of several conditions that can elevate CVP despite significant hypovolemia. An increase in CVP coupled with clinical improvement with volume loading corroborates fluid responsiveness but does not anticipate further effect.

PEARL

CVP is an unreliable surrogate for the prediction of volume status, preload, and response to fluid therapy.

Volumetric measures of preload, including stoke volume, right and global end-diastolic volume, and left ventricular end-diastolic area, can be obtained via several monitoring techniques. These volumetric surrogates of preload are intuitively more desirable, but they too have limited predictive value because discriminatory thresholds are imprecise and infrequent in clinical practice.[27,29-31] Serial volumetric data in response to therapy can assist in individual patient management, but the dynamic nature of cardiovascular function during critical illness confounds their ability to predict fluid responsiveness.

Fluid responsiveness is best predicted by dynamic indices of preload reserve. Respirophasic variation in stroke volume during positive-pressure mechanical ventilation is among the most reliable signs of preload responsiveness.[27] Positive-pressure ventilation induces cyclic alteration in preload. A resulting variation in systolic pressure, pulse pressure, and stroke volume greater than 13% identifies patients capable of augmenting stroke volume in response to fluid administration. Respiratory collapse of the inferior vena cava greater than 50% is another helpful indicator to evaluate volume responsiveness. Minimal variation in that vessel is associated with supranormal CVP and a low probability of fluid responsiveness.

PEARL

Respirophasic stroke volume variation is one of the most reliable signs of volume responsiveness but has specific requirements for interpretation:

- Positive-pressure ventilation with the patient passive on the ventilator
- >8 mL/kg tidal volume
- Regular rhythm

Passive leg raising is a provocative maneuver to test whether a reversible volume challenge is capable of improving stroke volume. This is an attractive option because it provides immediate information to guide therapy without the administration of potentially unnecessary fluid. Passive leg raising translocates venous blood from the lower extremities to the thorax to transiently augment preload. Volume-responsive patients respond with a temporary improvement in stroke volume greater than 15% over approximately 3 minutes. A sensitive bedside stroke volume monitor is required to recognize the response to this maneuver. Its sensitivity and specificity in predicting volume responsiveness are greater than 95% in a wide variety of patients, including ventilated and spontaneously breathing patients, as well as those with irregular cardiac rhythms.[32]

KEY POINTS

The solution to persistent hypoperfusion following initial fluid resuscitation is complex and warrants hemodynamic monitoring insight to guide therapy selection and dose.

In the absence of overt clinical hypovolemia, volume responsiveness should not be assumed and is best gauged by dynamic hemodynamic indices.

Overly aggressive fluid resuscitation and excess fluid balance increase patient morbidity.

Fluid Selection

The immediate goal of fluid resuscitation is vascular expansion to optimize stroke volume. Various fluid prescriptions are used for early resuscitation and correction of fluid and electrolyte deficits. Each possesses specific benefits and disadvantages in given clinical scenarios. The composition and distribution of crystalloids and colloids used in resuscitation are presented in Table 4-10. Randomized clinical trials of crystalloid versus col-

loid failed to prove clinical superiority of one agent, revealing comparable rates of mortality and lung dysfunction.[33-35]

KEY POINTS

The targeted end point used to guide the dose for fluid resuscitation is more important than the individual fluid product (ie, crystalloid versus colloid) selection.

Isotonic crystalloids remain the standard initial resuscitation fluid and confer significant cost advantage over colloid.

Crystalloid

Isotonic sodium-based crystalloids preferentially distribute to the extracellular compartment, which includes the vascular volume. Infusion of 1 liter of normal saline distributes approximately 250 mL into the vascular compartment. This is the basis for the 3:1 rule often cited for resuscitation in acute hemorrhagic shock. That ratio may more closely approximate 7:1 or 10:1 in patients with severe hemorrhage, owing to decreased COP secondary to hemorrhage, capillary leak, and crystalloid replacement.[36]

Fluid selection appears less important than volume dosage titrated to an appropriate therapeutic end point. Normal saline (0.9%) and lactated Ringer solution are the two most commonly used isotonic resuscitation solutions. Evidence of clinical

TABLE 4-10.

Intravenous fluid composition and distribution

| Solution | Electrolytes (mEq/L) | | | | | | | mOsm/L | pH | Distribution | |
	Na	K	Ca	Mg	Cl	HCO₃⁻	Lactate			Extra-cellular Fluid	Intra-cellular Fluid
Crystalloid											
0.9% NaCl	154				154			308	5	100%	
Lactated Ringer	130	4	2.7		109		28	273	6.5		
150 mEq NaHCO₃ (3 ampules) in 1 L water	130					130		260			
3% NaCl	513				513			1,027	5		
7.5% NaCl								2,400			
0.45% NaCl	77				77			154	5	67%	33%
0.20% NaCl	34				34			77	5		
D₅W								278	4	33%	67%
Colloid											
6% Hetastarch (Hextend)	143	3	5	1	124		28	307	5.9		
6% Hetastarch (HESpan)	154				154			310	5.5		
Human albumin, 5%	145				95			300			

superiority for either is lacking. However, the source of hypovolemia, associated electrolyte derangements, and volume requirements should influence fluid selection.

Normal saline supplies a supraphysiologic sodium and chloride load. The advantage of intravascular retention is countered by the induction of hyperchloremic metabolic acidosis when normal saline is administered in large volumes. Normal saline is preferred to correct volume and electrolyte (chloride) disturbances in patients with metabolic alkalosis, including those with loss of gastric secretion (associated with vomiting, gastric outlet obstruction, or nasogastric suctioning). In contrast, isotonic bicarbonate can be used for fluid resuscitation of patients with severe coexisting metabolic acidosis.

Lactated Ringer or Hartmann solution was introduced in the 1930s when sodium lactate was added as a buffer to Ringer solution for the treatment of metabolic acidosis. It is a more physiologic fluid, containing potassium and calcium in concentrations comparable to those in plasma. Compared with normal saline, lactated Ringer solution is slightly more hypotonic and should not be used in clinical situations in which maintenance of plasma osmolarity is a priority (eg, in patients with acute brain insult). Because of its more physiologic pH, lactated Ringer solution is often preferred for large-volume resuscitation. Calcium in the solution can bind to medications and the citrated anticoagulant in blood; therefore, lactated Ringer solution is not a compatible transfusion fluid.

Colloid

Colloid solutions are composed of electrolyte preparations fortified with large-molecular-weight (>30,000) molecules. The presence of these large molecules contributes to total oncotic pressure, which favors retention of fluid in the vascular space. The ideal colloidal solution has an oncotic pressure similar to that of plasma, which permits replacement of the plasma volume without distribution to other fluid compartments. The net effect and theoretic benefit of colloid infusion are intravascular

expansion without expansion of the interstitial compartment and a lower likelihood of pulmonary and interstitial edema. The potency of colloid solutions on plasma volume differs with individual fluids: the higher the COP, the greater the expansion of the plasma volume.

Human albumin and hydroxyethyl starch (HES) are the primary colloids used in the United States. Five percent albumin solution is iso-oncotic to plasma, and more than 70% of an infused volume is retained within the vascular space. It is recommended for resuscitation of patients with severe hypoalbuminemia and cirrhosis, but there is little outcome evidence to support this practice.[26,37] HES is a semisynthetic polymerized amylopectin available as a 6% isotonic solution. The average molecular weight of HES is equivalent to that of albumin, so it has a similar effect on COP and volume expansion as 5% albumin. The renal dysfunction and coagulopathy that complicated early-generation synthetic colloids do not appear clinically significant with new-generation HES solutions.

Vascular retention of colloids makes them efficient volume expanders. Although equally effective when titrated to the same clinical end points, crystalloid solutions require two to four times more volume for equivalent resuscitation. Dilutional hypoalbuminemia, transcapillary fluid shift, and interstitial and pulmonary edema are therefore limited with colloid use. However, if endothelial integrity is disrupted following injury or illness, macromolecules will not be restricted to the vascular compartment.[38]

Hypertonic Saline

Hypertonic sodium solutions, with sodium concentrations ranging from 3% to 7.5%, rapidly expand intravascular volume by mobilizing water from interstitial and intracellular spaces. Small infusions expand plasma by several times the infused volume without the resultant expansion of the interstitial fluid space and edema seen with crystalloid.[39] Additional benefits include improved cardiovascular function secondary to positive inotropic effects and pulmonary vasodilation, improved microcirculatory flow, and attenuation of the inflammatory response.[40] This combination of effects makes use of these so-

---

TABLE 4-11.

Limited volume resuscitation pending surgical control of bleeding: sources of life-threatening hemorrhage to consider

Ectopic pregnancy
Gastrointestinal bleeding
Major hemoperitoneum
Major hemothorax
Penetrating torso trauma
Postpartum hemorrhage
Ruptured abdominal aortic aneurysm
Severe pelvic fracture
Traumatic aortic injury

TABLE 4-12.

Parkland burn resuscitation formula to guide acute fluid therapy

24-hour fluid requirement = 4 mL × weight (kg) × % body surface area burn

- Half of the fluid calculation is administered over the first 8 hours after injury.
- The second half of the fluid calculation is administered over the subsequent 16 hours.
- Maintenance fluid calculations should be added to burn resuscitation estimates.
- Burn formulas estimate fluid requirements over the initial 24 hours of burn therapy.
- Volume requirements may substantially exceed formula approximation.

lutions attractive for volume expansion in trauma and septic patients alike. Used alone, however, the hemodynamic effects of hypertonic crystalloid are transient; therefore, hypertonic sodium solutions are generally used in combination with hyperoncotic colloid (6% dextran or 10% hetastarch). Currently, data are insufficient to conclude that hypertonic saline is better than isotonic crystalloid for the resuscitation of patients with burns, traumatic injuries, or sepsis. Animal sepsis models have shown that a single bolus of hypertonic sodium solutions produced sustained reduction in systemic and mesenteric oxygen extraction.[41] Traumatic brain injury remains the sole exception where some benefit is demonstrated.[42-44] The limited use of these solutions in the management of nontrauma patients limits clinical extrapolation beyond this population.

Hyperoncotic Albumin

Hyperoncotic albumin solutions (20% to 25% albumin) were developed in the 1940s for resuscitation of combat casualties. Infusion of hyperoncotic albumin results in vascular expansion more than two times the administered volume.[45] In addition to the obvious benefits of small-volume resuscitation, improved portability, and more rapid hemodynamic stabilization, hyperoncotic albumin offers other advantages. Synergistic interaction with administered drugs and primary antioxidant effects are hypothesized explanations for the reduction in morbidity and mortality linked to hyperoncotic albumin administered to patients with complicated hypoalbuminemic states, including decompensated end-stage liver disease.[46] Increased COP mobilizes interstitial edema, and the effects of hyperoncotic albumin are relatively long-lasting, persisting up to 12 hours after infusion. For this reason, hyperoncotic albumin is often matched with loop diuretic therapy to mobilize fluid in volume-overloaded patients.

Special Circumstances

Minimal Volume Resuscitation in Hemorrhagic Shock

Hemorrhagic shock poses the unique challenge of balancing the timing and type of resuscitation with the achievement of hemostasis. On one hand, hypotensive patients should be stabilized with rapid fluid infusion to maintain perfusion to essential organs. However, overly aggressive fluid resuscitation before control of the hemorrhage site can increase blood loss and the mortality rate. Aggressive fluid resuscitation increases blood pressure, decreases blood viscosity, and dilutes clotting factors, which are all associated with prevention of the formation of hemostatic plugs and the dislodgement of plugs that have formed.

The use of strategic, limited-volume resuscitation reemerged in the 1980s when the value of early prehospital fluid resuscitation in penetrating trauma was questioned.[47,48] A prospective trial by Bickell and colleagues, comparing immediate versus delayed fluid resuscitation in hypotensive patients with penetrating torso injuries, showed a reduced mortality rate, fewer complications, and a shorter hospital stay with delayed resuscitation.[49] The detrimental effects of aggressive volume resuscitation on normalization of blood pressure in laboratory experiments corroborate this concept. Limited resuscitation with judicious use of fluids may offer the optimal approach, with conventional resuscitation ensuing after surgical hemostasis is achieved (Table 4-11). The optimal degree and duration of permissive hypotension remain unclear, although current recommendations suggest a target SBP of 70 mm Hg.[24] Patients with concomitant brain injury are not candidates for this strategy.

Burn Resuscitation

Patients with second- and third-degree burns exhibit marked fluid shifts related to denuded skin, injured tissue, and systemic inflammatory response. Aggressive fluid resuscitation is necessary to restore intravascular volume and maintain end-organ perfusion. Early anticipation of these large fluid requirements prevents under-resuscitation. Initial fluid requirements are most commonly calculated according to the Parkland formula (Table 4-12).

Formula calculations should be based from the time of injury rather than from the time to medical attention and should incorporate prehospital fluid administration. Ringer lactate is the preferred crystalloid solution. Several formulas exist, but no single method is clearly superior.[50] *All formulas are intended*

TABLE 4-13.

Maintenance fluid estimate

Body Weight (kg)	Daily Maintenance (mL/day)	Hourly Maintenance (mL/hr)
1–10	100 mL/kg	5 mL/kg/hr
10–20	1,000 plus 50 mL/kg	40 plus 2 mL/kg/hr
20–80	1,500 plus 20 mL/kg[a]	60 plus 1 mL/kg/hr[a]

[a]To a maximum of 2,400 mL/day or 100 mL/hr

Sodium and chloride: 2–3 mEq/100 mL water

Potassium: 1–2 mEq/100 mL water

D_5 ¼ normal saline with 20 mEq KCl is a common maintenance solution for most euvolemic pediatric patients and provides 20% of daily calories at routine maintenance rate. Comorbid conditions and/or electrolyte abnormalities may necessitate modification.

to provide an initial guide for resuscitation requirements. Actual fluid needs may vary significantly, necessitating modifications based on individual status.[50] Strict adherence to a calculated number may result in over- or under-resuscitation. Over-administration of fluids is common and contributes to increased pulmonary complications and morbidity.[51,52] Maintenance fluid requirements should be allocated in addition to burn formula replacement. Urine output greater than 1 mL/kg/hr is a traditional end point for acute burn resuscitation and may be augmented by the perfusion end points discussed above.

Maintenance Fluid Therapy

In contrast to fluid resuscitation therapy, the goal of maintenance fluid therapy is to achieve normal body fluid composition and volume. Fluid orders anticipate daily fluid requirement, ongoing losses, and coexisting electrolyte abnormalities. Although the two therapies are often ordered concurrently, daily physiologic fluid requirements (true maintenance) should be consciously distinguished from therapy aimed to slowly replace an existing fluid deficit.

Routine water and electrolyte maintenance needs are based on normal energy expenditure, sensible loss from urine and stool, and insensible loss from the respiratory tract and skin. Calculations assume euvolemia and are adjusted for body mass (Table 4-13). Higher fluid requirements per kilogram in children are proportionate to total body water and metabolism. All maintenance prescriptions should be individualized. Energy expenditure, fluid losses, and electrolyte status vary with disease and dictate rate and electrolyte modifications. For example, exfoliative skin disease, increased work of breathing, and fever enhance insensible loss. Measurable nasogastric, fistula, ostomy, and urinary drainage can be estimated or replaced by drainage volume. Limitation of fluid and potassium is an important disease-specific modification for patients with renal insufficiency.

Hypotonic solutions with or without dextrose and potassium are popular fixed-combination maintenance solutions. Hospitalized patients often have impaired free-water excretion due to release of nonosmotic antidiuretic hormone, making them vulnerable to hyponatremia. The serum sodium concentration provides a simple and accurate marker of hydration status. Isotonic maintenance solutions should be considered in patients (including children) with a serum sodium concentration less than 138 mEq/L.[53,54] Glucose infusions are best formulated by adding dextrose to an electrolyte solution (ie, Ringer lactate, normal saline, 0.45 normal saline, or 0.2 normal saline) rather than using 5% dextrose, which behaves as electrolyte-free water on sugar metabolism.

Conclusion

Fluid therapy is provided to virtually all critically ill emergency department patients. Isotonic crystalloid solutions maximize extracellular fluid retention and remain the standard initial resuscitation fluid. Dynamic markers of volume responsiveness (eg, collapsibility of the inferior vena cava assessed with ultrasonography or respirophasic variation in stroke volume or pulse pressure) are superior to static markers in identifying patients likely to respond to fluid therapy. Importantly, normalization of vital signs does not indicate adequate resuscitation.

Rather, targeted end points such as lactate clearance and central venous oxygen saturation should be used to assess the adequacy of therapy in the critically ill emergency department patient.

References

1. Rivers E, Nguyen B, Havstad S, et al. Early goal-directed therapy in the treatment of severe sepsis and septic shock. *N Engl J Med.* 2001;345(19):1369-1377.
2. National Heart, Lung and Blood Institute Acute Respiratory Distress Syndrome (ARDS) Clinical Trials Network, Wiedmann HP, Wheeler AP, Bernard GR, et al. Comparison of two fluid-management strategies in acute lung injury. *N Engl J Med.* 2006;354(24): 2564-2575.
3. Orlinsky M, Shoemaker W, Reis ED, et al. Current controversies in shock and resuscitation. *Surg Clin North Am.* 2001;81(6):1217-1262.
4. Gravlee GP, Brockschmidt JK. Accuracy of four indirect methods of blood pressure measurement with hemodynamic correlations. *J Clin Monitor.* 1990;6:284-298.
5. Cohn JN. Blood pressure measurement in shock: mechanism of inaccuracy in ausculatory and palpatory methods. *JAMA.* 1967;199(13):118-122.
6. Carlson JE. Assessment of orthostatic blood pressure: measurement techniques and clinical applications. *South Med J.* 1999;92:167-173.
7. McGee S, Abernathy WB 3rd, Simel DL. The rational clinical examination: is this patient hypovolemic? *JAMA.* 1999;281:1022-1029.
8. Demetriades D, Chan LS, Bhasin P, et al. Relative bradycardia in patients with traumatic hypotension. *J Trauma.* 1998;45:534-539.
9. Hick JL, Rodgerson JD, Heegaard WG, et al. Vital signs fail to correlate with hemoperitoneum for ruptured ectopic pregnancy. *Am J Emerg Med.* 2001;19(6):488-491.
10. Rady MY, Smithline HA, Blake H, et al. A comparison of the shock index and conventional vital signs to identify acute, critical illness in the emergency department. *Ann Emerg Med.* 1994;24:685-690.
11. Birkhahn RH, Gaeta TJ, Terry D, et al. Shock index in diagnosing early acute hypovolemia. *Am J Emerg Med.* 2005;23:323-326.
12. Hyman SA, Smith DW, England R, et al. Pulmonary artery catheter introducers: do the component parts affect flow rate? *Anesth Analg.* 1991;73:573-575.
13. Jayanthi N, Harshad D. The effect of IV cannula length on the rate of infusion. *Injury.* 2006;37:41-45.
14. Stoneham MD. An evaluation of methods of increasing the flow rate of i.v. fluid administration. *Br J Anaesth* 1995;75:361-365.
15. LeDoux D, Astiz ME, Carpati CM, et al. Effects of the perfusion pressure on tissue perfusion in septic shock. *Crit Care Med.* 2000;28:2729-2732.
16. Tisherman SA, Barie P, Bokhari F, et al. Clinical practice guideline: endpoints of resuscitation. *J Trauma.* 2004;57:898-912.
17. Scalea TM, Hartnett RW, Duncan AO, et al. Central venous oxygen saturation: a useful clinical tool in trauma patients. *J Trauma.* 1990;30:1539-1543.
18. Davis JW, Parks SN, Kaups KL, et al. Admission base deficit predicts transfusion requirements and risk of complications. *J Trauma.* 1996;41(5):769-774.
19. Husain FA, Martin MJ, Mullenix PS, et al. Serum lactate and base deficit as predictors of mortality and morbidity. *Am J Surg.* 2003;185(5):485-491.
20. Abramson D, Scalea TM, Hitchcock R, et al. Lactate clearance and survival following injury. *J Trauma.* 1993;35(4):584-588.
21. Nguyen HB, Rivers EP, Knoblich BP, et al. Early lactate clearance is associated with improved outcome in severe sepsis and septic shock. *Crit Care Med.* 2004;32(8):1637-1642.
22. Kincaid EH, Miller PR, Meredith JW, et al. Elevated arterial base deficit in trauma patients: a marker of impaired oxygen utilization. *J Am Coll Surg.* 1998;187(4):384-392.
23. American College of Surgeons Committee on Trauma. *Advanced Trauma Life Support for Doctors.* 7th ed. Chicago, IL: American College of Surgeons; 2004.
24. Moore FA, McKinley BA, Moore EE. The next generation in shock resuscitation. *Lancet.* 2004;363:1988-1996.
25. Carcillo JA, Fields AI. Clinical practice parameters for hemodynamic support of pediatric and neonatal patients with septic shock. *Crit Care Med.* 2002;30(6):1365-1378.
26. Dellinger RP, Carlet JM, Masur H, et al. Surviving Sepsis Campaign guidelines for management of severe sepsis and septic shock. *Crit Care Med.* 2004;32:858-873.
27. Michard F, Teboul JL. Predicting fluid responsiveness in ICU patients. *Chest.* 2002;121:2000-2008.
28. Marik PE, Baram M, Vahid B. Does central venous pressure predict fluid responsiveness? *Chest.* 2008;134:172-178.
29. Osman D, Ridel C, Ray P, et al. Cardiac filling pressures are not appropriate to predict hemodynamic response to volume challenge. *Crit Care Med.* 2007;35(1):64-68.
30. Kumar A, Anel R, Bunnell E, et al. Pulmonary artery occlusion pressure and central venous pressure fail to predict ventricular filling volume, cardiac performance, or the response to volume infusion in normal subjects. *Crit Care Med.* 2004;32(3):691-699.
31. Coudray A, Romand J, Treggiari M, et al. Fluid responsiveness in spontaneously breathing patients: a review of indexes used in intensive care. *Crit Care Med.* 2005;33(2):2757-2762.

32. Monnet X, Rienzo M, Osman D, et al. Passive leg raising predicts fluid responsiveness in the critically ill. *Crit Care Med*. 2006;34(5):1402-1407.

33. Choi PT, Yip G, Quinonez LG, et al. Crystalloids vs colloids in fluid resuscitation: a systematic review. *Crit Care Med*. 1999;27:200-210.

34. Finfer S, Bellomo R, Boyce N, et al. A comparison of albumin and saline for fluid resuscitation in the intensive care unit. *N Engl J Med*. 2004;350:2247-2256.

35. Alderson P, Bunn F, Lefebvre C, et al. Human albumin solution for resuscitation and volume expansion in critically ill patients. *Cochrane Database Syst Rev*. 2002;(1):CD001208.

36. Rizoli SB. Crystalloids and colloids in trauma resuscitation: a brief overview of the current debate. *J Trauma*. 2003;54:S82-S88.

37. Cook C, Guyatt G. Colloid use for fluid resuscitation: evidence and spin. *Ann Intern Med*. 2001;135:205-208.

38. Fleck A, Raines G, Hawker G, et al. Increased vascular permeability: a major cause of hypoalbuminemia in disease and injury. *Lancet*. 1985;1:781-784.

39. Boldt J. Fluid choice for resuscitation of the trauma patient: a review of the physiological, pharmacological and clinical evidence. *Can J Anesth*. 2004;51(5):500-513.

40. Oliveira R, Velasco I, Soriano FG, et al. Clinical review: hypertonic saline resuscitation in sepsis. *Crit Care*. 2002;6(5):418-423.

41. Bunn F, Roberts I, Tasker R, et al. Hypertonic versus isotonic crystalloid for fluid resuscitation in critically ill patients. *Cochrane Database Syst Rev*. 2004;(3):CD002045.

42. Battison C, Andrews PG, Graham C, et al. Randomized, controlled trial on the effect of a 20% mannitol solution and a 7.5% saline/6% dextran solution on increased intracranial pressure after brain injury. *Crit Care Med*. 2005;33(1):196-202.

43. White H, Cook D, Venkatesh B. The role of hypertonic saline in neurotrauma. *Eur J Anesthesiol Suppl*. 2008;42:104-109.

44. Bhardwaj A, Ulatowski JA. Hypertonic saline solutions in brain injury. *Curr Opin Crit Care*. 2004;10(2):126-131.

45. Lamke LO, Liljedahl SO. Plasma volume expansion after infusion of 5%, 20% and 25% albumin solutions in patients. *Resuscitation*. 1976,5:85-92.

46. Jacob M, Chappell D, Conzen P, et al. Small-volume resuscitation with hyperoncotic albumin: a systematic review of randomized clinical trials. *Crit Care*. 2008;12(2):R34.

47. Aprahamian C, Thompson BM, Towne JB, et al. The effect of a paramedic system on mortality of major open intra-abdominal vascular trauma. *J Trauma*. 1983;23:687-690.

48. Kaweski SM, Sise MJ, Virgilio RW. The effect of prehospital fluids on survival in trauma patients. *J Trauma*. 1990;30:1215-1218.

49. Bickell WH, Wall MJ Jr, Pepe PE, et al. Immediate versus delayed fluid resuscitation for patients with penetrating torso injuries. *N Engl J Med*. 1994;331:1105-1109.

50. Hettiaratchy S, Papini R. Initial management of a major burn: II—assessment and resuscitation. *BMJ*. 2004;329(7457):101-103.

51. Ipaktchi K, Arbabi S. Advances in burn critical care. *Crit Care Med*. 2006;34:S239-S244.

52. Tricklebank S. Modern trends in fluid therapy for burns. *Burns*. 2009;35:757-767.

53. Shafiee MA, Bohn D, Hoorn EJ, Halperin ML. How to select optimal maintenance intravenous fluid therapy. *QJM*. 2003;96:601-610.

54. Moritz ML, Ayus JC. Prevention of hospital-acquired hyponatremia: a case for using isotonic saline. *Pediatrics*. 2003;11(2):227-230.

CHAPTER 5

Cardiac Arrest Updates

Benjamin J. Lawner and Joshua C. Reynolds

Introduction

Despite advances in resuscitation technology and the advent of new drug therapies, survival from sudden cardiac arrest has remained less than robust. Survival rates were dismal prior to the mid-1990s; most patients with an out-of-hospital cardiac arrest never saw the light of discharge.[1] Recent guidelines from the American Heart Association (AHA) on cardiopulmonary resuscitation (CPR) and emergency cardiovascular care (ECC) contain significant updates to existing guidelines on the care of the cardiac arrest patient. Renewed emphasis on early, high-quality uninterrupted chest compressions, rapid defibrillation, de-emphasis on immediate airway management and traditional advanced cardiovascular life support (ACLS) medications, and use of quantitative waveform capnography are just some of the recommendations contained in the 2010 AHA guidelines.[2] In addition to the AHA guidelines, recent emergency medicine literature has also borne witness to a sweeping paradigm shift in cardiac arrest care. The University of Arizona's Sarver Heart Center Cardiac Resuscitation research group has been instrumental in championing a "cardiocerebral resuscitation" (CCR) strategy.[3] In addition to the work by the University of Arizona, two rural EMS physicians in 2004 implemented protocols that emphasized high-quality compressions and delayed

ACLS interventions.[4] These treatment modalities form the basis of a CCR strategy. Communities using these protocols boasted neurologically intact survival rates in excess of 40%.[5,6] Using this research, along with the 2010 AHA guidelines on CPR and ECC, emergency physicians and EMS medical directors can implement protocols that favor an approach to resuscitation based on quality, uninterrupted compressions. CCR is one of the few interventions to result in improved neurologic outcomes and therefore demands serious consideration and integration into current resuscitation treatments. Even the latest randomized controlled trials fail to demonstrate the benefit of adherence to traditional and time-honored therapies. In 2009, Olasveengen et al conducted a study of 851 patients that randomized victims of cardiac arrest into groups that either received or did not receive intravenous drug therapy.[8] They found that patients receiving ACLS drug therapy did not have a statistically significant improvement in "survival to hospital discharge, quality of CPR, or long-term survival."[8]

Emergency care providers, as leaders of resuscitation teams, must take recent developments into account when orchestrating the response to a patient in cardiac arrest. There is an impressive arsenal of technologies available for deployment, but few of them are associated with any proven survival benefit. If the survival rates reported in communities implementing CCR are to be believed, it is reasonable to extrapolate that good neurologic outcome from cardiac arrest is predicated on a precious few interventions. As outlined in the 2010 AHA guidelines, these interventions consist of high-quality, uninterrupted chest compressions, rapid defibrillation, delayed ACLS interventions such as endotracheal intubation and drug administration, and a systematic approach to patients with return of spontaneous circulation (ROSC) that includes therapeutic hypothermia and early cardiac catheterization.[2] We feel that these essential interventions can be aptly termed the "critical C's of CPR":

1. Compressions (quality and uninterrupted)
2. Cardioversion (defibrillation)
3. CCR (delay of ACLS interventions)
4. Cooling (therapeutic hypothermia)
5. Cardiac catheterization

This chapter examines the best available evidence and assists emergency care providers in the complex medical decision-making process that takes place during resuscitation from cardiac arrest. It similarly addresses how the emergency department must interface with out-of-hospital providers and in-house specialists such as intensivists and cardiologists. Improved in-hospital communication and understanding are central to maintaining the newly minted chain of survival that spans the prehospital, emergency, and inpatient arenas and includes therapeutic hypothermia and post-arrest cardiac catheterization.

Evolving Physiology

The paradigm shift in resuscitation science and clinical practice has paralleled a revolution in the understanding of cardiac arrest physiology. Weisfeldt and Becker introduced a three-phase model of cardiac arrest in 2002 that describes this new understanding.[9] To effectively treat the cardiac arrest patient, emergency care providers must firmly grasp the dynamic nature of the condition while tailoring therapies appropriately (Figure 5-1).

The electrical phase (0–4 minutes) comprises the first minutes of cardiac arrest. The single most important intervention at this time is electrical defibrillation (assuming the patient presents with a shockable rhythm), which allows the heart to restore organized electrical activity. The highest probability of shock success lies within these first minutes, and nothing except patient or provider safety should delay this crucial intervention. The effectiveness of immediate defibrillation is best exemplified by the implantable cardiac defibrillator, which delivers a rescue shock within seconds and rarely fails to restore an organized rhythm. Initiatives to distribute automated external defibrillators and educate the public in their use are targeted at individuals with witnessed cardiac arrest. These devices have increased survival from out-of-hospital cardiac arrest.[10,11]

After the initial electrical phase, energy stores within the myocardium are depleted and the patient enters the circulatory phase (4–10 minutes). The goal of resuscitation during this stage is to restore energy substrates to the myocardium to render it more amenable to defibrillation. Electrical shocks delivered during this phase *without* prior chest compressions typically result in asystole or pulseless electrical activity. Continuous uninterrupted chest compressions are needed to reperfuse the myocardium and increase the likelihood of shock success. Nothing else, not even traditional ACLS interventions, must distract the resuscitation team leader from ensuring that high-quality compressions are provided. The circulation provided by high-quality compressions provides adequate coronary perfusion pressure, partially washes out inflammatory mediators, and restores energy substrates. However, even brief pauses in compressions (to perform other interventions) nullify their effectiveness.

KEY POINT

Nothing else, not even traditional ACLS interventions, must distract the resuscitation team leader from ensuring that high-quality compressions are provided.

The effectiveness of defibrillation and CPR rapidly declines during the metabolic phase (>10 minutes). Similar to the sepsis state, whole-body ischemia and reperfusion cause widespread tissue injury. Gut mucosal translocation of gram-negative bacteria results in widespread release of endotoxins and cytokines.

FIGURE 5-1.

A timeline for increasing the likelihood of neurologically intact survival after cardiac arrest

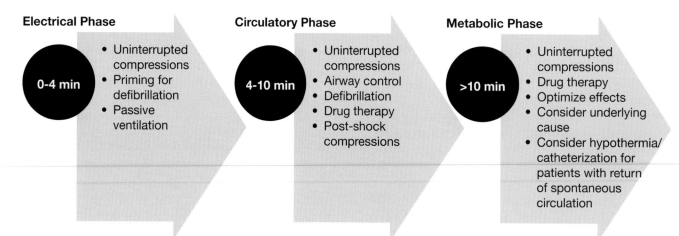

Electrical Phase

0-4 min
- Uninterrupted compressions
- Priming for defibrillation
- Passive ventilation

Circulatory Phase

4-10 min
- Uninterrupted compressions
- Airway control
- Defibrillation
- Drug therapy
- Post-shock compressions

Metabolic Phase

>10 min
- Uninterrupted compressions
- Drug therapy
- Optimize effects
- Consider underlying cause
- Consider hypothermia/ catheterization for patients with return of spontaneous circulation

Cellular reperfusion itself exacerbates these injuries as a result of the initiation of apoptosis and accelerated cell death. Interventions such as hypothermia-mediated attenuation of reperfusion injury, extracorporeal membrane oxygenation, and the use of various apoptosis inhibitors and other biochemical interventions are areas of ongoing research to combat the pathophysiology of this final phase.

Reorganizing

Historically, emergency care providers have been satisfied with return of spontaneous circulation (ROSC) alone as an acceptable outcome in cardiac arrest. Survival to emergency department arrival or hospital admission can no longer be acceptable in our efforts to improve the results of resuscitation after cardiac arrest. The benchmark to which we hold our interventions must be nothing short of neurologically intact survival to hospital discharge.

The mantra of ACLS has been "ABC" (airway, breathing, circulation). The care provider is instructed to first check the patient's airway and, if necessary, establish its patency, and then deliver rescue breaths. Only then is the provider directed to check for signs of circulation and, if necessary, begin chest compressions. These chest compressions are then interrupted for the delivery of additional rescue breaths, defibrillation, pulse checks, and other ACLS interventions such as establishment of venous access, delivery of vasoactive medications, and definitive airway management. This prioritization of tasks has been shown time and time again to delay and interfere with the two most crucial interventions in cardiac arrest resuscitation: continuous uninterrupted chest compressions and defibrillation. As a result, the 2010 AHA guidelines for CPR and ECC change the traditional mantra of "ABC" to "CAB" (compressions, airway, breathing).[2] This reversal to CAB is the foundation of CCR. We will examine each component of cardiac arrest care and, based on the latest available evidence, attempt to optimize it and place it in the proper sequence to maximize neurologically intact survival to hospital discharge.

PEARL
The new mantra for cardiac arrest is "CAB" (compressions, airway, breathing) for adults and pediatric patients.

Airway

The airway is traditionally the foundation of all resuscitative efforts. Conventional wisdom is that, without the establishment of a patent, stable, and definitive airway through which oxygenation and ventilation can be provided, resuscitation efforts are typically for naught. As such, airway management is usually of utmost importance for emergency care providers and is one of the defining skills of our specialty. However, because the first few minutes of cardiac arrest resuscitation are crucial to neurologically intact survival, resuscitation team leaders cannot afford to waste precious time on advanced airway management. Nearly 25% of all interruptions in chest compressions are accounted for by endotracheal intubation.[12] Instead, the first phase of resuscitation must focus on the delivery of continuous, high-quality chest compressions and rapid defibrillation. If there is a need to stabilize an airway early in resuscitation,

the use of a supraglottic airway device is a rapid and recommended alternative to endotracheal intubation.[2] In addition to supraglottic devices, commercially available airways adjuncts can safely be deployed to secure the unstable airway.[13] If endotracheal intubation is required, the use of cricoid pressure is no longer recommended.[2] Once an endotracheal tube has been placed, the 2010 AHA guidelines recommend the use of quantitative waveform capnography for monitoring endotracheal tube placement.[2]

KEY POINT
The first phase of resuscitation must focus on the delivery of continuous, high-quality chest compressions and rapid defibrillation.

Breathing

One of the tenets of bystander CPR is the provision of positive-pressure mouth-to-mouth ventilations. Increasing evidence shows that the lay public is reluctant to perform this intervention, and this reluctance often precludes the provision of any assistance whatsoever, including chest compressions. Bystanders are fearful of contracting a disease and of doing harm to the person in cardiac arrest. Interestingly, this long-accepted intervention may not even be necessary.

The average patient experiencing cardiac arrest (that is clearly not respiratory in origin) begins with an oxygen saturation near 100%. Based on the extraction and depletion of the central oxygen saturation during CPR, additional oxygen is not required for at least several minutes. Chest compressions alone result in chest wall recoil, which provides passive ventilation with 21% FIO_2. Exhaled air supplied during bystander mouth-to-mouth ventilations has an FIO_2 much less than 21%. Mouth-to-mouth ventilation actually depletes the central oxygen saturation more quickly than passive ventilation with room air provided by chest compressions alone.

KEY POINT
Mouth-to-mouth ventilation depletes the central oxygen saturation more quickly than passive ventilation with room air provided by chest compressions alone.

Health care providers deliver ventilations via bag-valve-mask and an attached reservoir of 100% FIO_2. Traditionally, compressions and ventilations are provided in an alternating fashion at a fixed ratio. However, even these brief pauses in compressions to deliver intermittent positive-pressure rescue breaths detract from the beneficial effects of CPR. Passive ventilation alone with an oxygen facemask provides sufficient oxygen delivery for the first minutes of resuscitation and does not detract from continuous chest compressions. There is increasing evidence[14] that passive ventilation could even be superior to positive-pressure ventilation in witnessed cardiac arrest with a shockable rhythm—ventricular fibrillation (VF) or ventricular tachycardia (VT). The appropriate FIO_2 for ventilation during cardiac arrest remains controversial because of concern about free-radical–induced damage from cellular reperfusion with 100% FIO_2.[15] This remains an ongoing area of scientific inquiry.

Compressions

The cornerstone of successful cardiac arrest resuscitation is truly continuous, high-quality, uninterrupted chest compressions. The resuscitation team leader must take steps to ensure their delivery, such as rotating providers every few minutes to reduce fatigue and using continuous feedback devices that optimize both rate and depth with audiovisual cues. The 2010 AHA guidelines recommend a depth of at least 2 inches for adult victims of cardiac arrest.[2] For pediatric patients, a depth of approximately 1.5 inches for most infants and 2 inches for most children is recommended.[2] In addition to providing compressions of appropriate depth, it is also important to allow complete recoil of the chest between compressions.[2] The quality of chest compressions can also be assessed with end-tidal CO_2 monitoring or arterial pressure during the relaxation phase of compression.[2] Compressions are so vital because they restore both cerebral and coronary perfusion pressure, which washes out inflammatory mediators and renews energy substrates. This is especially crucial for cerebral tissue because it is sensitive to hypoxic-ischemic injury and ultimately plays a primary role in meaningful neurologic recovery.

Compressions restore adequate coronary perfusion pressure (CPP), but only if they are truly continuous. Even brief pauses in compressions result in a dramatic drop-off of CPP, and the provider must essentially start over to build and maintain it. There is a threshold CPP that must be reached for successful defibrillation and resuscitation.[16] Preserving CPP is important because it improves the likelihood of shock success. Since there is so much at stake when ensuring this crucial intervention, there has been movement to automate and standardize it. Private industry has manufactured an array of mechanical devices that provide continuous uninterrupted compressions, and they may have a larger role in the future of cardiac arrest resuscitation.[17] To date, however, no device has been shown to be superior to manual CPR.[2]

PEARL

Even brief pauses in compressions result in a dramatic drop-off of CPP, and the provider must essentially start over to build and maintain it.

Defibrillation

Defibrillation stuns the heart, allowing viable cardiac pacemaker tissue to resume normal firing. In a witnessed cardiac arrest when the patient is still in the electrical phase, early defibrillation is critical. Implantable cardiac defibrillators and automated external defibrillators are a testament to this. However, once the myocardial energy substrates have been depleted, attempting defibrillation without first providing circulation via chest compressions typically results in pulseless electrical activity or asystole. Even if an organized electrical rhythm is restored, the myocardium itself does not contract sufficiently to generate forward flow. The myocardium first has to be "primed" to receive the electrical shock. Optimal timing of defibrillation can be guided by the appearance of the VF waveform. Several mathematical calculations are used to analyze the "coarseness" of the waveform to yield a calculated value that reliably predicts shock success.[18]

FIGURE 5-2.

Sample EMS protocol for cardiocerebral resuscitation. The protocol starts with passive insufflation via a nonrebreather mask. From: SHARE Program: Cardiocerebral Resuscitation (CCR) for EMS Providers. Phoenix, Arizona Department of Health Services, 2010. http://www.azshare.gov/ccr_share.html. Used with permission of the Arizona Sarver Heart Center.

Cardiocerebral Resuscitation (CCR)

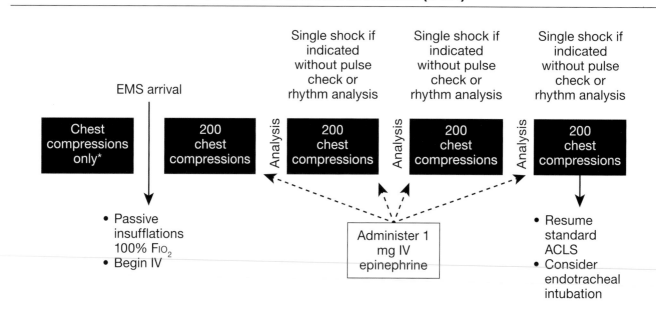

*If adequate bystander chest compressions are provided, EMS providers perform immediate rhythm analysis.

Any pause in chest compressions undermines their benefit, even the traditional pause for a "pulse check" after defibrillation. It can take up to a minute for the organized electrical activity in a functioning myocardium to generate forward blood flow sufficient to be palpated as a pulse. Continuous chest compressions augment this restoration of circulation. To even further reduce "hands-off time," providers may consider performing "hands-on defibrillation." There is increasing evidence that providers can safely continue compressions during the delivery of an electrical shock with a *biphasic* defibrillator. Lloyd et al[19] found that the amount of current experienced by study participants was below the threshold of perceptibility.

Venous Access

The establishment of venous access is a time-consuming process, even for the most experienced providers. With limited personnel and resources (ie, in the prehospital setting), this intervention should be de-emphasized and should not interfere with chest compressions. Instead, prehospital emergency care providers should look to adjuncts such as intraosseous devices that can be deployed rapidly and easily without distracting from crucial chest compressions.[20]

Medications

Much time and energy have been devoted to the use of vasoactive and antiarrhythmic medications such as epinephrine, atropine, vasopressin, amiodarone, lidocaine, and magnesium sulfate during cardiac arrest. As they are currently used, they increase the number of patients that achieve ROSC and survive to emergency department arrival or hospital admission, but none has been shown to affect neurologically intact survival to hospital discharge.[8] In fact, atropine is no longer recommended in the 2010 AHA guidelines for CPR and ECC for patients with pulseless electrical activity or asystole.[2]

Overall, these vasoactive and antiarrhythmic drugs carry no proven benefit in cardiac arrest. Perhaps this is because they are given late during resuscitation. After out-of-hospital cardiac arrest, prehospital care providers typically arrive during the circulatory phase and drugs are not administered until well into the metabolic phase. Yet, these same drugs have been used in

animal models with moderate success.[21] Aside from the obvious differences in species, medications are given in animal models during the circulatory phase, when the primary task is to augment coronary and cerebral perfusion pressures and restore energy substrates to the myocardium. Perhaps these medications will one day contribute to neurologically intact survival in humans, but only if they are delivered in a timely manner that does not prevent compression delivery.

Prehospital Considerations

Emergency physicians are often tasked with providing online and offline medical control to emergency medical technicians, paramedics, and other prehospital professionals. It is no longer sufficient to ensure that practicing paramedics maintain current certification in ALS. Indeed, emergency physicians must lead the way in educating our EMS colleagues about the importance of basic life support (BLS). Despite clear outcomes data, current prehospital literature is replete with instances of sustained interruptions in CPR and poor-quality compressions.[22,23] The relevance of quality compressions to improved outcome was described over a decade ago in Norway, when patients receiving quality bystander CPR experienced an unheard-of survival-to-discharge rate of 23%.[24] Current technologies provide real-time feedback on both the quality and timing of compressions. Automated compression devices completely remove the variable of fatigue from the resuscitation equation. Newer technologies certainly require an investment of funds. At the very least, paramedics and other "lead" prehospital care providers should be trained about the imperatives of early compressions, early defibrillation, and consideration of a delay in intubation. Without question, the focus on prehospital CPR has shifted away from "packaging" a patient with intravenous access and placement of an advanced airway. Embracing BLS is not without precedent. EMS systems led by resuscitation trailblazers such as Valenzuela, Kern, and Kellum have implemented a CCR-based approach.[25] The Arizona Department of Health, through its Save Hearts in Arizona Registry & Education (SHARE) program, has posted a public version of its *statewide* prehospital cardiac arrest protocol (Figure 5-2).[26]

TABLE 5-1.

Prehospital termination of resuscitation rules[a]

Prehospital resuscitation should be terminated if none of the following applies:

Advanced Life Support	Basic Life Support
Arrest witnessed by EMS	Arrest witnessed by EMS
Shock delivered	Shock delivered
ROSC at any point during resuscitation at the scene	ROSC prior to transport
Arrest witnessed by bystander	
Bystander compressions	

[a]Exclusion criteria: age <18 years, presumed noncardiac cause of arrest, patient "obviously dead" (ie, decapitation, rigor mortis)

Prehospital termination of resuscitation has been a controversial topic. However, recent evidence sheds light on this difficult task. There are now validated prehospital termination-of-resuscitation rules that are 100% specific for both BLS and ALS prehospital personnel.[27,28] The BLS rules recommend that prehospital resuscitation be terminated if none of the following three criteria is present: 1) there was ROSC prior to transport, 2) the arrest was witnessed by EMS personnel, and 3) a shock was delivered. Exclusion criteria for these rules are age less than 18 years, a presumed noncardiac cause of the arrest, or the patient is "obviously dead" according to local guidelines (ie, decapitation or rigor mortis). The ALS rules recommend that prehospital resuscitation should be terminated if none of the following five criteria is present: 1) the arrest was witnessed by EMS personnel, 2) a shock was delivered, 3) there was ROSC at any point during the resuscitation attempt at the scene, 4) bystander chest compressions were performed, and 5) the arrest was witnessed by a bystander (Table 5-1).

Regionalization of Arrest Care

A testament to the reevaluation of cardiac arrest care is the development of regionalized cardiac arrest centers.[29] Regardless of post-arrest ECG findings, patients who exhibit ROSC can benefit from direct transport to a facility with the resources for percutaneous coronary intervention (PCI).[30] The cost of poor neurologic outcomes is enormous; it may be wise to consider a progressive approach to resuscitation that optimizes chances for the best outcome. A cardiac arrest survival system built on the foundations of excellent BLS care, early defibrillation, cooling, and catheterization can positively influence survival rates. Political, economic, and geographic considerations pose considerable challenges to a systems-based approach. A cardiac arrest center is a logical extension of a regional PCI or STEMI center.[31]

Although performing cardiac catheterization on patients with ROSC is a progressive and currently revolutionary strategy, it is definitely an intervention associated with improved outcomes.[30] Theoretically, designated cardiac arrest centers would provide the post-arrest victim with a variety of resources, including induced hypothermia, PCI, and a dedicated critical care system.[32] Emergency physicians engaged in medical direction must be actively involved in the regionalization discussion. In 2010, an expert panel with members from the American College of Emergency Physicians, the National Association of Emergency Medical Services Physicians, and the American Heart Association urged communities to explore coordinated systems of survival. In its policy statement, the panel stated, "We believe that the time has come for a call to develop and implement standards for regional systems of care for those with restoration of circulation after out-of-hospital cardiac arrest."[33]

The call for directed transport is far from revolutionary, although the discussion of how best to allocate critical care resources is ongoing. It is clear, however, that an evidence-based and state-of-the-art chain of survival must now incorporate links such as compression-only bystander CPR, quality BLS, early defibrillation, cooling, and cardiac catheterization.

PEARL

An evidence-based and state-of-the-art chain of survival must incorporate links such as compression-only bystander CPR, quality BLS, early defibrillation, cooling, and cardiac catheterization.

Special Considerations in Cardiac Arrest Management

It is well known that cardiac arrest algorithms are far from inclusive. The CCR approach has improved outcomes, but it is structured around a witnessed arrest from VF or VT. Ischemic disease and lethal arrhythmia are the most common causes of out-of-hospital cardiac arrest in adults, but it is imperative to maintain a broad-based and inclusive differential when treating pediatric patients, trauma patients, and victims of overdose.

Traumatic Cardiac Arrest

Out-of-hospital traumatic cardiac arrest has a dismal prognosis.[34] Victims of hemorrhagic shock require blood and blood products, which are usually not immediately available. Therefore, an approach to traumatic cardiac arrest is predicated on achieving hemostasis and delivering the patient to definitive care. The lessons learned on the battlefields of Afghanistan and Iraq have direct patient care implications. Front-line combat casualty care emphasizes simple and immediately executable strategies. Military medicine has seen a resurgence in tourniquet use; long-standing bias and perhaps overestimated concerns about ischemic complications have given way to a more liberal approach that favors tourniquets in the setting of life-threatening hemorrhage.[35,36] Commercially available tourniquets, patterned after military tools, are designed to minimize deleterious complications while optimizing hemorrhage control.

Although the imperative of hemostasis is a long-standing pillar of trauma care, volume expansion with crystalloid intravenous fluids has fallen out of favor. The risks of hemodilution and metabolic derangement have resulted in the abandonment of indiscriminate infusion of intravenous Ringer lactate or normal saline. In the setting of life-threatening bleeding, volume should be replaced with packed red blood cells and fresh frozen plasma. The optimum ratio of blood to blood products has been a source of controversy; current clinical practices favor a 1-to-1 infusion ratio.[37,38] A smaller subset of patients may benefit from crystalloid infusions titrated to fluid loss or a predetermined mean arterial pressure. Patients with crush injuries, massive musculoskeletal injuries, and burns benefit from vigorous crystalloid infusion. Poor outcome is linked to hypotension in patients with isolated head trauma. Aggressive intravenous fluid administration and early neurosurgical intervention should be considered when managing head-injured patients. A sensible and aggressive approach to the patient in traumatic cardiac arrest incorporates high ratios of packed red blood cells to fresh frozen plasma, hemorrhage control, permissive hypotension, and early surgical consultation. (See Chapter 15, "The Crashing Trauma Patient.")

Cardiac Arrest Management in the Poisoned Patient

Clearly, resuscitation of the critically ill patient is often undertaken without the benefit of a complete history. Therefore, consideration of underlying causes is of prime importance. Certain toxidromes are associated with high patient mortality rates, myocardial depression, and lethal arrhythmia. In specific cases, the administration of a particular ACLS drug can counteract a poison's deleterious effects. Consider consultation with a regional poison control center when appropriate. Discuss any suspicious patient presentations with prehospital care providers. (See Chapter 14, "The Critically Ill Poisoned Patient.")

Cardiac Arrest in the Pediatric Patient

Emergency physicians, as resuscitation professionals, need to maintain proficiency in pediatric emergency skills. Pediatric cardiac arrest rarely results from lethal arrhythmia. It usually results from hypoxic insult, so special attention to airway priorities is of extreme importance. Pediatric resuscitation strategies emphasize airway control and correction of underlying pathology. In many cases, effective airway control is achieved with use of a bag-valve mask. Advantages such as airway protection and prevention of aspiration have been associated with tracheal intubation; however, improved patient outcomes have not been consistently documented in the literature.[39] Protracted resuscitation attempts could necessitate placement of a more definitive airway. Cuffed endotracheal tubes form a superior airway seal and have not been associated with a concurrent rise in airway complications. Provided that cuff pressure is reliably measured, current guidelines support the use of cuffed endotracheal tubes for pediatric airway management.[40] Ideally, providers are trained to recognize signs of impending circulatory collapse. Effective strategies in the management of pediatric arrest are predicated on the recognition and subsequent prevention of shock states.

Even though children are not "small adults," emergency department resuscitation protocols for adults and children share several common priorities. The value of quality compressions and BLS cannot be overstated. Lengthy attempts to establish intravenous access are discouraged in favor of quicker modalities such as intraosseous needle insertion. Devices such as the E-Z IO drill (Vidacare, Shavano Park, TX) minimize the technical difficulty of placing a catheter into the bone marrow. Children with ROSC benefit from therapeutic hypothermia. Some tertiary care centers have reported favorable results with extracorporeal membrane oxygenation in victims of refractory arrest.[41] This technology can enhance the resuscitation armamentarium in hospitals with specialized personnel and equipment.

Finally, adequate preparation and training are essential. Pediatric supplies must be readily accessible and familiar to all providers charged with leading resuscitation. Weight-based drug regimens and color-coded kits containing appropriately sized equipment can minimize stress during an arrest scenario.

On the Horizon: New and Emerging Technologies

The uptick in survival rates has contributed to a resurgence of resuscitation research. From EMS systems exploring new protocols for witnessed arrest to the idea of suspended animation, the future of resuscitation science is bright. New paradigms in cardiac arrest management can produce system-wide reforms. Areas ripe for continued exploration include the following:

- Appropriate resuscitation situations amenable to extracorporeal membrane oxygenation
- "Suspended animation" protocols and the use of ice-cold saline infusion to induce cardioplegia and markedly reduce, or suspend, metabolic demand
- New defibrillator/monitor technologies that afford rescuers real-time feedback about compression quality and timing. Although costly, this technology is currently available. Feedback-enabled devices permit real-time quality improvement as well as in-depth case review of cardiac arrest care.
- Defibrillator analysis of VF waveform characteristics to predict likelihood of shock success

Research is ongoing into specific neuroprotective agents that could limit the deleterious effects of cerebral ischemia. Pharmacologic agents such as terlipressin have been associated with ROSC in several case reports of in-hospital pediatric cardiac arrest.[42] Other protocols have investigated the utility of inhalational anesthetics.[43]

References

1. Ewy GA. A new approach for out-of-hospital CPR: a bold step forward. *Resuscitation.* 2003;58:271-272.
2. Neumar RW, Otto CW, Link MS, et al. Part 8: adult advanced cardiovascular life support: 2010 American Heart Association Guidelines for Cardiopulmonary Resuscitation and Emergency Cardiovascular Care. *Circulation.* 2010;122(suppl 3):S729–S767.
3. Ewy GA. Cardiocerebral resuscitation: the new cardiopulmonary resuscitation. *Circulation.* 2005;111:2134-2142.
4. Davis DP. Cardiocerebral resuscitation: a broader perspective. *J Am Coll Cardiol.* 2009;53:158-160.
5. Garza AG, Gratton MC, Salomone JA, et al. Improved patient survival using a modified resuscitation protocol for out-of-hospital cardiac arrest. *Circulation.* 2009;119:2597-2605.
6. Kellum MJ, Kennedy KW, Ewy GA. Cardiocerebral resuscitation improves survival of patients with out-of-hospital cardiac arrest. *Am J Med.* 2006;119:335-340.
7. Eisenberg MS. Improving survival from out-of-hospital cardiac arrest: back to the basics. *Ann Emerg Med.* 2007;49:314-316.
8. Olasveengen TM, Sunde K, Brunborg C, et al. Intravenous drug administration during out-of-hospital cardiac arrest. *JAMA.* 2009;302:2222-2229.
9. Weisfeldt ML, Becker LB. Resuscitation after cardiac arrest: a 3-phase time-sensitive model. *JAMA.* 2002;288:3035-3038.
10. ECC Committee, Subcommittee and Task Forces of the American Heart Association. 2005 American Heart Association Guidelines for Cardiopulmonary Resuscitation and Emergency Cardiovascular Care. Part 5: Electrical therapies: automated external defibrillators, defibrillation, cardioversion, and pacing. *Circulation.* 2005;112:IV-35–IV-46.
11. Sanna T, La Torre G, de Waure C, et al. Cardiopulmonary resuscitation alone vs. cardiopulmonary resuscitation plus automated external defibrillator use by non-healthcare professionals: a meta-analysis on 1583 cases of out-of-hospital cardiac arrest. *Resuscitation.* 2008;76:226-232.
12. Wang HE, Simeone SJ, Weaver MD, et al. Interruptions in cardiopulmonary resuscitation from paramedic endotracheal intubation. *Ann Emerg Med.* 2009;54:645-652.
13. Guyette FX, Greenwood MJ, Neubecker D, et al. Alternate airways in the prehospital setting (resource document to NAEMSP position statement). *Prehosp Emerg Care.* 2007;11:56-61.
14. Bobrow BJ, Ewy GA, Clark L, et al. Passive oxygen insufflation is superior to bag-valve-mask ventilation for witnessed ventricular fibrillation out-of-hospital cardiac arrest. *Ann Emerg Med.* 2009;54:656-662.
15. Hazelton JL, Balan I, Elmer GI, et al. Hyperoxic reperfusion after global cerebral ischemia promotes inflammation and long-term hippocampal neuronal death. *J Neurotrauma.* 2010;27:753-762.
16. Reynolds JC, Salcido DD, Menegazzi JJ. Coronary perfusion pressure and return of spontaneous circulation after prolonged cardiac arrest. *Prehosp Emerg Care.* 2010;14(1):78-84.

17. Wigginton JC, Isaacs SM, Kay JJ. Mechanical devices for cardiopulmonary resuscitation. *Curr Opin Crit Care.* 2007;13:273-279.

18. Callaway CW, Sherman LD, Holt E, et al. Ventricular fibrillation waveform predicts defibrillation success by automatic external defibrillators. [SAEM abstract 038] *Acad Emerg Med.* 2000;7:438.

19. Lloyd MS, Heeke B, Walter PF, Langberg JJ. Hands-on defibrillation: an analysis of electrical current flow through rescuers in direct contact with patients during biphasic external defibrillation. *Circulation.* 2008;117:2510-2514.

20. Guyette FX, Rittenberger JC, Platt T, et al. Feasibility of basic emergency medical technicians to perform selected advanced life support interventions. *Prehosp Emerg Care.* 2006;10:518-521.

21. Reynolds JC, Rittenberger JC, Menegazzi JJ. Drug administration in animal studies of cardiac arrest does not reflect human clinical experience. *Resuscitation.* 2007;74(1):13-26.

22. Valenzuela TD, Kern KB, Clark LL, et al. Interruptions of chest compressions during emergency medical systems resuscitation. *Circulation.* 2005;112:1259-1265.

23. Wik L, Kramer-Johansen J, Myklebust H, et al. Quality of cardiopulmonary resuscitation during out-of-hospital cardiac arrest. *JAMA.* 2005;293:299-304.

24. Wik L, Steen PA, Bircher NG. Quality of bystander cardiopulmonary resuscitation influences outcome after prehospital cardiac arrest. *Resuscitation.* 1994;28:195-203.

25. Kern KB, Valenzuela TD, Clark LL, et al. An alternative approach to advancing resuscitation science. *Resuscitation.* 2005;64:261-268.

26. SHARE Program: Cardiocerebral Resuscitation (CCR) for EMS Providers. Phoenix, Arizona Department of Health. 2010. Available at http://www.azshare.gov/ccr_share.html. Accessed on June 1, 2010.

27. Sasson C, Hegg AJ, Macy M, et al. Prehospital termination of resuscitation in cases of refractory and out-of-hospital cardiac arrest. *JAMA.* 2008;300:1423-1438.

28. Morrison LJ, Verbeek PR, Zhan C, et al. Validation of a universal prehospital termination of resuscitation clinical prediction rule for advanced and basic life support providers. *Resuscitation.* 2009;80:324-328.

29. Spaite DW, Stiell IG, Bobrow BJ, et al. Effect of transport interval on out-of-hospital cardiac arrest survival in the OPALS study: implications for triaging patients to specialized cardiac arrest centers. *Ann Emerg Med.* 2009;54:248-255.

30. Reynolds JC, Callaway CW, El Khoudary SR, et al. Coronary angiography predicts improved outcome following cardiac arrest: propensity-adjusted analysis. *J Int Care Med.* 2009;24:179-186.

31. Kahn JM, Branas CC, Schwab CW, et al. Regionalization of medical critical care: what can we learn from the trauma experience? *Crit Care Med.* 2008;36:3085-3088.

32. Rittenberger JC, Callaway CW. Transport of patients after out-of-hospital cardiac arrest: closest facility or most appropriate facility? A*nn Emerg Med.* 2009;54:256-257.

33. Nichol G, Aufderheide TP, Eigel B, et al. Regional systems of care for out-of-hospital cardiac arrest: a policy statement from the American Heart Association. *Circulation.* 2010;121(5):709-729.

34. Lockey D, Crewdson K, Davies G. Traumatic cardiac arrest: who are the survivors? *Ann Emerg Med.* 2006;48:240-244.

35. Welling DR, Burris DG, Hutton JE, et al. A balanced approach to tourniquet use: lessons learned and relearned. *J Am Coll Surg.* 2006;203:106-115.

36. Kragh JF Jr. Use of tourniquets and their effects on limb function in the modern combat environment. *Foot Ankle Clin.* 2010;15:23-40.

37. Beekley AC. Damage control resuscitation: a sensible approach to the exsanguinating surgical patient. *Crit Care Med.* 2008;36(7 suppl):S267-S274.

38. Zink KA, Sambasivan CN, Holcomb JB, et al. A high ratio of plasma and platelets to packed red blood cells in the first six hours of massive transfusion improves outcomes in a large multicenter study. *Am J Surg.* 2009;197(5):565-570.

39. Bingham RM, Proctor LT. Airway management. *Pediatr Clin North Am.* 2008;55:873-886.

40. Weiss M, Dullenkopf A, Fisher JE, et al. Prospective randomized controlled multi-centre trial of cuffed or uncuffed endotracheal tubes in small children. *Br J Anaesth.* 2009;103:867-873.

41. Hickey RW, Nadkarny V. Future directions in cardiocerebral resuscitation. *Pediatr Clin North Am.* 2008;55:1051-1064.

42. Anton JG, Lopez-Herce J, Morteruel E, et al. Pediatric cardiac arrest refractory to advanced life support: is there a role for terlipressin? *Pediatr Crit Care Med.* 2010;11:139-141.

43. Derwall M, Timper A, Kottman K, et al. Neuroprotective effects of the inhalational anesthetics isoflurane and xenon after cardiac arrest in pigs. *Crit Care Med.* 2008;36[suppl]:S492-S495.

CHAPTER 6

Post–Cardiac Arrest Management

Evie G. Marcolini and Michael C. Bond

Introduction

There is perhaps nothing more gratifying to an emergency physician than successfully resuscitating a patient from sudden cardiac death. Albeit exciting, the initial enthusiasm at the return of spontaneous circulation is quickly tempered by the realization of the challenges of the immediate post-cardiac arrest period. With the persistent national epidemic of hospital and intensive care unit (ICU) crowding, no longer can emergency physicians successfully resuscitate patients from sudden cardiac death and expeditiously transfer them to the appropriate ICU. In fact, many of these patients remain in the emergency department for exceedingly long periods of time awaiting an ICU bed. As a result, emergency physicians become responsible for the immediate phase of critical care that follows resuscitation from cardiac arrest. Thus, it is imperative that emergency physicians be knowledgeable in the management of these critically ill patients.

This chapter focuses on the critical care of emergency department patients successfully resuscitated from sudden cardiac death. Essential elements in the care of these patients include mechanical ventilation, circulatory support, invasive and non-invasive hemodynamic monitoring, neuroprotective strategies, and appropriate supportive care. Armed with this information, emergency physicians can deliver effective and efficient care to the post–cardiac arrest patient, thereby reducing morbidity and ultimately influencing outcome.

Definition

The term *post-resuscitation disease* was coined in the 1970s, when Dr. Vladimir Negovsky attempted to describe the unique pathophysiology of patients resuscitated from cardiopulmonary arrest.[1,2] In 2008, the International Liaison Committee on Resuscitation (ILCOR) used the term *post–cardiac arrest syndrome* (PCAS) to differentiate it from the resuscitation of patients with sepsis or shock caused by other critical illnesses. PCAS consists of four general processes: post-cardiac arrest brain injury, post-cardiac arrest myocardial dysfunction, systemic ischemia and reperfusion syndrome, and the overall response to cardiac arrest.

Cardiopulmonary arrest can be thought of as the ultimate shock state, resulting in markedly impaired oxygen delivery and extraction, endothelial activation, systemic inflammation, multi-organ failure, and death. Once return of spontaneous circulation is achieved, care of the post-cardiac arrest patient ultimately is directed to reversing these detrimental pathophysiologic processes (Figure 6-1).

FIGURE 6-1.

Summary of emergency department management of patients after resuscitation from cardiac arrest

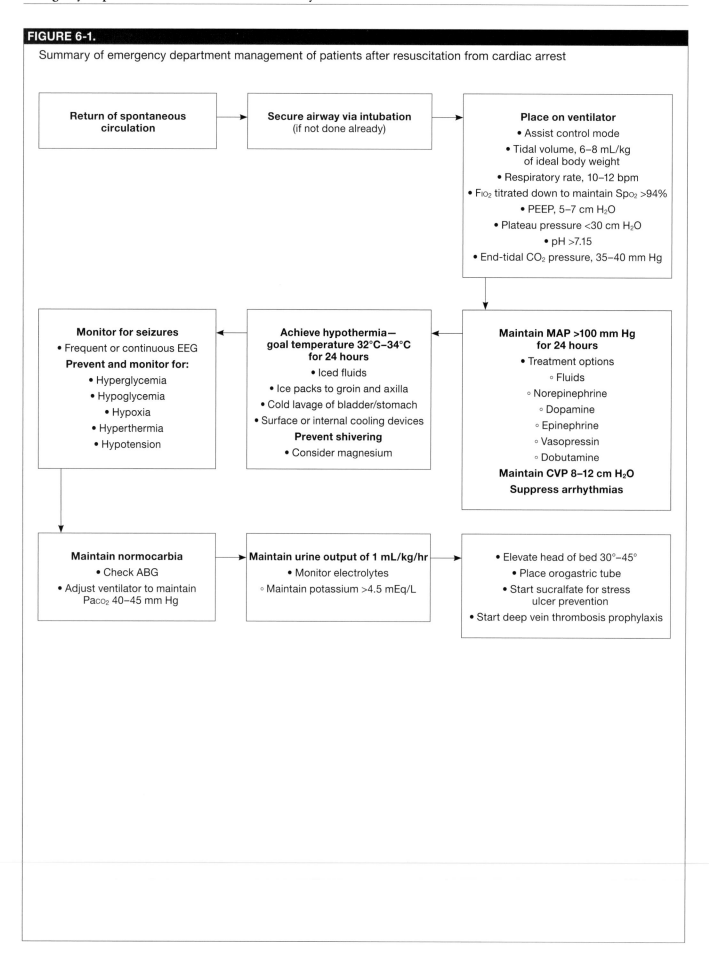

Management of the Post–Cardiac Arrest Patient

Oxygenation and Ventilation

Intubate the patient who is successfully resuscitated from sudden cardiac death and initiate mechanical ventilation. Ventilating the patient is of primary importance to prevent hypoxia and maintain normocapnia. Mechanical ventilation, like any medical intervention, can injure a patient if it is not applied and managed correctly. *Ventilator-induced lung injury* is a term used to describe a series of pathophysiologic mechanisms such as alveolar overdistention (volutrauma), sheer stress from repeated opening and closing of alveolar units (atelectrauma), barotrauma, and the systemic release of inflammatory mediators (biotrauma). Initially, for the post–cardiac arrest patient, the ventilator should be set to limit ventilator-induced lung injury by achieving lower and safer alveolar distending pressures. These initial settings (Figure 6-1) are a starting point for ventilatory support. Adjustments are made based on serial measurements of pH, $Paco_2$, and plateau pressures.

A natural consequence of using these initial settings to limit lung injury is limiting the accumulation of carbon dioxide. Hypercapnia can increase intracranial pressure (ICP) and exacerbate existing acidosis. Similarly, hypocapnia can propagate cerebral injury by causing cerebral vasoconstriction, leading to ischemia. Given the emphasis on neuroprotective strategies in the PCAS patient, the ventilator should be adjusted to achieve a $Paco_2$ between 40 and 45 mm Hg. Capnography can be a useful tool to maintain the neuroprotective goal for $Paco_2$.[3] End-tidal carbon dioxide values should be maintained between 35 and 40 mm Hg.[3]

Circulatory Support

All PCAS patients should receive continuous cardiac monitoring and pulse oximetry, a Foley catheter for measuring urine output, and serial laboratory diagnostic testing that includes cardiac enzymes, lactate, and arterial blood gases. Most patients with PCAS have tenuous cardiovascular status at best. Hemodynamic instability in these patients can be caused by hypovolemia, impaired vasoregulation, myocardial dysfunction, dysrhythmias, or even iatrogenic sources such as the initiation of therapeutic hypothermia.

Achieving an adequate circulating volume is the first priority in many PCAS patients. Administering intravenous fluids is the first strategy for correcting intravascular volume depletion. Although the debate over crystalloid versus colloid therapy seems endless, isotonic crystalloids are currently the recommended fluid of choice in PCAS patients.[4] Current recommendations state that fluid therapy should be titrated to achieve a central venous pressure (CVP) between 8 and 12 mm Hg.[4] These recommendations are based on the principles of early goal-directed therapy,[5] not on formal studies of CVP goals for PCAS patients. It is important to recognize the limitations of CVP in the assessment of volume status: it can be altered by tricuspid valve disease, arrhythmias, pericardial effusion, right ventricular dysfunction, or simply the reference level of the transducer. As a result, volume status should be monitored by additional means.

One option is the use of bedside ultrasonography to measure the diameter of the inferior vena cava during the "sniff test." Another well-described method for assessing volume status and determining the likelihood of response to the administration of intravenous fluids is the monitoring of pulse pressure variation, as measured on a tracing from an arterial line. Finally, monitoring urine output can also assist in the titration of fluid therapy. A urine output of at least 0.5 mL/kg/hr should be achieved and maintained when titrating fluid therapy in these patients.

PEARL

It is important to recognize the limitations of CVP in the assessment of volume status: it can be altered by tricuspid valve disease, arrhythmias, pericardial effusion, right ventricular dysfunction, or simply the reference level of the transducer.

Maintaining adequate oxygen delivery to vital organs is essential in the treatment of patients following cardiac arrest. Oxygen delivery to the tissues depends directly on organ perfusion pressure. The best physiologic estimate of organ perfusion pressure is mean arterial pressure (MAP), which must be monitored continuously in patients after cardiac arrest. Human data show that an elevated MAP significantly correlates with improved neurologic outcome in PCAS patients.[6] It is postulated that after cardiac arrest, cerebral blood flow requires elevated MAPs to maintain adequate cerebral perfusion. Although the optimal MAP has yet to be prospectively defined, current recommendations state that in the first 24 hours following return of spontaneous circulation, MAP should be maintained near 100 mm Hg.[4] If the goal MAP cannot be achieved with intravenous fluids alone, vasopressor medications should be initiated. At this point, the blood pressure should be monitored continuously with the use of an arterial line.

The efficacy of the various vasopressors in the management of PCAS has not been studied formally. Based on the authors' experience, norepinephrine is a reasonable first-line agent because it increases MAP through vasoconstriction and has minimal effects on heart rate and cardiac index. In addition, norepinephrine improves renal perfusion and lactate clearance.[7] Dopamine is also a reasonable first-line vasopressor medication; however, its effect of increasing the heart rate and contractility can increase myocardial workload in an already compromised situation. Phenylephrine is, at best, a second-line agent because it increases MAP without increasing heart rate or cardiac index. Continuous infusion of epinephrine has been used since it will increase MAP through increases in heart rate and systemic resistance. Unfortunately, in comparison with other vasopressor medications, epinephrine results in a greater degree of impaired splanchnic perfusion and increases in lactate levels. Vasopressin is a hormone that acts synergistically with other catecholamines to increase MAP by increasing systemic vascular resistance. Similar to epinephrine, it has the potential to decrease splanchnic perfusion and can thereby increase lactate levels. It should be used as a last resort after first-line agents have been unsuccessful, and care must be taken to ensure that intravascular volume is adequate.

If fluid therapy and vasopressor medications are unsuccessful, inotropic therapy can be used to achieve hemodynamic goals. Inotrope-responsive myocardial stunning can be present for as long as 72 hours in survivors of cardiac arrest.[8] The duration of myocardial stunning correlates to the length of cardiac arrest; echocardiography can help determine cardiac function.[8] Dobutamine has been the inotrope of choice and can be used to support hemodynamics either by itself on in conjunction with norepinephrine. It can produce up to a 50% increase in cardiac index as well as an increase in cardiac oxygen consumption, with a concomitant decrease in pulmonary artery occlusion pressure. However, dobutamine can exacerbate tachycardia in hypovolemic patients; therefore, adequate fluid resuscitation should continue.

While intravenous fluids, vasopressor medications, and inotropic therapy are provided, the success of resuscitation should be monitored via serial laboratory assessments. Lactate values have been studied extensively and can be used as a marker of the success of therapeutic efforts. The time to lactate clearance has a direct correlation with outcome in PCAS patients.[9] Lactate should be measured every 3 to 4 hours in the management of these critically ill patients. In addition to lactate, central venous oxygen saturation has been proposed as an endpoint for resuscitation in the critically ill. This parameter has been studied primarily in patients with severe sepsis and septic shock, with the goal of achieving a central venous oxygen saturation of more than 70%. Although it has been found useful in the management of sepsis, there are no studies to date that support its routine use in the management of PCAS patients.

For patients who remain hemodynamically unstable despite fluid, vasopressor medications, and inotropic therapy, the placement of an intra-aortic balloon pump, the initiation of extracorporeal membrane oxygenation, or the placement of a transthoracic ventricular assist device should be considered. These potentially life-saving therapies require appropriate consultation and resources and may not be possible in many emergency departments.

Neuroprotective Strategies

Brain injury is the most common cause of death in patients who survive a cardiac arrest.[10] Therapeutic hypothermia, the only therapy shown to increase survival in the PCAS population, has been shown in two randomized, unblinded trials and a meta-analysis to improve short-term neurologic recovery and survival after PCAS of presumed cardiac origin.[11-15] The number needed to treat for one survivor to leave the hospital with good neurologic function is between 4 and 13. Animal studies show that earlier implementation leads to better outcomes.[16]

Therapeutic hypothermia consists of induction, maintenance, and rewarming phases. Methods to achieve goal temperatures include administration of ice-cold intravenous fluids, applications of ice packs to the groin and axilla, and the use of surface or internal cooling devices. There is no evidence for the superiority of one method of induction over another. Studies are based on cooling patients to 32°C to 34°C for 12 to 24 hours.[11,12,15] Sedation and neuromuscular blockade can be used to prevent shivering; human data show that warming the skin will reduce the core-temperature threshold for shiver-

ing.[17] During the induction and rewarming phases, fluid and electrolyte shifts occur and must be monitored. Decreased core temperatures cause vasoconstriction with increased CVP and subsequent diuresis, which will reverse upon rewarming. The maintenance phase of treatment requires continuous feedback of temperature to avoid significant temperature fluctuation. Rewarming can be regulated by most cooling devices. Current recommendations are to rewarm at 0.25°C to 0.5°C per hour to minimize rapid changes in electrolyte concentrations, metabolic rate, and hemodynamic stability.[18]

Patients in whom therapeutic hypothermia is being induced must be monitored and treated for shivering. Adequate sedation can be achieved using benzodiazepines or propofol. If shivering continues despite titration of sedative medications, neuromuscular blocking agents should be used. However, neuromuscular blockers have a longer duration of action in the setting of hypothermia, and continuous electroencephalographic (EEG) monitoring may be necessary to watch for seizure activity. Sedation and hypothermia are both neuroprotective in that they decrease oxygen consumption. Magnesium sulfate has been shown in human research to increase the shivering threshold. In animal studies, magnesium has been shown to provide added neuroprotection during therapeutic hypothermia.[19,20] It also increases the cooling rate via vasodilation.

Contraindications to therapeutic hypothermia include severe systemic infection, preexisting coagulopathy, and established multi-organ failure.[21] Complications include infection, hemodynamic instability, decreased cardiac output, arrhythmias (most commonly bradycardia), coagulopathy, hyperglycemia, increased amylase, hypophosphatemia, hypocalcemia, hypokalemia, and hypomagnesemia.

In addition to therapeutic hypothermia, other neuroprotective strategies should be used in the PCAS patient. Seizures should be aggressively treated with standard medications such as benzodiazepines, phenytoin, valproate, propofol, and barbiturates. The most common adverse effect of these medications— hypotension—must be avoided. Myoclonus is best treated with clonazepam. Electroencephalography should be used frequently or continuously to monitor the patient for subclinical seizure activity. Hyperthermia, hypoxemia, and hyperglycemia should be avoided because they worsen neurologic outcome. Each degree increase in temperature increases the risk of a poor outcome with an odds ratio of 2.26.[9]

PEARL

Each degree increase in temperature increases the risk of a poor outcome with an odds ratio of 2.26.[9]

Thrombolytic Therapy

In a retrospective review of medical examiner cases, massive pulmonary embolus was found to be the second leading cause of death in nontraumatic out-of-hospital deaths.[22] Smaller pulmonary emboli can lead to hypoxemic cardiac arrest, manifesting an electromechanical dissociation rhythm that is responsive to adequate oxygenation. Although thrombolysis after cardiac arrest has been shown to be safe, prospective studies of thrombolytics demonstrated no improvement in outcomes.[23,24]

Cardiac arrest results in endothelial dysfunction, causing an increase in fibrin generation and impaired anticoagulation.[25] In a retrospective study of PCAS patients who survived ventricular fibrillation arrest, 27% received thrombolytics and had a good neurologic recovery.[26] Clear prospective data are lacking, but it is reasonable to consider treating suspected pulmonary embolus with the administration of thrombolytics.

KEY POINT
Consider thrombolytic therapy in patients with suspected massive pulmonary embolism.

Supportive Care

Prevent Ventilator-Associated Pneumonia

Ventilator-associated pneumonia is defined as pneumonia occurring more than 48 hours after intubation. It is a leading cause of morbidity and mortality in the ICU population. Mortality rates for this disastrous complication range from 20% to 50%. Intubated PCAS patients are at risk for ventilator-associated pneumonia, but several low- to no-cost interventions markedly decrease the risk. These include semi-recumbent positioning (head of bed elevated 30° to 40°, if there are no contraindications), frequent suctioning of the oropharynx, maintaining adequate endotracheal cuff pressures to prevent aspiration (between 20 and 30 cm H_2O), oral care with chlorhexidine rinses, and gastric decompression with an orogastric tube.[27,28]

Prevent Stress-Related Mucosal Injury

Stress-related mucosal injury is present in up to 75% of intubated patients on arrival in the ICU. Clinically significant bleeding occurs in up to 25% of this patient group, with hemorrhage requiring transfusion occurring in 2% to 5%. As a result, initiation of stress ulcer prophylaxis in the emergency department is indicated for intubated PCAS patients at high risk for gastrointestinal hemorrhage. Indicators of high risk for bleeding and thus for prophylaxis include duration of mechanical ventilation for more than 48 hours; a history of peptic ulcer disease, gastritis, or gastrointestinal hemorrhage; and coagulopathy. Other patients at risk include those with sepsis, severe head injury, renal failure, hepatic failure, hypotension, and multisystem trauma.

Maintain Adequate Hemoglobin Levels

Goals for hemoglobin concentration have not been well studied in PCAS patients. In septic patients, early goal-directed therapy guidelines recommend maintaining a hematocrit of 30% during the initial 6 hours of resuscitation.[5] This value has not been widely accepted. However, because most PCAS patients have a cardiac cause of the arrest, it is reasonable to maintain hematocrit above 30% to prevent myocardial ischemia.

KEY POINT
Maintain hematocrit above 30%.

Prevent Deep Venous Thrombosis

Prophylaxis against deep venous thrombosis is recommended early and in all ICU patients. In PCAS patients who do not have a high risk of bleeding, low-dose heparin, low-molecular-weight heparin, or mechanical compression devices are recommended, depending on patient comorbidities, medication allergies, presence of bleeding, and clinical stability.[29]

KEY POINT
Administer deep venous thrombosis prophylaxis.

Monitor Glucose Concentrations

Retrospective data have shown that the blood glucose level is independently associated with survival in PCAS patients.[30] Tight glucose control has improved outcomes in surgical and medical ICU patients, while moderate control has resulted in a lower incidence of hypoglycemia in patients resuscitated from ventricular fibrillation.[31–33] Observational human data show a direct correlation between hyperglycemia and poor neurologic outcome in patients with PCAS.[34] The optimal glucose concentration has not been defined. Given the available evidence, current recommendations are to maintain glucose concentrations between 144 and 180 mg/dL.[3,35] A standard protocol for managing hyperglycemia has not been prospectively validated. Discussion with ICU physicians and establishment of institutional protocols is advised until additional evidence clarifies the ideal glucose target and appropriate insulin protocol.

KEY POINT
Monitor glucose concentrations and maintain levels between 144 and 180 mg/dL.

Manage Acute Coronary Syndrome

Acute myocardial infarction is the most common cause of sudden cardiopulmonary arrest.[36] Standard therapy with antiplatelet medication and anticoagulation should be started in patients who have suspected acute coronary syndrome. Ideally, this would be coordinated with the cardiologist who will be involved in the care of the patient. It is reasonable to withhold anticoagulation until all central venous access or arterial lines are placed in order to prevent bleeding complications.

Use caution starting β-blockers in patients who already have a labile blood pressure or might require vasopressor support. It is imperative to maintain an adequate MAP to ensure an adequate cerebral perfusion pressure. Although β-blockers can be protective and decrease long-term mortality rates in patients with acute coronary syndrome, the hypotension they can cause in the short term can have detrimental effects on the patient's neurologic recovery.

Data support early angiography along with hypothermia treatment for PCAS patients who likely arrested secondary to sequelae from coronary artery disease.[13] The challenge in such a protocol is inclusion/exclusion criteria, since there are no reliable indicators of acute myocardial infarction in PCAS patients. Taking into consideration all other physiologic factors of the patient, it is reasonable to begin hypothermia treatment and consider early angiography. Thrombolytic therapy has been recommended for PCAS patients if percutaneous coronary intervention is not available, although this has not been studied in patients in whom therapeutic hypothermia is induced.

Possible risks include ineffectiveness of thrombolysis and/or hemorrhage. As with any patient with ST elevation myocardial infarction, coronary artery bypass grafting is recommended in those with left main coronary artery thrombosis or three-vessel disease.

KEY POINTS

Start administration of an antiplatelet medication.

Start anticoagulation with heparin or low-molecular-weight heparin if it is not contraindicated.

Consider reperfusion therapy with percutaneous coronary intervention or thrombolytics in patients with acute myocardial infarction.

Conclusion

Until recently, the return of spontaneous circulation has been the hallmark of a "successful" resuscitation. There is now a heightened appreciation and data to show that the delivery of care via protocol has a significant influence on the outcome of PCAS.[12] Many disciplines of health care will be involved in the care of a patient with PCAS, including emergency medicine, critical care medicine, and subspecialties such as cardiology, neurology, and nephrology. By implementing a standardized approach, we can build on the work that has been done so far to achieve return of spontaneous circulation and further improve the long-term outcomes of this patient population.

References

1. Negovsky VA, Gurvitch AM. Post-resuscitation disease—a new nosological entity: its reality and significance. *Resuscitation.* 1995;30:23-27.

2. Negovsky VA. The second step in resuscitation: the treatment of the 'post-resuscitation disease.' *Resuscitation.* 1972;1:1-7.

3. Peberdy MA, Callaway CW, Neumar RW, et al. Part 9: post–cardiac arrest care: 2010 American Heart Association Guidelines for Cardiopulmonary Resuscitation and Emergency Cardiovascular Care. *Circulation.* 2010;122(suppl 3):S768-S786.

4. Neumar RW, Nolan JP, Adrie C, et al. Post–cardiac arrest syndrome: epidemiology, pathophysiology, treatment, and prognostication: a consensus statement from the International Liaison Committee on Resuscitation (American Heart Association, Australian and New Zealand Council on Resuscitation, European Resuscitation Council, Heart and Stroke Foundation of Canada, InterAmerican Heart Foundation, Resuscitation Council of Asia, and the Resuscitation Council of Southern Africa); the American Heart Association Emergency Cardiovascular Care Committee; the Council on Cardiovascular Surgery and Anesthesia; the Council on Cardiopulmonary, Perioperative, and Critical Care; the Council on Clinical Cardiology; and the Stroke Council. *Circulation.* 2008;118:2452-2483.

5. Rivers E, Nguyen B, Havstad S, et al. Early goal-directed therapy in the treatment of severe sepsis and septic shock. *N Engl J Med.* 2001;345:1368-1377.

6. McIntyre LA, Fergusson DA, Hutchison JS, et al. Effect of a liberal versus restrictive transfusion strategy on mortality in patients with moderate to severe head injury. *Neurocrit Care.* 2006;5:4-9.

7. Balk RA, Casey LC. *Sepsis and Septic Shock.* Philadelphia, PA: W.B. Saunders; 2000.

8. Laurent I, Monchi M, Chiche JD, et al. Reversible myocardial dysfunction in survivors of out-of-hospital cardiac arrest. *J Am Coll Cardiol.* 2002;40:2110-2116.

9. Donnino MW, Miller J, Goyal N, et al. Effective lactate clearance is associated with improved outcome in post–cardiac arrest patients. *Resuscitation.* 2007;75:229-234.

10. Fink MP. *Textbook of Critical Care.* 5th ed. Philadelphia, PA: Elsevier Saunders; 2005.

11. Hypothermia after Cardiac Arrest Study Group. Mild therapeutic hypothermia to improve the neurologic outcome after cardiac arrest. *N Engl J Med.* 2002;346:549-556.

12. Bernard SA, Gray TW, Buist MD, et al. Treatment of comatose survivors of out-of-hospital cardiac arrest with induced hypothermia. *N Engl J Med.* 2002;346:557-563.

13. Sunde K, Pytte M, Jacobsen D, et al. Implementation of a standardised treatment protocol for post resuscitation care after out-of-hospital cardiac arrest. *Resuscitation.* 2007;73:29-39.

14. Nolan JP, Morley PT, Hoek TL, Hickey RW. Therapeutic hypothermia after cardiac arrest: an advisory statement by the Advanced Life Support Task Force of the International Liaison Committee on Resuscitation. *Resuscitation.* 2003;57:231-235.

15. Holzer M, Bernard SA, Hachimi-Idrissi S, et al. Hypothermia for neuroprotection after cardiac arrest: systematic review and individual patient data meta-analysis. *Crit Care Med.* 2005;33:414-418.

16. Kuboyama K, Safar P, Radovsky A, et al. Delay in cooling negates the beneficial effect of mild resuscitative cerebral hypothermia after cardiac arrest in dogs: a prospective, randomized study. *Crit Care Med.* 1993;21:1348-1358.

17. Cheng C, Matsukawa T, Sessler DI, et al. Increasing mean skin temperature linearly reduces the core-temperature thresholds for vasoconstriction and shivering in humans. *Anesthesiology.* 1995;82:1160-1168.

18. Arrich J. Clinical application of mild therapeutic hypothermia after cardiac arrest. *Crit Care Med.* 2007;35:1041-1047.

19. Wadhwa A, Sengupta P, Durrani J, et al. Magnesium sulphate only slightly reduces the shivering threshold in humans. *Br J Anaesth.* 2005;94:756-762.

20. Zhu H, Meloni BP, Moore SR, et al. Intravenous administration of magnesium is only neuroprotective following transient global ischemia when present with post-ischemic mild hypothermia. *Brain Res.* 2004;1014:53-60.

21. Soar J, Nolan JP. Mild hypothermia for post cardiac arrest syndrome. *BMJ.* 2007;335:459-460.

22. Courtney DM, Kline JA. Identification of prearrest clinical factors associated with outpatient fatal pulmonary embolism. *Acad Emerg Med.* 2001;8:1136-1142.

23. Bottiger BW, Bode C, Kern S, et al. Efficacy and safety of thrombolytic therapy after initially unsuccessful cardiopulmonary resuscitation: a prospective clinical trial. *Lancet.* 2001;357:1583-1585.

24. Abu-Laban RB, Christenson JM, Innes GD, et al. Tissue plasminogen activator in cardiac arrest with pulseless electrical activity. *N Engl J Med.* 2002;346:1522-1528.

25. Gando S, Kameue T, Nanzaki S, Nakanishi Y. Massive fibrin formation with consecutive impairment of fibrinolysis in patients with out-of-hospital cardiac arrest. *Thromb Haemost.* 1997;77:278-282.

26. Schreiber W, Gabriel D, Sterz F, et al. Thrombolytic therapy after cardiac arrest and its effect on neurological outcome. *Resuscitation.* 2002;52:63-69.

27. Rello J, Diaz E, Roque M, Valles J. Risk factors for developing pneumonia within 48 hours of intubation. *Am J Respir Crit Care Med.* 1999;159:1742-1746.

28. Gaussorgues P, Gueugniaud PY, Vedrinne JM, et al. Bacteremia following cardiac arrest and cardiopulmonary resuscitation. *Intensive Care Med.* 1988;14:575-577.

29. Geerts W, Selby R. Prevention of venous thromboembolism in the ICU. *Chest.* 2003;124(6 suppl):357S-363S.

30. Skrifvars MB, Pettila V, Rosenberg PH, Castren M. A multiple logistic regression analysis of in-hospital factors related to survival at six months in patients resuscitated from out-of-hospital ventricular fibrillation. *Resuscitation.* 2003;59:319-328.

31. Van den Berghe G, Wilmer A, Hermans G, et al. Intensive insulin therapy in the medical ICU. *N Engl J Med.* 2006;354:449-461.

32. Van den Berghe G, Schoonheydt K, Becx P, et al. Insulin therapy protects the central and peripheral nervous system of intensive care patients. *Neurology.* 2005;64:1348-1353.

33. Oksanen T, Skrifvars MB, Varpula T, et al. Strict versus moderate glucose control after resuscitation from ventricular fibrillation. *Intensive Care Med.* 2007;33:2093-2100.

34. Mullner M, Sterz F, Binder M, et al. Blood glucose concentration after cardiopulmonary resuscitation influences functional neurological recovery in human cardiac arrest survivors. *J Cereb Blood Flow Metab.* 1997;17:430-436.

35. Losert H, Sterz F, Roine RO, et al. Strict normoglycaemic blood glucose levels in the therapeutic management of patients within 12h after cardiac arrest might not be necessary. *Resuscitation.* 2008;76:214-220.

36. Huikuri HV, Castellanos A, Myerburg RJ. Sudden death due to cardiac arrhythmias. *N Engl J Med.* 2001;345:1473-1482.

Deadly Arrhythmias: Recognition and Resuscitative Management

Peter P. Monteleone, Mark R. Sochor, and William J. Brady

IN THIS CHAPTER

Bradyarrhythmias: bradycardia and atrioventricular block
Sinus bradycardia
Junctional bradycardia
Idioventricular rhythm (bradycardia)
Atrioventricular block

Tachyarrhythmias: narrow complex tachycardia
Paroxysmal supraventricular tachycardia
Atrial fibrillation and atrial flutter

Tachyarrhythmias: wide complex tachycardia
Ventricular tachycardia
Ventricular tachycardia versus supraventricular tachycardia with aberrant conduction

Wolff-Parkinson-White syndrome

Introduction

Abnormal heart rhythms, arrhythmias, are commonly encountered in emergency department settings. At times, the arrhythmia is of limited or no consequence, for example, in the patient with upper respiratory infection and chronic atrial fibrillation (AF) with controlled ventricular response. At other times, the arrhythmia is of major concern and significantly involved in the presentation, as in the patient with ST-segment elevation myocardial infarction (STEMI) and unstable ventricular tachycardia (VT). Arrhythmias can be simple, such as in the young woman with paroxysmal supraventricular tachycardia (PSVT), for whom the diagnosis and management are usually straightforward and the outcome favorable. They can also be complex, such as in the overdose patient with wide complex tachycardia (WCT), convulsions, and hypotension—clearly, a complex rhythm in a complex situation.

Regardless of the arrhythmia, appropriate management can occur only if the correct diagnosis is made in a timely fashion. A correct diagnosis is, of course, based on a sound understanding of the electrocardiogram (ECG) and the various features of the individual arrhythmias. Furthermore, the rhythm must be diagnosed in the context of the patient's presentation. Specific patient characteristics such as age and medical history must be considered in the evaluation. For instance, the elderly patient who had a myocardial infarction (MI) in the past and who is now demonstrating a WCT is probably experiencing VT; advanced age and a history of MI favor that diagnosis. Perhaps more important, the patient's hemodynamic stability must be assessed and determined. In a general sense, unstable arrhythmias require a more urgent evaluation and management plan, whereas a stable presentation allows a more comprehensive evaluation, consideration of treatment, and eventual initiation of therapy.

A focused evaluation of the patient should be done early in the emergency department evaluation. In the advanced cardiovascular life support guidelines, the American Heart Association (AHA) suggests that the following descriptors should be considered in the assessment of instability: hypotension or systemic hypoperfusion, altered mentation, ischemic chest pain, and respiratory distress (Table 7-1).[1]

Chest pain and dyspnea represent other instability considerations. In this context, chest pain results from coronary hypoperfusion and dyspnea from pulmonary edema; in both cases, some objective supporting evidence is usually detected (eg, ST-segment abnormality, rales on examination, or low oxygen saturation). Another potential instability criterion involves extremely rapid heart rates. As the ventricular rate approaches 300 beats/min, systemic hypoperfusion becomes more extensive. In addition, the R-R interval narrows proportionally, increasing the opportunity for an R-on-T phenomenon and ventricular fibrillation. Any complex resuscitation scenario is best interpreted by the clinician at the bedside.

Bradyarrhythmias: Bradycardia and Atrioventricular Block

Bradyarrhythmia is a descriptive term for bradycardic rhythms with a ventricular rate slower than 60 beats/min in the adult. Age-related norms define pediatric bradyarrhythmias. Bradyarrhythmias include bradycardia and atrioventricular (AV) block. The bradycardias include sinus bradycardia, junctional rhythm, and idioventricular rhythm as well as AF with a slow ventricular response and the sinoventricular rhythm of pronounced hyperkalemia. Bradyarrhythmias are the result of sinus node dysfunction or AV conduction disorders; these in turn are affected by diseases (eg, myocardial ischemia), conditions (eg, hypothermia), or drugs (eg, digoxin) that affect the automaticity and refractoriness of cardiac cells and the conduction of impulses within the system. In fact, the pathophysiology of the various bradyarrhythmias includes a range of factors related in complex fashion, including heightened autonomic tone, coronary hypoperfusion, myocardial ischemia, systemic hypoxia, and adverse toxic-metabolic effects.

KEY POINT

The vast majority of bradyarrhythmias are secondary events, that is, they are external to the cardiac pacemaker–conduction system.[2]

In a review of prehospital patients with unstable bradycardia or AV block, 80% were found to have a secondary cause of the rhythm abnormality.[3,4] The most frequently identified secondary causes were acute coronary syndrome (ACS) and toxicologic events; multifactorial events (eg, hypoxia with hypoperfusion) were frequently encountered as well.[3,4] In this same series, bradycardias were encountered significantly more often than AV block. In fact, two thirds of patients demonstrated sinus bradycardia, junctional bradycardia, or idioventricular bradycardia; sinus (41% of bradycardic rhythms) and junctional bradycardias (44%) were seen equally often, while idioventricular bradycardia (15%) was much less common. The vast majority of AV blocks seen in this population were third-degree heart blocks (82% of AV blocks); first- and second-degree AV blocks were seen much less commonly, representing only 18% of all AV conduction blocks.[3,4] Among patients with ACS, sinus bradycardia and third-degree AV block were the most common bradyarrhythmias encountered.

Management issues in the bradyarrhythmic patient can include the administration of various medications, electrical therapy in the form of cardiac pacing, general supportive issues (eg, oxygen delivery, intravenous fluids), and specific therapeutic concerns (eg, treatment of hyperkalemia).[1] Medications used in the bradycardic patient include atropine, glucagon, and adrenergic agonists.

In many cases, the first agent used in the treatment of symptomatic bradyarrhythmias is atropine, which enhances the automaticity of the sinoatrial (SA) node and AV nodal conduction, both via a direct vagolytic mechanism. For patients not in cardiac arrest, the clinical indications for atropine include symptomatic sinus bradycardia and AV block.

KEY POINT

In adults, the initial dose of atropine is 0.5 mg to 1 mg intravenously, repeated every 3 to 5 minutes to a maximum total dose of 3 mg[5]; the pediatric dose is 0.02 mg/kg.[6]

Generally, patients are more likely to respond to the first dose than to subsequent doses of atropine; furthermore, bradycardia responds more readily than does AV block to atropine administration.[2–4]

The medical literature reports several concerns with atropine administration that are largely theoretical or based on very limited evidence. The issues include the potentiation of ischemia in patients with active ACS, the development of malignant ventricular arrhythmias in ACS patients, and the worsening of AV block in patients with high-grade AV conduction block. Certainly, atropine might exacerbate ischemia if given during an acute coronary event; systemic and coronary hypoperfusion from an unstable bradyarrhythmia can adversely affect outcome as well.[2–4] The development of malignant ventricular arrhythmias after administration of atropine for unstable bradyarrhythmia is infrequent in the prehospital setting, reported at an incidence of 2% to 4%.[3,4,7]

PEARL

A paradoxic slowing of the heart rate after administration of atropine for unstable bradyarrhythmia has been found, rarely, in patients with infranodal AV block, namely, Mobitz type II second-degree AV block and third-degree AV block with a wide QRS complex. Most patients with these rhythms do not manifest this paradoxic reaction. The emergency physician should be aware of these possible, yet uncommon, adverse effects in this subgroup of bradyarrhythmias.

Glucagon, a naturally occurring hormone, has both positive inotropic and chronotropic effects. Glucagon has been used most extensively in patients with cardioactive medication overdose or overexposure, in particular, in patients experiencing bradyarrhythmias related to calcium channel antagonists and β-blocker overdoses.[8,9] Recommended dose ranges in the setting of toxicity from these drugs are variable; generally, an

TABLE 7-1.

Instability considerations in the arrhythmic patient

Hypotension and/or hypoperfusion
Altered mental status
Ischemic chest discomfort
Dyspnea resulting from pulmonary edema
Extremely rapid rate, approaching 300 beats/min

initial intravenous bolus of 2 to 10 mg is suggested, with continuous infusion, if necessary, at 2 to 5 mg/hr. In infants and small children, the bolus dose is 50 mcg/kg. Adverse effects include nausea, emesis, hypokalemia, and inconsequential hyperglycemia. Glucagon has also been used successfully in patients with bradycardia unrelated to poisoning.

Adrenergic agents, administered intravenously via rapid bolus and sustained infusion, have been proposed as potential agents in the management of compromising bradyarrhythmias. These agents include dopamine, epinephrine, and isoproterenol. They are potent chronotropes and thus can increase the heart rate in certain situations; they also increase conduction velocity within the AV node and the intraventricular conduction system. Unfortunately, these agents also markedly increase myocardial work and oxygen demand, among other negative effects, in patients with conditions such as ACS. These agents should be considered temporary measures, providing a medical bridge to more definitive management via transcutaneous or transvenous cardiac pacing. In some patients, the administration of one of these agents in conjunction with atropine and other resuscitative interventions will correct the bradyarrhythmia, restoring an adequate heart rate and appropriate rhythm; in these cases, ongoing therapy is not indicated.

KEY POINT

The administration of dopamine, epinephrine, and isoproterenol should be considered temporary therapy, providing a medical bridge to more definitive management via transcutaneous or transvenous cardiac pacing.[5]

Cardiac pacing is accomplished either transcutaneously or transvenously. Transcutaneous pacing is markedly easier to perform, is frequently quite effective, but is quite uncomfortable for the patient unless pain medication or sedation is administered. This technique is used only under emergency conditions, for unstable patients, and the administration of sedative-hypnotic agents is problematic in terms of worsening perfusion or compromising an already jeopardized airway. In contrast, transvenous pacing is highly effective yet quite invasive. It requires considerable expertise for placement and specific equipment for insertion, making it a difficult intervention for the emergency physician. Both pacing modalities can be applied in a prophylactic sense or an active pacing mode. From a precautionary approach, cardiac pacing can be prepared but not activated if the physician is concerned about the development of a hemodynamically compromising rhythm or the worsening of an already-present bradycardia. If active pacing is required, then either modality can be used, resulting in electrical capture and mechanical pacing. "Electrical capture" is manifested by the pacing unit producing a paced rhythm, and "mechanical pacing" is determined if a pulse is felt corresponding to the paced electrical rhythm.

Transcutaneous cardiac pacing is easily performed and is often the initial form of pacing employed in patients with compromising bradyarrhythmias. Like the adrenergic agents, it should be viewed as an interim therapy. The endpoint of transcutaneous pacing is correction/resolution of the bradycardia, establishment of transvenous pacing, or patient death. Transcutaneous pacemakers generally have two connections to the patient: a set of pads for delivering the pacing current and leads for monitoring the patient. Most units allow both defibrillation and pacing through the same pads. The placement of the pads is generally anterior/posterior, with the anterior pad placed as close as possible to the point of maximum cardiac impulse and the posterior pad placed directly opposite the anterior, in the left perithoracic region. Two variables require adjustment: the energy output required to pace the patient and the rate at which pacing occurs. Complications include pain, minor local tissue injury, and failure to detect underlying ventricular arrhythmias.

Transvenous cardiac pacing allows more controlled pacing of the heart compared with transcutaneous pacing. This technique is, of course, invasive, yet the amount of current required to pace the heart is better tolerated by most patients than with the transcutaneous method. Central venous access is required; it is best established via the right internal jugular vein or the left subclavian vein.

PEARL

The right internal jugular route is preferred for transvenous cardiac pacing so that the left central veins remain "device free" in case permanent cardiac pacing is needed.

The following discussion focuses on the placement of the transvenous pacing wire in the patient with a perfusing cardiac rhythm (ie, the patient is not in cardiac arrest).

Optimally, the transvenous wire is placed with fluoroscopic guidance, but that technology is often not available in the emergency department. Therefore, the pacing wire is usually placed in a "blind" fashion using a balloon-tipped catheter (this technique should be used only for the patient in extremis). The balloon-tipped catheter (pacing wire) is inserted into the central line and advanced approximately 10 cm. At this point, the pulse generator is activated in the "sense" mode. The pacing wire is further advanced into the ventricle until cardiac electrical activity is sensed. At this time, the balloon is deflated, the generator is switched to the "pace" mode, and the current is increased from a minimal setting used during the first phase (eg, <0.2 mA) to a setting that is likely to electrically capture the ventricle (eg, 4 to 5 mA). The monitor is then watched for electrical capture as the wire is advanced up to 10 cm further. If capture does not occur, the wire should be withdrawn back to the initial 10-cm mark and the process repeated. If available, ultrasonographic guidance can be employed.

Sinus Bradycardia

Sinus bradycardia (SB) is a very common arrhythmia. The pacemaker of the rhythm remains the SA node, with normal impulse formation and transmission through the atria, AV node, and beyond to the ventricles—a normal association of P wave to QRS complex. The abnormal feature of SB is the rate; it occurs when the rate is less than 60 beats/min in the adult patient; age-adjusted rates are used in infants and children.

SB is seen in a number of different scenarios. It is frequent in early ACS presentations; an inferior wall STEMI usually presents with SB caused by heightened parasympathetic tone.

Adverse medication effect, whether unintentional exposure or purposeful ingestion, is another common scenario. Further, the ECG must be interpreted within the context of the individual patient presentation. Rates less than 60 beats/min are not always pathologic. For instance, highly trained endurance athletes can have a resting heart rate in the range of 40 to 50 beats/min. For them, SB is likely not of clinical concern. Conversely, in a patient with ACS or cardiotoxic ingestion, it is a compromising rhythm, suggesting impending cardiovascular collapse.[2-4] The presence of worrisome symptoms or signs, however, produces a clinical situation in which the bradyarrhythmia can require urgent to emergent therapy.

ECG Diagnosis

SB is defined as sinus rhythm with a rate less than 60 beats/min in an adult. All other characteristics of this rhythm are normal: P wave, the PR interval, and P-QRS relationship. The P wave is upright in the limb leads. The PR interval is fixed in length; it can be normal or abnormally prolonged with a first-degree AV block. Importantly, however, the P-wave-to-QRS-complex relationship is normal, with all sinus-node–originated P waves conducted to the ventricles with a resultant QRS complex (Figure 7-1).

Specific Management Considerations

As noted, SB is a frequent rhythm in early ACS presentations, particularly in patients with inferior-wall STEMI. In these situations, atropine has demonstrated significant efficacy via its direct vagolytic action on the SA node; its use should be considered early in patients with symptomatic SB related to ACS. A dose of 0.5 to 1 mg, administered intravenously, should be used, followed by three additional doses at 3- to 5-minute intervals if compromise continues, for a total dose of 3 mg.[5] Larger individual doses, larger cumulative amounts, and more frequent use of atropine have demonstrated prompt, beneficial response in this clinical scenario. SB responds appropriately to atropine more often than do other bradycardias.[3,4]

PEARL

SB is a frequent rhythm in early ACS presentations, particularly in patients with inferior-wall STEMI.

General supportive care, including appropriate volume resuscitation, vasopressor support for perfusion, and adequate oxygenation, is also important in the early management of SB, regardless of the underlying pathophysiology.

Junctional Bradycardia

The site of origin of this bradyarrhythmia is most often the AV node. On occasion, the proximal bundle of His is the focus. In either case, the resulting QRS complex is narrow. The AV node can be considered the first default pacemaker if the sinus node is nonfunctional for whatever reason. The AV node provides "pacemaking function" and an escape rhythm—the junctional rhythm. As with SB, the junctional rhythm is commonly

---

FIGURE 7-1.

Sinus bradycardia is defined as the presence of sinus rhythm with a rate slower than 60 beats/min. The P wave is upright in the limb leads and in leads I, II, and III. The PR interval is fixed in length; it can be normal or abnormally prolonged with a coexisting first-degree AV block. Importantly, however, the P-wave-to-QRS-complex relationship is normal, with all sinus-node–originated P waves conducted to the ventricles, with a resultant QRS complex. Image courtesy of Ulrich Luft, MD.

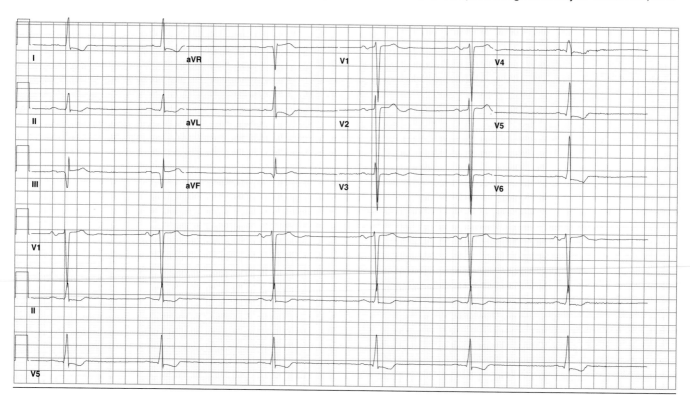

seen in patients with ACS and toxicologic exposures. In highly trained athletes, a junctional rhythm can be nonpathologic.[2-4]

ECG Diagnosis

A junctional rhythm demonstrates a regular, narrow QRS complex at a rate of roughly 40 to 60 beats/min (Figure 7-2). Junctional rhythms originate from the AV node, usually with a ventricular rate of 45 to 60 beats/min. Slower junctional rhythms (35 to 45 beats/min) have been found to originate in the proximal bundle of His; the QRS complex remains narrow in these presentations.[3] P waves are usually not present; if a P wave is seen, it will be retrograde. "Retrograde" refers to conduction from, rather than to, the AV node; the AV nodal impulse moves in retrograde fashion back into the atria, producing this type of P wave. The retrograde P wave can be found before, during, or after the QRS complex; frequently, it is inverted.

Specific Management Considerations

Junctional bradycardia is the second most common arrhythmia in patients with ACS, after SB, and responds reasonably well to atropine, again via the drug's direct vagolytic action. Junctional bradycardic rhythms are also frequently seen in poisoned patients. They are less likely to respond in appropriate fashion to atropine than are ACS-mediated rhythms, but such therapy is still recommended.[3,4] Thus, when managing a patient with a compromising junctional rhythm, the clinician should consider atropine therapy while other targeted treatments are prepared. The junctional rhythm can originate from either

within (rates of 45 to 60 beats/min) or below (rates of 35 to 45 beats/min) the AV node.

PEARL

Atropine is more likely to work at the AV-node level of the conduction system; it is less likely to be effective if the rhythm originates below the AV node.

Idioventricular Rhythm (Bradycardia)

An idioventricular rhythm results from a pacemaker site located in the distal intraventricular conduction system or the ventricular myocardium. In either case, this type of rhythm should be considered a secondary default pacemaker, after failure of both the SA and AV nodes. With rates of less than 40 beats/min, the idioventricular rhythm will support marginal perfusion at best. This rhythm is seen less frequently in patients with intact perfusion (ie, with a pulse); it is more common in those with electrical activity on the cardiac monitor yet no palpable pulse.

ECG Diagnosis

An idioventricular rhythm is a very slow rhythm with a rate that is usually between 30 and 40 beats/min; however, the rate can range from 20 to 50 beats/min. The QRS complexes are abnormally widened if the pacemaker site is found in the more distal portions of the ventricular conduction system or the ventricular myocardium itself. If the pacemaker site is in the ventricular septum, the complexes may be only minimally

FIGURE 7-2.

A junctional rhythm demonstrates a regular, narrow QRS complex at a rate of roughly 40 to 60 beats/min. Slower junctional rhythms (35–45 beats/min) have been found to originate in the bundle of His. The QRS complex remains narrow in these presentations. P waves are usually not present. Image courtesy of Ulrich Luft, MD.

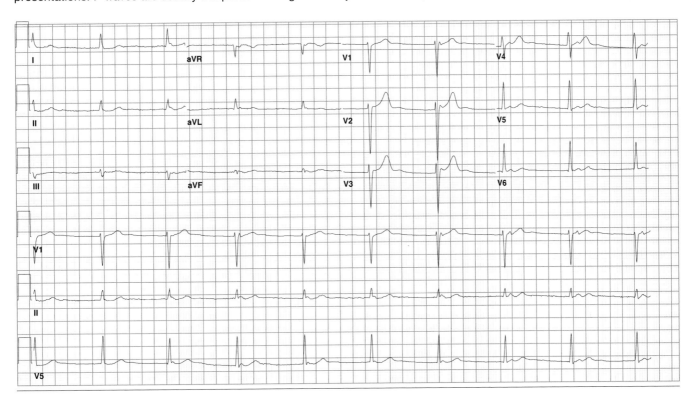

widened. In either case, the QRS complexes occur at a regular frequency. Preexisting intraventricular conduction delay (ie, bundle-branch block) accompanied by a junctional escape rhythm is indistinguishable from a more rapid idioventricular rhythm. Management of both rhythms remains the same.[10]

Specific Management Considerations

Atropine and other medications are much less likely to be effective in compromising idioventricular rhythms. Thus, cardiac pacing is more likely necessary in these presentations. General resuscitative management is crucial in this particular rhythm scenario; adequate oxygenation, appropriate intravascular volume status, and sufficient perfusion are key considerations in patients with idioventricular rhythm. Furthermore, specific therapies, such as attention to hyperkalemia or specific cardioactive medication poisonings, should also be considered.

PEARL

Atropine and other medications are much less likely to be effective in compromising idioventricular rhythms.

Atrioventricular Block

AV conduction blocks are seen frequently in the emergency department. These bradyarrhythmias induce hemodynamic compromise much less often than those discussed heretofore. The site of the block is related to its potential to progress to complete AV block. Proximal locations are less likely to be problematic; distal locations tend to be more ominous. More proximal locations of block (at or above the AV node) are usually seen with first-degree and second-degree type I AV block and are lower-risk presentations. Distal sites of dysfunction (within or below the AV node) are encountered in second-degree type II and third-degree AV block.

Certain forms of AV block can be considered benign. First-degree AV block is rarely, if ever, symptomatic or worrisome. In fact, it is considered a normal variant condition; a patient with first-degree AV block who lacks symptoms, signs, or a troubling clinical presentation needs no further attention or therapy for the conduction issue. The same is true for second-degree type I AV block. Extreme caution is advised, however, in the interpretation of these forms of AV block and the clinical situation.

KEY POINT

Patients with ACS, metabolic abnormality, or cardioactive medication ingestion who demonstrate new-onset first-degree or second-degree type I AV block should be considered at risk of progression to complete heart block and managed accordingly.

Second-degree type II and third-degree AV block should always be considered pathologic. In most cases, these forms of AV block are present in patients who are acutely ill and compromised hemodynamically. Patients with second-degree type II AV block have a high risk of progression to complete heart block. These "high-grade" forms of AV block are seen frequently in patients with STEMI, both inferior and anterior. In fact, the presence of third-degree AV block is predictive of STEMI in chest pain patients.[3,4]

FIGURE 7-3.

First-degree AV block, showing fixed prolongation of the PR interval. Note that the normal PR interval is 0.12 to 0.2 seconds. The PR interval does not change appreciably from beat to beat. The P-wave-to-QRS-complex relationship is normal, with each P wave producing a QRS complex. Image courtesy of Ulrich Luft, MD.

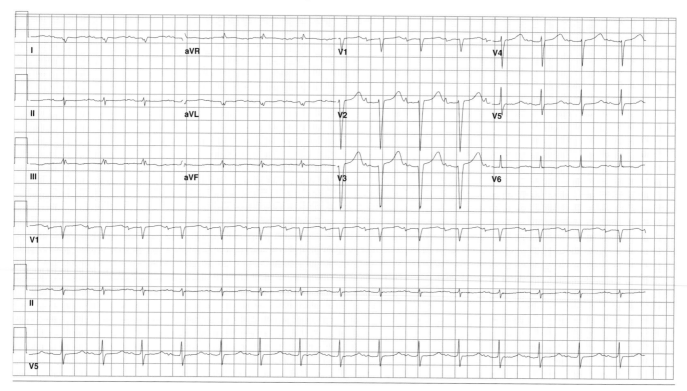

ECG Diagnosis

From the electrocardiographic perspective, AV block is diagnosed based on the PR interval and the relationship of the P wave to the QRS complex. In *first-degree AV block* (Figure 7-3), the PR interval is prolonged (the normal PR interval is 0.12 to 0.2 seconds). The prolongation is fixed and unchanging; minimal variability can be seen because of changes in heart rate and autonomic tone. Each P wave is associated with a QRS complex. The rhythm is regular with uniform, consistent P-P and R-R intervals.

Second-degree AV block is usually, but not always, an irregular rhythm. There are two types of second-degree AV block: Mobitz type I and Mobitz type II. Both feature intermittent failure of atrial impulses to reach the ventricles (ie, some of the P waves are not followed by QRS complexes). *Second-degree type I AV block* is characterized by an initially normal PR interval that progressively lengthens (Figure 7-4). At first, each P wave is associated with a QRS complex. The PR interval lengthening occurs until a beat is not conducted to the ventricle. A P wave will be noted without an associated QRS complex for this beat. As this pattern progresses, the R-R interval shortens. This pattern then repeats itself at varying intervals. Grouped beating of Wenckebach is observed in this form of AV block. Grouped beating is seen when the QRS complexes occur in groups separated by a pause, yielding the apparent irregularity of the rhythm. The morphology of the P waves and the QRS complexes is generally normal.

Second-degree type II AV block (Figure 7-5) also features intermittently blocked P waves but with a different pattern. In this form of AV block, the PR interval is fixed and non-changing; it can be normal or prolonged. Each P wave is associated with a QRS complex and unchanging PR interval. This pattern continues until, ultimately, a P wave occurs without conduction to the ventricle; thus, no QRS complex is seen. As with type I block, the pattern then repeats itself at varying intervals. Most patients with type II AV block have an associated bundle-branch block, meaning the block is distal to the bundle of His, producing a widened QRS complex; less often, the block is intra-Hisian or in the AV node, demonstrating a narrow QRS complex.

The magnitude of AV block is expressed as a ratio of P waves to QRS complexes (the conduction ratio). When the conduction ratio is 2:1, it is impossible to differentiate the two types of second-degree AV block, since the conduction of every other P wave is blocked and therefore the PR interval cannot be assessed for lengthening. A 2:1 AV block is a generally regular rhythm. If the conduction ratio is other than 2:1, then the rhythm can appear irregular with grouping of conducted beats separated by the nonconducted beat. The descriptor "high-grade" is applied when more than one P wave is nonconducted.

Third-degree AV block (complete heart block) is called *complete atrioventricular dissociation* (Figure 7-6). In this case, the atria and ventricles are working independently of one another without any electrical communication. The SA node usually produces regularly occurring P waves; thus, the P-P intervals are

---

Second-degree type I AV block. Progressive prolongation of PR interval until a beat is not conducted (ie, a QRS complex is dropped). Image courtesy of Amal Mattu, MD.

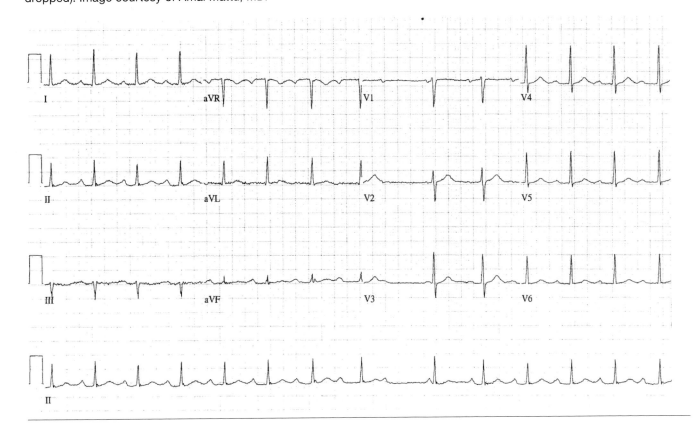

constant and unchanging. In complete heart block, the atrial pacemaker can be either sinus or ectopic and may be tachycardic or bradycardic, but it is faster than the escape pacemaker, which can be either junctional or ventricular. Thus, the atrial rate is faster than the ventricular rate. The escape rhythm most often occurs in regular fashion as well, again with constant and unchanging R-R intervals. Depending on the site of the conduction block, the escape rhythm can be either junctional (narrow QRS complex) or idioventricular (wide QRS complex). The PR interval is variable, constantly changing without consistent pattern, due to the complete lack of electrical communication between the atria and the ventricles.

Specific Management Considerations

First-degree AV block itself rarely requires intervention. The sole instance of concern regarding this block is the patient with an acute clinical condition that can affect cardiac conduction (eg, ACS or overdose). In this case, the first-degree AV block is not of concern in and of itself; rather, its presence can be predictive of a more significant conduction abnormality, particularly if the conduction disturbance is of new onset. In this situation, the clinician should consider increasing the level of surveillance of the patient and prepare for more aggressive resuscitative therapy. The same statements can be made about second-degree type I AV block.

The "high-grade" AV blocks (second-degree type II and third-degree AV blocks) can require treatment to reduce their negative effect on perfusion. Medications such as atropine are less likely to be of benefit in these situations. Cardiac pacing can be indicated if the patient is compromised. At the least, transcutaneous pacing pads can be applied, but not activated, in the asymptomatic patient with these blocks. Other causes, such as hyperkalemia, must be considered, with empiric therapy initiated at the discretion of the treating clinician.[2]

Tachyarrhythmias: Narrow Complex Tachycardia

The term *narrow complex tachycardia* (NCT) refers to a broad range of tachycardias with a narrow or normal QRS complex width.[11] In a very basic sense, NCT is defined as a cardiac rhythm with a ventricular rate higher than 100 beats/min and a QRS complex width less than or equal to 0.08 seconds in the adult patient. It is not unreasonable to include tachycardias with QRS complex widths of 0.08 to 0.1 seconds in this definition. As with other electrocardiographic diagnoses, the pediatric population has age-appropriate rates and widths for NCT. NCTs span the realm of acute care medicine with a multitude of arrhythmias, causes of rhythm disturbances, acuity levels, natural histories, management strategies, and outcomes. Rhythms in the NCT category include the following: sinus tachycardia (ST), PSVT, AF, atrial flutter, multifocal atrial tachycardia, various atrial tachycardias, and pre-excited (ie, related to the Wolff-Parkinson-White [WPW] syndrome) NCT. Each of these rhythm disturbances can present as cardiovascular collapse, directly related to the arrhythmia or its causative syndrome. For instance, the patient with PSVT can

---

FIGURE 7-5.

Second-degree type II AV block. Fixed PR interval with sudden dropped beat. The ventricular depolarization can be a narrow or wide QRS complex. Image courtesy of Amal Mattu, MD.

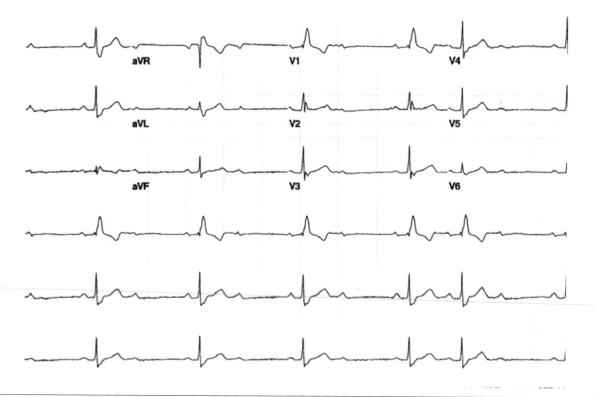

present with significant hypotension, the circulatory shock being a result of the rhythm itself. Conversely, a patient with significant hypotension secondary to gastrointestinal hemorrhage can present with ST, the circulatory shock being a result of the hemorrhage, with the rhythm solely a manifestation of the hemodynamic compromise.

KEY POINT
The management of NCTs is based on the rhythm, the patient's presentation, and related clinical issues.

Certain tachyarrhythmias require urgent rhythm-specific therapy, while others need treatment aimed at the underlying cause(s) of the dysrhythmia. Determination of patient stability, or lack thereof, will guide early management decisions. In a very general sense, NCTs can be approached with the following therapies: intravenous fluids, supplemental oxygen, vagal maneuvers, adenosine, β-blockers, calcium channel blockers, and electrical cardioversion. It must be stressed, however, that the list of interventions above does not apply to all NCTs. Basic supportive therapy in most patients involves an intravenous fluid bolus to expand the circulating intravascular volume; this can be the sole necessary intervention or one component of management. Supplemental oxygen, administered by nasal cannula, face mask, or endotracheal tube, is another important intervention in the patient with NCT.

For some NCTs, the first appropriate treatment is the vagal maneuver. This intervention can be considered in the patient with PSVT, AF, or WPW-related NCT. Vagal maneuvers can be curative if delivered correctly and early in the PSVT patient's clinical course. In fact, if performed early, vagal maneuvers will convert the rhythm in approximately 20% of such presentations.

PEARL
Vagal maneuvers should be considered in the patient with PSVT, AF, or WPW-related NCT.

For PSVT and WPW-related NCT, adenosine is the next most appropriate therapeutic agent. It is unlikely to be of therapeutic benefit in other NCT presentations. In atrial flutter, it can temporarily halt conduction, revealing the flutter waves and aiding in the rhythm diagnosis. Adenosine is a very short-acting agent that blocks the AV node and interrupts the reentrant circuit. It is generally a safe choice with an excellent record of successful arrhythmia termination in this setting. It should be given initially as a rapid 6-mg IV bolus; if that is unsuccessful, a 12-mg rapid bolus is given and may be repeated if no response occurs. Dosing for children is 0.1 mg/kg, with a maximum first dose of 6 mg; a second dose of 0.2 mg/kg, with a maximum of 12 mg, may be administered if the first is unsuccessful in terminating the arrhythmia.[6]

It is important to define a "failure" in the administration of adenosine. The serum half-life of the drug is very short. Thus, its AV nodal blocking effect is transient and brief, even though quite profound. A brief period of AV nodal blockade with near-immediate recurrence of the PSVT is not, in fact, a treatment

FIGURE 7-6.

Third-degree AV block, also known as complete heart block. There is a complete lack of electrical communication between the atria and the ventricles. Note the regular rates of both the P waves and QRS complexes, with the atrial rate exceeding the ventricular rate. At times, the P wave is "lost" within the larger QRS complex. Image courtesy of Ulrich Luft, MD.

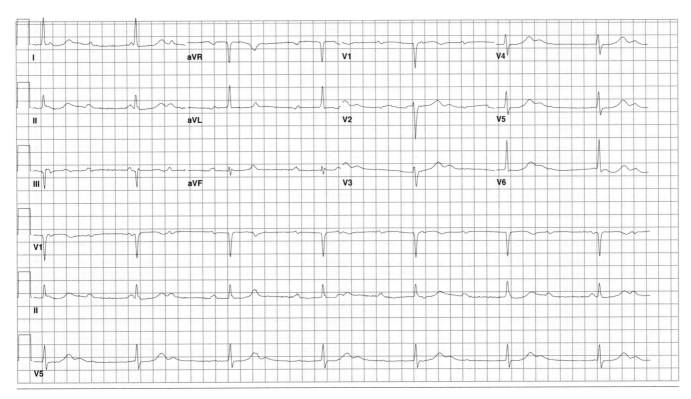

failure, but a consequence of the medication's brief duration of effect. In such situations, repeat dosing of adenosine at the same dose likely will not be successful; a higher dose should be given, if possible. Alternatives include the combination of adenosine with another AV nodal blocking agent, such as a β-blocker or calcium channel blocker, with repeat administration of adenosine.[12]

If adenosine ultimately fails, then other longer-acting AV nodal blocking agents such as β-blockers and calcium channel blockers may be given intravenously. These two medication classes may be considered when direct control of the ventricular rate is a desired goal, as in PSVT, AF, atrial flutter, and WPW-related NCT. Metoprolol is a reasonable β-blocker for such situations. It is given intravenously at a dose of 5 mg and can be repeated two additional times at appropriate intervals if the desired effect is not observed. Esmolol, a parenteral β-blocker with a relatively short duration of effect, can be used in place of the longer-duration agents. Diltiazem, administered at a dose of 0.25 mg/kg IV over several minutes, is an appropriate calcium channel blocker for such arrhythmias. If the desired clinical response does not occur, it can be repeated at a dose of 0.35 mg/kg IV.[5]

Electrical cardioversion can be considered in patients with PSVT, AF, atrial flutter, and WPW-related NCT who are unstable at presentation or who have not responded to initial pharmacologic measures. Caution regarding hemodynamic stability must be exercised here; not all patients who are unstable and present with one of these arrhythmias require electrical cardioversion. AF, for example, can be the primary cause of hemodynamic instability but, more often, it is a manifestation of instability rather than its cause. Therefore, electrical cardioversion is not required in all unstable AF presentations.

KEY POINT

If electrical cardioversion is considered, its use should be coupled with administration of a sedative with or without analgesic effect.

Paroxysmal Supraventricular Tachycardia

PSVT is the second most common pathologic supraventricular tachycardia (SVT) in the emergency department population, after AF.[13] Although younger patients are more likely to experience PSVT in the absence of known cardiovascular disease, no definitive conclusions can be drawn regarding the influence of age or sex on the mechanism of the tachycardia. In a population of 485 patients with NCT without overt electrocardiographic evidence of preexcitation, Brembilla-Perrot and associates determined that AV nodal reentrant tachycardia (AVNRT) was the most common mechanism of SVT in all age groups, from teenage to elderly, and that age was not a reliable predictor of tachycardia mechanism.[14]

With regard to sex, the incidence of PSVT is relatively evenly distributed between men and women; however, in the specific case of AVNRT, there appears to be a higher prevalence of disease among women, with the prevalence ranging from 68% to 76% in three studies. The reason for this unbalanced

FIGURE 7-7.

Paroxysmal supraventricular tachycardia: rapid, regular, narrow QRS complex tachycardia without evidence of P waves. Image courtesy of Ulrich Luft, MD.

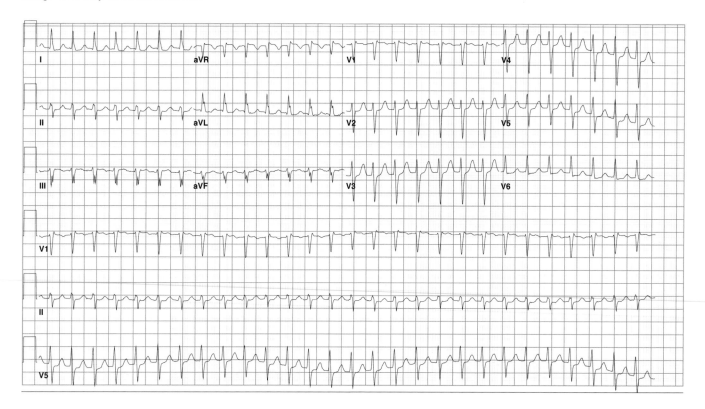

distribution is unclear. Regardless of the rhythm mechanism, in most instances of PSVT the rhythm can largely be considered a nuisance and not a threat to life. The vast majority of patients with PSVT do not have an underlying causative illness. Management of the arrhythmia, as described above, is all that is required. The rare patient will present with PSVT as a manifestation of an underlying issue and will thus require management of the arrhythmia and the causative problem.[13]

Approximately 80% of patients with PSVT have an arrhythmia focus in the AV node; the remaining patients have PSVT with an atrial focus. It is estimated that 2% to 3% of PSVT-appearing arrhythmias are, in fact, WPW-related NCT, the narrow-complex AVRT. Because the vast majority of PSVT cases result from a problem in the AV node, it is not surprising that adenosine and other AV nodal blocking agents are successful in rhythm management and ultimate conversion.

ECG Diagnosis

PSVT is a narrow QRS complex tachycardia. The QRS complex is of normal width, usually less than 0.08 seconds in duration. On occasion, the QRS complex can be minimally widened to no more than 0.1 seconds. PSVT is rapid and regular. In the adult patient, the rate is usually 170 to 180 beats/min but can range from as low as 130 beats/min to as high as 300 beats/min. In children, the rate can approach 240 to 260 beats/min, particularly in infants.

P waves are usually not seen. Because atrial and ventricular depolarizations usually occur almost simultaneously, the P waves are frequently buried in the QRS complex and totally obscured. In fact, in 70% of PSVT cases, the P wave is not observed on the ECG. In a minority of presentations, the so-called retrograde P wave is noted. As with junctional bradycardia, "retrograde P waves" refers to conduction from, rather than to, the AV node. The AV nodal impulse moves in retrograde fashion back into the atria. The retrograde P wave can be found before, during, or after the QRS complex. Frequently, it is inverted in the limb leads. If the P wave occurs after the QRS complex, it can distort the terminal portion of the complex, producing a "pseudo" S wave in the inferior leads and a "pseudo" R wave in V_1. PSVT and rapid ST can be compared in Figures 7-7 and 7-8.

Specific Management Considerations

PSVT is usually managed with favorable patient outcome. In most cases, vagal maneuvers and intravenous adenosine are curative. It is the uncommon patient who requires a β-blocker or calcium channel blocker. In such cases, the patient has not responded to intravenous adenosine, likely because of its ultra-short serum half-life. The use of an agent with a longer serum half-life can assist in the conversion to sinus rhythm; this therapy can be used in full dose or partial dose combined with repeat adenosine administration. In patients with recalcitrant PSVT or unstable presentations, electrical cardioversion can be employed.[13]

FIGURE 7-8.

Sinus tachycardia with a rate of 150 beats/min. The rapid rhythm was a manifestation of the primary event. Appropriately, the arrhythmia did not receive focused therapy. Sinus tachycardia should be considered a "reactive rhythm." Image courtesy of Ulrich Luft, MD.

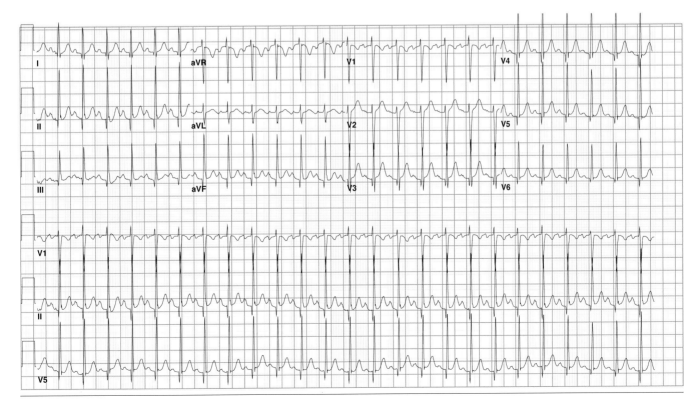

Atrial Fibrillation and Atrial Flutter

AF remains the most prevalent form of NCT. In the United States, 2.3 million individuals carry this diagnosis and 0.2% of emergency department visits were attributed to AF between 1993 and 2004.[15] Patients can present to the emergency department with worsening of their chronic AF as a result of poorly controlled ventricular rates; with paroxysmal AF associated with hyperthyroidism, hypokalemia, or hypomagnesemia; or following excessive ethanol intoxication (the holiday heart syndrome).[16] The mechanism of AF appears to be multiple micro-reentrant wavelets in the atria. Paroxysms of AF can be triggered by preceding alterations in autonomic tone[17] or ectopic foci, which are frequently located in or around the pulmonary veins.[18] AF is the second most common tachycardia in patients with WPW syndrome, occurring in 20% to 25% of these patients.

Atrial flutter is most commonly caused by a macro-reentrant circuit within the right atrium. It shares many etiologic features with AF. Indeed, it may often be confused with "coarse" AF.

ECG Diagnosis

AF is usually easily diagnosed via an ECG. The rhythm is irregular in an irregular fashion. P waves are absent. The baseline can be isoelectric or exhibit fibrillatory waves of varying morphology at a rate of 400 to 700 beats/min. The amplitude of the fibrillatory waves is suggestive of the underlying pathology. Fine fibrillatory waves, defined as amplitude of less than 0.5 mm, are associated with ischemic heart disease, while coarse waves, greater than 0.5 mm in amplitude, signify left atrial enlargement likely related to chronic hypertension. The ventricular rate varies, but most often a ventricular response of approximately 170 beats/min is seen, representing the "natural" rate of atrial fibrillation (ie, not altered by another disease state or medications). The QRS complex is narrow in most presentations. Preexisting bundle-branch block or rate-related bundle dysfunction can produce a widened QRS complex (Figure 7-9).

Atrial flutter can be regular or irregular. P waves are present and are of a single morphology. Typically, the P waves appear as downward deflections, called flutter waves, which resemble a saw blade and have a "sawtooth" appearance. These waves are best seen in the inferior leads and lead V₁. Most commonly, the atrial rate is regular, usually at 300 beats/min, with a range from 250 to 350 beats/min. Less commonly, atrial rates can vary from 340 to 430 beats/min. Some form of AV block is usually present, although 1-to-1 conduction is possible. The ventricular rhythm is frequently regular and is a function of the AV block. Two-to-one AV block, which is most common, will produce a ventricular rate around 150 beats/min, while a 3-to-1 AV block will result in a ventricular rate of 100 beats/min. The degree of AV block is often fixed, but it can be variable, yielding an irregular ventricular response. An NCT that is regular, occurring at an approximate rate of 150 beats/min, should strongly suggest atrial flutter with 2-to-1 conduction. This is the "natural" rate for atrial flutter unaffected by other disease states or medications. As with AF, the QRS complex is narrow. Preexisting bundle-branch block or rate-related bundle dysfunction can produce a widened QRS complex and thus a WCT.

FIGURE 7-9.

Atrial fibrillation: ECG demonstrating an irregularly irregular rhythm with wide complexes secondary to left bundle-branch block. Image courtesy of Ulrich Luft, MD.

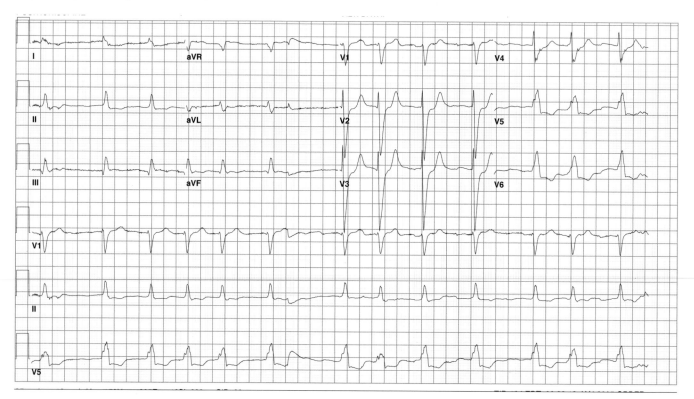

Specific Management Considerations

In patients who have new-onset AF and are profoundly unstable, urgent electrical cardioversion is the most appropriate therapy. Fortunately, this scenario is uncommon. More often, new-onset AF presents less dramatically, with a rapid ventricular response and a potential range of symptoms, including weakness, dizziness, palpitations, chest discomfort, and dyspnea. In fact, hemodynamic instability is not a "yes or no" issue. Rather, stability must be considered along an AF spectrum ranging from an asymptomatic patient with the arrhythmia discovered incidentally to the individual with new-onset tachyarrhythmia in profound shock caused by a rapid ventricular response. Emergency physicians must consider numerous factors in this situation, including the clinical data characterizing the specific presentation as well as the patient's comorbidity, particularly the presence of mitral valve disease, left atrial dilation, and left ventricular function. These features influence treatment decisions in two important areas: the choice of therapeutic agents for rate control and the probability of success of cardioversion.

An important consideration in assessing a patient with AF is how to control the ventricular response (by gaining control of the AV node). The symptoms most often associated with AF result primarily from the rapid rate. Rate control by itself significantly reduces related symptoms. The continued presence of AF at a controlled rate, however, can still produce unwanted clinical manifestations. Recall that an organized atrial contraction contributes to left ventricular filling. The loss of this "atrial kick" can continue to produce unpleasant manifestations despite adequate rate control.

KEY POINT
Adequate rate control should be a primary issue for emergency physicians to address in all AF scenarios.

The unstable patient may also be treated urgently with rate control rather than cardioversion initially. Rate control can be achieved relatively easily with calcium channel blockade or β-adrenergic blockade; additional agents include digoxin, magnesium, and amiodarone.

The final consideration for emergency physicians regarding AF focuses on cardioversion. The primary question here is whether emergency physicians should consider cardioversion in patients with new-onset AF. In the unstable presentation related directly to AF with rapid ventricular response, the answer to the question is relatively straightforward: Yes, urgent electrical cardioversion is most likely required. The question is less easily answered in other, more common scenarios such as in new-onset arrhythmia without significant adverse clinical effects. Numerous studies suggest that a significant portion of patients with new-onset AF spontaneously convert to sinus rhythm within 24 hours after onset and evaluation.[19-22] This high rate of spontaneous conversion coupled with the results of numerous AF trials demonstrates that rate control is similar to rhythm control in regard to several key endpoints.[21,22] The AFFIRM and RACE trials demonstrated no significant differences between rate control and rhythm control groups in the occurrence of study endpoints representing quality of life issues, control of symptoms, and the occurrence of adverse events.[21,22] As such, patients with new-onset AF who are stable can be managed with rate control alone, as either inpatients or outpatients.

Tachyarrhythmias: Wide Complex Tachycardia

Ventricular Tachycardia

VT is a potentially malignant rhythm disturbance that originates from any part of the myocardium or conduction system below the AV node. In most instances, VT presents as a wide QRS complex (>0.12 seconds) and a rate greater than 120 beats/min. In rare cases, VT presents as a "normal appearing" QRS complex; examples are children with an age-related "narrow" QRS complex width and adults with cardiac glycoside toxicity, the so-called fascicular tachycardia, a very rare rhythm disorder.[23,24] VT is frequently encountered as a complication of coronary artery disease, related to active ischemia or the presence of scar tissue, which can create a substrate for ventricular arrhythmias.

Patients with cardiomyopathy are the second most frequently encountered group experiencing VT. Medications, particularly type IA antiarrhythmic agents, can produce ventricular arrhythmias. Other drugs that can cause VT include digoxin, phenothiazines, tricyclic antidepressants, and the sympathomimetic agents. In addition, electrolyte disorders, particularly abnormalities of potassium, can produce VT.

VT can be considered from a range of perspectives: 1) sustained versus nonsustained, based on its persistence; 2) stable versus unstable, based on its hemodynamic impact; and 3) monomorphic versus polymorphic, based on the appearance of the QRS complex. Furthermore, the term *wide complex tachycardia* describes the rhythm scenario characterized by a broad QRS complex (>0.12 seconds) and a ventricular rate over 100 beats/min. The electrocardiographic differential diagnosis of WCT classically includes VT and SVT with aberrant intraventricular conduction.

ECG Diagnosis

Monomorphic VT is usually regular, with rates between 120 and 300 beats/min, most often in the 140 to 180 beats/min range (Figure 7-10A). Certain medications such as amiodarone can slow the rate of VT. Patients chronically receiving medications such as amiodarone can present with ventricular rates of 110 to 130 beats/min. On rare occasions, monomorphic VT presents as an irregular rhythm.

Polymorphic VT is defined as a VT with an unstable (frequently varying) QRS complex morphology in any single ECG lead (Figure 7-10B). Variations in the R-R interval and electrical axis are also noted features of this ventricular arrhythmia. Torsade de pointes is identified when polymorphic VT occurs in the setting of delayed myocardial repolarization manifested on the sinus rhythm ECG by a prolongation of the QT interval. Torsade de pointes, thus, is one subtype of polymorphic VT and not a synonym for the category of polymorphic VT. The literal translation of the French term (ie, "twisting of the points") describes the appearance of the QRS complex (Figure 7-10C).

FIGURE 7-10.

Ventricular tachycardia. A. Monomorphic ventricular tachycardia. B. Polymorphic ventricular tachycardia. C. Polymorphic ventricular tachycardia, torsade de pointes subtype. Images courtesy of Amal Mattu, MD.

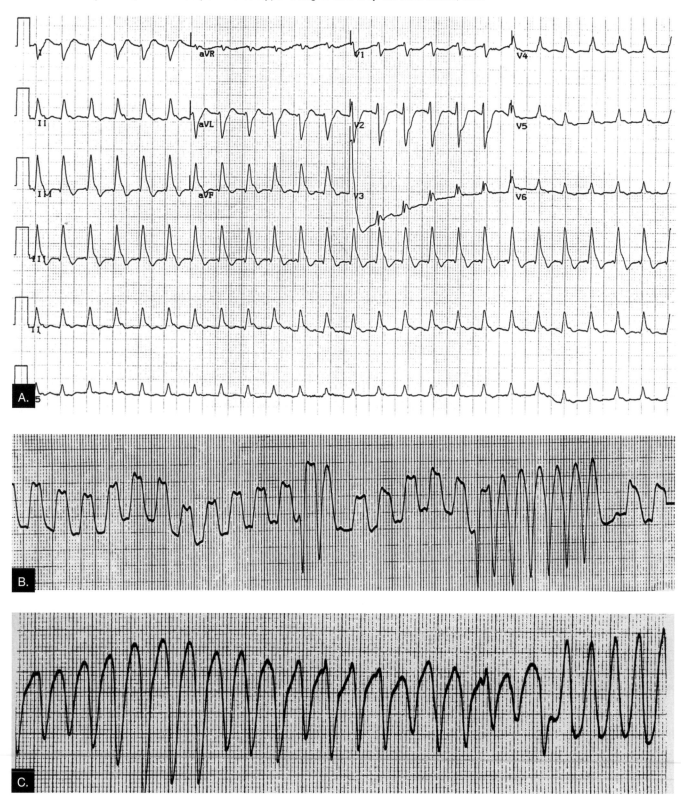

Specific Management Considerations

The management of VT is similar to that of many of the NCTs. Treatment decisions are based on the patient's presentation and related clinical issues. Hemodynamic instability should prompt the consideration of electrical cardioversion coupled with administration of a sedative with or without analgesic effect. Pharmacologic agents may be considered for certain unstable patients, based on the presenting features and active medical issues.

In the stable patient, pharmacologic agents may be considered first-line therapy. These agents include procainamide, amiodarone, lidocaine, and magnesium.[5] Procainamide is an effective agent for stable VT patients with preserved left ventricular function. Procainamide will terminate most cases of stable VT and is superior to amiodarone and lidocaine. In fact, in the 2010 AHA guidelines, procainamide is preferred over amiodarone, sotalol, and lidocaine for the treatment of stable monomorphic VT.[5] Procainamide is given at 20 to 50 mg/min until the arrhythmia terminates or one of the following criteria is achieved: hypotension (systolic blood pressure <90 mm Hg); the QRS complex duration is prolonged by 50% from its original duration; the tachycardia accelerates; or a total of 17 mg/kg has been given.[5] An alternative dosing protocol requires 10 minutes for the maximum dose of 10 mg/kg; in this regimen, procainamide is administered at 100 mg/min until a maximum of 10 mg/kg or one of the above criteria is reached. Procainamide should not be used in patients with a prolonged QT interval.[5] If the patient has a tenuous hemodynamic status, amiodarone is the antiarrhythmic of choice, with lidocaine as the acceptable alternative. In such patients, amiodarone is given as a dose of 150 mg IV over 10 minutes, and lidocaine is given as a bolus of 1.5 mg/kg IV over 2 minutes. Magnesium can also be considered as a primary antiarrhythmic agent, but its use should be reserved for various "niche" applications, such as in patients with known hypomagnesemia, QT interval prolongation, or polymorphic VT. Magnesium can be given at a dose of 1 to 2 grams (8 to 16 mEq) IV over 20 to 30 minutes to a stable patient and more rapidly in an unstable patient. Its main adverse effect is altered mentation with respiratory depression. Regardless of the agent used, very careful cardiovascular monitoring is required.

In addition to these medications, the 2010 AHA guidelines state that adenosine may be used for undifferentiated, regular, monomorphic WCT.[5] If used, adenosine is dosed similarly to the treatment of PSVT as described above.[5] The rationale for adenosine use in this scenario is to aid in the detection of SVT with aberrancy because adenosine can slow or convert this rhythm to sinus rhythm (see next section). Note that adenosine can also convert VT ("adenosine-sensitive VT"), so great caution should be used if adenosine is administered. Adenosine should not be given to patients with irregular or polymorphic VT.[5]

If pharmacologic interventions are unsuccessful, then sedation-assisted electrical cardioversion may be used. Regardless of ventricular function, synchronized cardioversion is the next treatment of choice in the event of antiarrhythmic drug failure or if the patient has ongoing ACS or becomes unstable. Attention should also be given to underlying inciting issues, including electrolyte disorders (potassium and magnesium), medication toxicities, acute coronary ischemia, genetic issues (long QT syndrome), and other cardiac and noncardiac ailments.

Ventricular Tachycardia versus Supraventricular Tachycardia with Aberrant Conduction

A wide QRS complex tachycardia, defined electrocardiographically in the adult patient as an arrhythmia with a QRS complex of more than 0.12 seconds in duration and a ventricular rate faster than 120 beats/min, presents diagnostic challenges for the emergency physician. The electrocardiographic differential diagnosis of WCT classically includes VT versus SVT with aberrant ventricular conduction. Aberrant ventricular conduction of an SVT can be caused by a preexisting bundle-branch block; a functional (rate-related) bundle malfunction resulting in a widened QRS complex when the heart rate exceeds a characteristic maximum for that patient; or accessory atrioventricular conduction, as encountered in preexcitation syndromes such as that described by Wolff, Parkinson, and White. Other clinical syndromes less frequently encountered in this WCT differential include rapid sinus tachycardia with preexisting bundle-branch block configuration, sodium channel blockade (eg, tricyclic antidepressant ingestion), and hyperkalemia. If one considers all patients encountered with WCT from the perspective of the cardiologist, approximately 80% will be diagnosed with VT. This preponderance of VT probably reflects referral bias of difficult cases to electrophysiology centers.[25-29] Emergency physicians likely encounter a much broader range of causes in undifferentiated WCT presentations.

Consideration must be given to the effect of the ECG on clinical decision making. As in any presentation in clinical medicine, it is vital for the physician to interpret the diagnostic study within the context of the clinical presentation. Although any WCT is abnormal, differences in the presentation will dictate markedly disparate early diagnostic and management strategies. Both VT in a middle-aged man with STEMI and AF with bundle-branch block in an elderly woman with urosepsis-related hypotension involve a WCT, but the initial treatment is typically quite different.

A significant portion of patients presenting to the emergency department with WCT are diagnosed with VT. Numerous strategies aimed at assisting the clinician with the proper diagnosis of WCT have been proposed, emphasizing various data, including patient age and cardiovascular history,[29,30] the physical examination findings, the ECG,[31-36] and the response to therapeutic interventions. Although these principles are useful, they have largely centered on criteria suggestive of VT.

KEY POINT

Aberrantly conducted SVT is often the default diagnosis in the event that none of the criteria for VT is met—a major flaw in medical decision making with the potential for serious adverse consequences.[27,28,37,38]

For instance, the use of an AV nodal blocking agent such as diltiazem in a VT patient incorrectly diagnosed with aberrant SVT can cause cardiovascular collapse and death. The clinician can be misled by the hemodynamically stable presentation of a

VT patient; the error results from the assumption that stability is associated with aberrantly conducted SVT, again subjecting the VT patient to the potentially severe adverse effects of various medications.

Of the various clinical features, patient age, medical history, and the ECG are most useful, yet they serve only as guides, not specific diagnostic criteria. VT is a more likely diagnosis in older individuals with WCT. For instance, age greater than 50 years is a reasonably strong predictor that the WCT is VT. Furthermore, a WCT patient who had an MI in the past and who has significant left ventricular dysfunction is also more likely to experience VT.[29,30] Again, it must be emphasized that these two features in the presentation are not absolute criteria for a VT diagnosis—they only support a statistically more likely VT diagnosis in patients with WCT.

In the patient with WCT, electrocardiographic features that strongly suggest the correct rhythm diagnosis are irregularity, AV dissociation, fusion and capture beats, and QRS complex concordance. VT is usually very regular; if the rhythm is irregular, the degree of irregularity is minimal. Marked irregularity is strongly suggestive of AF with bundle-branch block; of course, polymorphic VT is also irregular, but this particular rhythm diagnosis is usually quite apparent. The presence of the remaining features is strongly suggestive of VT.

AV dissociation can be quite useful in this diagnostic consideration and can help "rule in" VT. In cases of VT without retrograde conduction to the atria, the sinus node continues to initiate atrial depolarization. Since atrial depolarization is completely independent of ventricular activity; the resulting P waves will be dissociated from the QRS complexes, that is, no association of the P wave with the QRS complex will be noted. Nonetheless, AV dissociation is not common; it is noted in only 5% to 10% of patients with WCT diagnosed with VT.

Capture and fusion beats in the patient with WCT suggest VT. In the patient with VT, an independent atrial impulse can occasionally cause ventricular depolarization via the normal conducting system. Such a supraventricular impulse, if conducted and able to trigger a depolarization within the ventricle, will result in wide QRS complex beats—QRS complex morphology different from the other wide QRS complex beats. If the resulting QRS complex occurs earlier than expected and is narrow, the complex is called a *capture beat*. The supraventricular impulse electrically captures the ventricle, producing a narrow complex. The presence of capture beats strongly supports a diagnosis of VT. Fusion beats occur when a sinus beat conducts to the ventricles via the AV node and joins, or fuses, with a ventricular beat originating from the abnormal ectopic focus. These two electrical "beats" combine, resulting in a QRS complex of intermediate width and differing morphology compared with the other beats of monomorphic VT. The presence of fusion beats is strongly suggestive of VT. Fusion and capture beats occur infrequently and are seen in fewer than 10% of patients with VT.

Lastly, QRS concordance can assist with rhythm diagnosis. Its presence is suggestive of VT. Concordance addresses the relationship of the polarity of the QRS complexes across the precordium. Concordance of the QRS complexes in the chest leads that are either predominantly positive or negative suggests

FIGURE 7-11.

WPW (ventricular preexcitation) syndrome. Image courtesy of Ulrich Luft, MD.

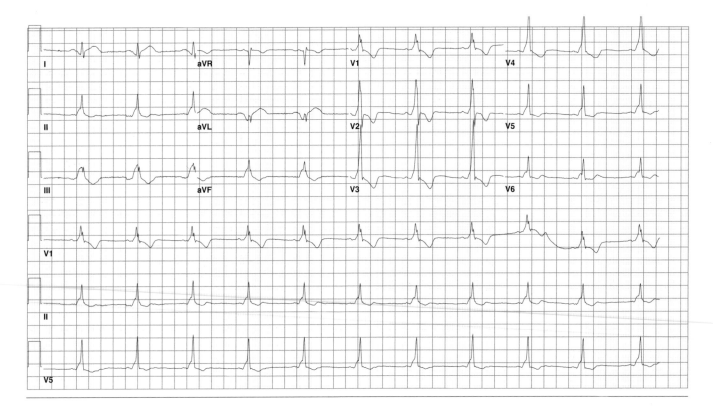

a ventricular origin of the tachycardia.

In many ways, the management of arrhythmic patients is rather simple if the clinician maintains a focus on *treating the entire patient, not just the ECG.* Simultaneously, the clinician must realize that not all WCT presentations are arrhythmias requiring antiarrhythmic agents or urgent electrical therapy.

Wolff-Parkinson-White Syndrome

WPW syndrome is a form of ventricular preexcitation involving an accessory conduction pathway between the atria and the ventricles. In the patient with WPW syndrome, the accessory pathway bypasses the AV node, creating a direct electrical connection between the atria and ventricles and thereby removing the protection against excessively rapid rates that is provided by the AV node in patients without this condition. Furthermore, the accessory pathway will conduct any impulse that presents itself (ie, non-decremental conduction), again in marked contrast to the AV node. WPW patients are prone to a variety of supraventricular tachyarrhythmias. Most patients with preexcitation syndromes remain asymptomatic throughout their lives. When symptoms do occur, they are usually secondary to tachyarrhythmias, including reentrant tachyarrhythmias (PSVT [narrow and wide QRS complex tachycardias], 70%), AF (25%), and VF (rare).[39]

The diagnosis of WPW syndrome relies on the electrocardiographic features listed in Table 7-2. The PR interval is shortened because the impulse progressing down the accessory pathway is not subjected to the physiologic slowing that occurs in the AV node. Thus, the ventricular myocardium is activated by two pathways, resulting in a fused, or widened, QRS complex (Figure 7-11). The initial part of the complex, the delta wave, represents aberrant activation through the accessory pathway, while the terminal portion of the QRS represents normal activation through the His-Purkinje system from impulses having traveled through both the AV node and the accessory pathway.

The most frequently encountered rhythm disturbance seen in the WPW patient is AV reciprocating tachycardia (AVRT). In the setting of AVRT, the ventricle is activated through either the normal conduction system or the accessory pathway, with return of the impulse to the atrium by the other pathway. Such AVRT is referred to as either orthodromic (anterograde conduction via the AV node) or antidromic (retrograde conduction via the AV node). Orthodromic, or anterograde, AVRT is a reentrant tachycardia in which the atrial stimulus is conducted to the ventricle through the AV node, with return of the impulse to the atria through the accessory pathway. Such tachycardia represents approximately 90% of AVRT seen in WPW patients.

In approximately 10% of AVRT patients with WPW, an antidromic (retrograde) reciprocating tachycardia is observed. In this instance, the reentrant circuit conducts in the opposite direction, with anterograde conduction down the accessory pathway and return of the impulse retrograde to the atria via the AV node. With this pathway, the QRS complexes appear wide (essentially, an exaggeration of the delta wave) and the 12-lead ECG displays a very rapid WCT that is nearly indistinguishable from VT.

PEARL
AF occurs more frequently in patients with WPW syndrome than in the general population.

AF is found in up to 20% of WPW patients with symptomatic arrhythmia.[40] As with the two forms of AVRT, the accessory pathway lacks the feature of slow, decremental conduction; therefore, the pathway can conduct atrial beats at a rate of 300 beats/min or more, subjecting the ventricle to very rapid rates. The electrocardiographic features of this rhythm include the rapid ventricular response (much too rapid for conduction down the AV node); the wide, bizarre QRS complexes; and the delta wave. Significant beat-to-beat variation is seen in the QRS complex morphologies, owing to a combination of the two impulses arriving at the ventricle and fusing to form a composite depolarization and thus potentially different QRS complex configurations from one beat to the next.

The initial treatment of all three arrhythmias (narrow QRS complex AVRT, wide QRS complex AVRT, and AF) in the WPW patient depends on the patient's clinical stability and the electrocardiographic features of the arrhythmia.

KEY POINT
Electrical cardioversion should be applied to all patients with hemodynamic instability, regardless of the features of the tachyarrhythmia.

In the hemodynamically stable patient, the next step must include consideration of the QRS complex width and the regularity of the rhythm. In patients with a regular narrow QRS complex tachycardia (ie, orthodromic AVRT) who are stable, the first therapeutic intervention is performance of the vagal maneuvers. If this intervention fails, the next step would be administration of adenosine, a short-acting agent that blocks the AV node and interrupts the reentrant circuit. Adenosine is generally a safe choice and has an excellent record of successful arrhythmia termination in this setting. It should be given initially as a rapid 6-mg IV bolus; if that is unsuccessful, a 12-mg rapid bolus is given and may be repeated if no response occurs. If adenosine fails, then other longer-acting AV nodal blocking agents may be given intravenously such as β-blockers and calcium channel blockers. The final medication that can be considered is procainamide, which blocks the accessory conduction pathway. It acts more slowly than the calcium channel antago-

TABLE 7-2.

Electrocardiographic features of WPW syndrome

PR interval <0.12 seconds

Slurring and slow rising of the initial segment of the QRS complex (a delta wave)

Widened QRS complex with total duration >0.12 seconds

Secondary repolarization changes reflected in ST-segment/T-wave changes that are generally directed opposite (discordant) to the major delta wave and QRS complex

---

nists and β-adrenergic blocking agents. If all medications fail in this setting, the patient can be electrically cardioverted after appropriate sedation.

In patients with a wide QRS complex tachycardia, either regular (ie, orthodromic AVRT) or irregular (AF), who are stable, the first therapeutic maneuver should be administration of procainamide. If that is unsuccessful, electrical cardioversion after appropriate sedation should be considered. AV nodal blocking interventions and agents such as vagal maneuvers, adenosine, amiodarone, β-blockers, and calcium channel blockers should be avoided. Such therapy can potentiate conduction via the accessory pathway, with the development of extremely rapid ventricular rates and, ultimately, cardiovascular decompensation.

Conclusion

Critically ill emergency department patients often manifest arrhythmias. For some, the arrhythmia is the primary reason for critical illness, while for others it can be a reflection of illness severity. Regardless, the emergency physician must be expert at ECG interpretation and diagnosis of potentially lethal arrhythmias. Furthermore, the emergency physician must be able to rapidly initiate lifesaving therapy for critically ill patients with a bradyarrhythmia or tachyarrhythmia. Quite simply, these are quintessential skills in emergency critical care.

References

1. Sinz E, Navarro K. *Advanced Cardiovascular Life Support Provider Manual*. Dallas, TX: American Heart Association; 2011.
2. Brady WJ, Harrigan RA. Diagnosis and management of bradycardia and atrioventricular block associated with acute coronary ischemia. *Emerg Med Clin North Am*. 2001;19:371-384.
3. Brady WJ, Swart G, DeBehnke DJ, et al. The efficacy of atropine in the treatment of hemodynamically unstable bradycardia and atrioventricular block: prehospital and emergency department considerations. *Resuscitation*. 1999;41:47-55.
4. Swart G, Brady WJ, DeBehnke DJ, Ma OJ, Aufderheide TP. Acute myocardial infarction complicated by hemodynamically unstable bradyarrhythmia: prehospital and emergency department treatment with atropine. *Am J Emerg Med*. 1999;17:647-652.
5. Neumar RW, Otto CW, Link MS, et al. Part 8: adult advanced cardiovascular life support: 2010 American Heart Association Guidelines for Cardiopulmonary Resuscitation and Emergency Cardiovascular Care. *Circulation*. 2010;122(suppl 3):S729-S767.
6. Kleinman ME, Chameides L, Schexnayder SM, et al. Part 14: pediatric advanced life support: 2010 American Heart Association Guidelines for Cardiopulmonary Resuscitation and Emergency Cardiovascular Care. *Circulation*. 2010;122(suppl 3):S876-S908.
7. Richman S. Adverse effect of atropine during myocardial infarction. *JAMA*. 1974;228:1414-1416.
8. Fernandes CM, Daya MR. Sotalol-induced bradycardia reversed by glucagon. *Can Fam Phys*. 1995;41:659-660.
9. Love JN, Howell JM. Glucagon therapy in the treatment of symptomatic bradycardia. *Ann Emerg Med*. 1997;29:181-183.
10. Chou T, Knilans TK. *Electrocardiography in Clinical Practice: Adult and Pediatric*. 4th ed. Philadelphia, PA: WB Saunders; 1996.
11. Borloz MP, Mark DG, Pines JM, Brady WJ. Electrocardiographic differential diagnosis of narrow QRS complex tachycardia: an ED-oriented algorithmic approach. *Am J Emerg Med*. 2010;28:378-381.
12. Brady WJ, DeBehnke DJ, Wickman LL, Lindbeck G. Treatment of out-of-hospital supraventricular tachycardia: adenosine vs. verapamil. *Acad Emerg Med*. 1996;3:574-585.
13. Luber S, Brady WJ, Joyce T, Perron AD. Paroxysmal supraventricular tachycardia: outcome after emergency department care. *Am J Emerg Med*. 2001;19:40-42.
14. Brembilla-Perrot B, Houriez P, Beurrier D, et al. Influence of age on the electrophysiological mechanism of paroxysmal supraventricular tachycardias. *Int J Cardiol*. 2001;78:293-298.
15. McDonald AJ, Pelletier AJ, Ellinor PT, Camargo CA. Increasing US emergency department visit rates and subsequent hospital admissions for atrial fibrillation from 1993 to 2004. *Ann Emerg Med*. 2008;51:58-65.
16. Crozier I, Melton I, Pearson S. Management of atrial fibrillation in the emergency department. *Int Med J*. 2003;33:182-185.
17. Bettoni M, Zimmerman M. Autonomic tone variations before the onset of paroxysmal atrial fibrillation. *Circulation*. 2002;105:2753-2759.
18. Haïssaguerre M, Jaïs P, Shah DC, et al. Spontaneous initiation of atrial fibrillation by ectopic beats originating in the pulmonary veins. *N Engl J Med*. 1998;339:659-666.
19. Ergene U, Ergene O, Fowler J, et al. Must antidysrhythmic agents be given to all patients with new-onset atrial fibrillation? *Am J Emerg Med*. 1999;17:659-662.
20. Digitalis in Acute Atrial Fibrillation (DAAF) Trial Group. Intravenous digoxin in acute atrial fibrillation: results of a randomized, placebo-controlled multicentre trial in 239 patients. *Eur Heart J*. 1997;18:649-654.
21. Olshansky B, Rosenfeld LE, Warner AL, et al. The atrial fibrillation follow-up investigation of rhythm management (AFFIRM) study. *J Am Coll Cardiol*. 2004;43:1209-1210.
22. Hagens VE, Van Gelder IC, Crijins HJ, et al. The RACE study in perspective of randomized studies on management of persistent atrial fibrillation. *Card Electrophysiol Rev*. 2003;7:118-121.
23. Hudson KB, Brady WJ, Chan TC, et al. Electrocardiographic features of ventricular tachycardia. *J Emerg Med*. 2003;25:303-314.
24. Meldon SW, Brady WJ, Berger S, Mannenbach M. Pediatric ventricular tachycardia: a report of three cases with a review of the acute diagnosis and management. *Pediatr Emerg Care*. 1994;10:294-300.
25. Steinman RT, Herrera C, Schluger CD, et al. Wide QRS tachycardia in the conscious adult: ventricular tachycardia is the most frequent cause. *JAMA*. 1989;261:1013-1016.
26. Morady F, Baerman JM, DiCarlo LA, et al. A prevalent misconception regarding wide complex tachycardias. *JAMA*. 1985;254:2790-2792.
27. Stewart RB, Bardy GH, Greene HL. Wide complex tachycardia: misdiagnosis and outcome after emergent therapy. *Ann Intern Med*. 1986;104:766-771.
28. Akhtar M, Shenasa M, Jazayeri M, et al. Wide QRS complex tachycardia: reappraisal of a common clinical problem. *Ann Intern Med*. 1988;109:905-912.
29. Tchou P, Young P, Mahmud R, et al. Useful clinical criteria for the diagnosis of ventricular tachycardia. *Am J Med*. 1988;84:53-56.
30. Baerman JM, Morady F, DiCario LA, de Buitleir M. Differentiation of ventricular tachycardia from supraventricular tachycardia with aberration: value of the clinical history. *Ann Emerg Med*. 1987;16:40-43.
31. Falk RH, Knowlton AA, Bernard SA, et al. Digoxin for converting recent-onset atrial fibrillation to sinus rhythm. *Ann Intern Med*. 1987;106:503-506.
32. Levitt MA. Supraventricular tachycardia with aberrant conduction versus ventricular tachycardia: differentiation and diagnosis. *Am J Emerg Med*. 1988;6:273-277.
33. Antunes E, Brugada J, Steurer G, et al. The differential diagnosis of a regular tachycardia with a wide QRS complex on the 12-lead ECG: ventricular tachycardia, supraventricular tachycardia with aberrant intraventricular conduction, and supraventricular tachycardia with anterograde conduction over an accessory pathway. *Pacing Clin Electrophysiol*. 1994;17:1515-1524.
34. Wellens HJ, Bar FW, Lie KI. The value of the electrocardiogram in the differential diagnosis of a tachycardia with a widened QRS complex. *Am J Med*. 1978;64:27-33.
35. Steurer G, Gursoy S, Frey B, et al. The differential diagnosis on the electrocardiogram between ventricular tachycardia and preexcited tachycardia. *Clin Cardiol*. 1994;17:306-308.
36. Brugada P, Brugada J, Mont L, et al. A new approach to the differential diagnosis of a regular tachycardia with a wide QRS complex. *Circulation*. 1991;83:1649-1659.
37. Drew BJ, Scheinman MM. ECG criteria to distinguish between aberrantly conducted supraventricular tachycardia and ventricular tachycardia: practical aspects for the immediate care setting. *Pacing Clin Electrophysiol*. 1995;18:2194-2208.
38. Herbert ME, Votey SR, Mortan MT, et al. Failure to agree on the electrocardiographic diagnosis of ventricular tachycardia. *Ann Emerg Med*. 1996;27:35-38.
39. Mark DG, Brady WJ, Pines JM. Pre-excitation syndromes: diagnostic consideration in the emergency department. *Am J Emerg Med*. 2009;27:878-888.
40. Wellens HJ, Durrer D. Wolff-Parkinson-White syndrome and atrial fibrillation. Relation between refractory period of AP and ventricular rate during atrial fibrillation. *Am J Cardiol*. 1974;34:777-782.

CHAPTER 8

Cardiogenic Shock

Jehangir Meer and Amal Mattu

IN THIS CHAPTER

Defining cardiogenic shock, reviewing its pathophysiology and various causes

Discussing the initial resuscitation and stabilization of patients in cardiogenic shock

Understanding that reperfusion therapy is the definitive therapy for most patients

Knowing when to employ mechanical support devices
Intraaortic balloon pump
Ventricular assist devices
Extracorporeal life support

Reviewing the current evidence for experimental therapies

Exploring special causes and treatments of cardiogenic shock

Introduction

Cardiogenic shock represents the extreme end of the spectrum of cardiac disorders resulting from left ventricular (LV) or right ventricular (RV) failure leading to a shock state; the left ventricle is the site of failure in 97% of cases.[1] It is defined as a state of end-organ hypoperfusion (Table 8-1) induced by heart failure after correcting hypovolemia and arrhythmias.[2]

Patients presenting in cardiogenic shock can be extremely challenging for emergency physicians to manage, as they often require multiple, time-dependent interventions. In the past, the mortality rate associated with cardiogenic shock was 80% to 90%, but with recent advances in treatment, the mortality rate has decreased, although it remains high at 50%.[3]

The most common cause of cardiogenic shock is acute coronary syndrome (ACS), specifically ST-segment elevation myocardial infarction (STEMI). Cardiogenic shock complicates 7% to 10% of cases of acute STEMI and 2.5% of non-STEMIs and is the most common cause of death in patients with acute myocardial infarction (AMI).[4,5] In select cases, aggressive treatment with reperfusion therapy and surgical treatment is lifesaving. Patients who survive to hospital admission have an excellent chance of long-term survival and good functional status.[6]

The pathogenesis of cardiogenic shock is thought to occur simultaneously along macrocellular and microcellular levels. Patients who develop cardiogenic shock classically have had a large anterior myocardial infarction (MI) or a reinfarction, resulting in a substantial area of nonfunctioning myocardium, which causes a significant decrease in stroke volume and arterial pressure and a modest depression in ejection fraction. It is thought that a series of neurohormonal responses then becomes activated, with the sympathetic nervous system and renin-angiotensin systems signaling peripheral vasoconstriction and salt and water retention. In addition, a systemic inflammatory response state develops, with release of cytokines and excessive nitric oxide production, further depressing myocardial function. These pathways lead to a vicious cycle of further myocardial ischemia and necrosis, resulting in lower arterial pressure, anaerobic metabolism, lactic acidosis, multi-organ failure, and death.[7,8]

The timing of shock after MI varies. A few patients (10%–15%) are in cardiogenic shock when they arrive in the emergency department. Shock develops in most patients within 48 hours after the onset of infarction.[8] In some cases, onset is delayed for as much as 2 weeks.[9] Patients in whom shock develops early tend to have a lower 30-day mortality rate than those in whom it emerges later.[8]

The most common cause of cardiogenic shock is myocardial

FIGURE 8-1.

Algorithm demonstrating the general approach to a patient presenting in cardiogenic shock

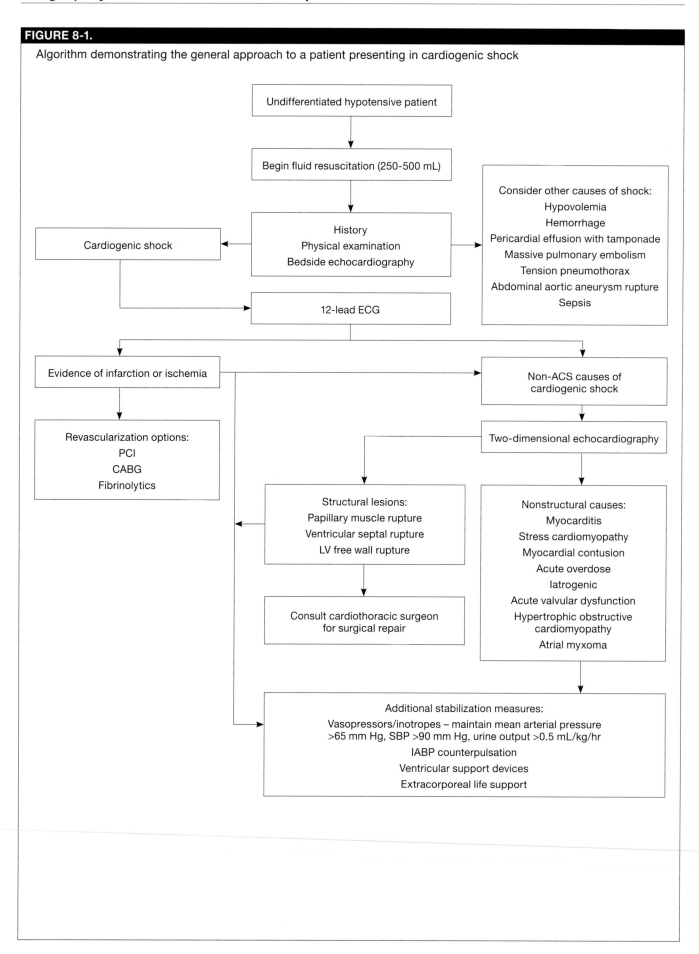

depression from an AMI or ACS. Other causes are presented in Table 8-2. In most cases, the cause can be established by interpretation of a 12-lead ECG tracing.

Initial Resuscitation and Stabilization

When assessing patients in cardiogenic shock, emergency physicians must rapidly determine if the cause is pump failure or if it is of a hypovolemic, hemorrhagic, obstructive, distributive, or septic nature (Figure 8-1). Because many patients present in extremis, the available history is often limited, but descriptions of chest pain or its anginal equivalents (eg, dyspnea, diaphoresis, presyncope, arm pain) should be elicited. Information from emergency medical services personnel or family members is often very helpful. On physical examination, these patients often have abnormal vital signs such as tachycardia, rapid and faint pulses, hypotension, and tachypnea (caused by congestive heart failure or respiratory compensation for metabolic acidosis). They can appear agitated or confused. The cardiovascular examination can reveal jugular venous distention and pulmonary rales, found in LV pump failure; or jugular venous distention and absent rales, found in RV failure. Third or fourth heart sounds may be heard. The presence of a systolic murmur suggests mechanical complications such as ventricular septal rupture or acute mitral regurgitation.[7]

A 12-lead ECG should be obtained urgently on the patient's arrival, looking for evidence of STEMI or ACS (Table 8-3). Patients should be placed on continuous cardiac monitoring to look for the presence of arrhythmias or atrioventricular blocks. Tachyarrhythmias should be treated with electrical cardioversion as antiarrhythmic medications can worsen hypotension. Bradycardic rhythms should be treated with atropine and transcutaneous or transvenous pacing. In addition, blood samples should be drawn for laboratory analysis of cardiac biomarkers, serum lactate level, coagulation studies, complete blood count (CBC), and chemistries. A portable chest film should be ordered. If the emergency department is equipped with ultrasound and the treating physician is trained in bedside ultrasonography, a focused, limited echocardiogram should be obtained and assessed for global contractility and other causes of shock (pericardial effusion with tamponade, dilated aortic root or detection of intimal flap, or RV dilatation). Several studies have shown that emergency physicians can, with little training, accurately identify depressed LV contractility using bedside ultrasound.[10,11] Of course, if it is available, a formal echocardiogram (transthoracic or transesophageal) performed

by a cardiologist can help to rule out structural causes of cardiogenic shock. Although the use of pulmonary artery catheters is a class I recommendation by the American College of Cardiology/American Heart Association (ACC/AHA) in patients with hypotension not responding to fluid administration, their use has declined in many centers. They have largely been replaced with two-dimensional echocardiography.[12,13]

PEARL
To identify cardiogenic shock, look for evidence of pump failure and rule out other causes of shock. Limited bedside echocardiography performed by an emergency physician can confirm pump failure (by showing decreased global contractility) and exclude other causes of shock (pericardial effusion with tamponade and massive pulmonary embolism).

KEY POINTS
Place all patients in whom cardiogenic shock is suspected on cardiac monitors for the evaluation of arrhythmias.

Treat tachyarrhythmias with electrical cardioversion; antiarrhythmic medications may worsen hypotension.

Treat symptomatic bradycardia with atropine and transcutaneous or transvenous pacing.

Initial resuscitation should focus on the ABCs. Patients who are hypoxic or in significant respiratory distress require respiratory support with positive-pressure, noninvasive ventilation or mechanical ventilation. Because of the nature of shock (pump failure), most resuscitation efforts will be directed at improving circulation, with the aim of keeping systolic arterial pres-

TABLE 8-1.

Clinical markers of hypoperfusion[6]

Cool extremities

Decreased urine output (<0.5 mL/kg/hr)

Change in mental status

Hypotension (SBP <90 mm Hg) for at least 30 minutes

Decreased cardiac index (<2.2 L/min/m²)

TABLE 8-2.

Causes of cardiogenic shock

Myocardial ischemia/infarction
- Mechanical complications of AMI
  - Acute mitral regurgitation secondary to papillary muscle rupture
  - Ventricular septal rupture
  - LV free wall rupture

Nonischemic depression of myocardial contractility
- Myocarditis
- Takotsubo (stress-induced) cardiomyopathy
- Sepsis
- Myocardial contusion
- Acute overdose of cardiotoxic drug (β-blockers, calcium channel blocker, digoxin)
- Iatrogenic
- Post-cardiotomy shock

Valvular pathology
- Acute aortic regurgitation
- Aortic and mitral stenosis

LV outflow tract obstruction
- Hypertrophic obstructive cardiomyopathy
- Left atrial myxoma

sure above 90 mm Hg, mean arterial pressure above 65 mm Hg, and urine output more than 0.5 mL/kg/hr. An initial fluid bolus should be given to optimize preload and improve ventricular filling. This is particularly true in patients with RV failure (eg, those with RV infarction, who are preload dependent), in whom additional fluid may be required and in whom nitrates, β-blockers, and morphine should be avoided. Unlike in the management of sepsis, the amount of intravenous fluid administered should be monitored cautiously. Most patients require some type of inotrope or vasopressor in combination (Table 8-4), and placement of a central line is recommended. The ACC/AHA recommend dobutamine as a first-line agent (an inotrope with selective β-agonist and arterial dilator properties) if the systolic blood pressure (SBP) is above 90 mm Hg. If the systolic pressure is below 90 mm Hg, then dopamine (which has both inotropic and vasopressor properties) should be started and titrated to maintain adequate pressure. If the response to dopamine is insufficient, norepinephrine (which has stronger vasopressor action than dopamine) may be added. The smallest possible dose of these inotropes/vasopressors should be administered. Although these agents improve contractility and increase arterial pressure, they also increase myocardial oxygen demand and can worsen ischemia and arrhythmias. Pure vasopressors such as phenylephrine should be avoided because they increase myocardial oxygen demand without improving contractility.

KEY POINT

Pure vasopressors such as phenylephrine should be avoided because they increase myocardial oxygen demand without improving contractility.

Additional medications to consider include aspirin, intravenous heparin, and glycoprotein IIb/IIIa (GpIIb-IIIa) inhibitors. No randomized trials have evaluated the use of GpIIb-IIIa inhibitors in the setting of cardiogenic shock, yet they are commonly used as adjunctive therapy.[7] Clopidogrel should be given only after consultation with an interventional cardiologist because its administration prior to percutaneous coronary intervention (PCI) is controversial.[7] About one fourth of patients in cardiogenic shock have severe triple-vessel disease or left main coronary artery disease that requires urgent coronary artery bypass grafting (CABG). The administration of clopidogrel before CABG has been associated with increased perioperative bleeding and morbidity.[7]

Medications to avoid in patients in cardiogenic shock include nitroglycerin, β-blockers, calcium channel blockers, and diuretics because they are likely to worsen hypotension.

KEY POINTS

Initial treatment of cardiogenic shock

- Correct hypotension with judicious use of fluids (250- to 500-mL bolus; more if RV infarction is suspected).
- Add vasopressors/inotropes early to keep mean arterial pressure >65 mm Hg, SBP >90 mm Hg, and urine output >0.5 mL/kg/hr.

Reperfusion Therapy

Since ischemia is the most common cause of cardiogenic shock, it is logical that reperfusion therapy would be a cornerstone of its management. Several trials have examined whether PCI is superior to fibrinolytic therapy or CABG in improving outcomes among patients in cardiogenic shock.

The first large-scale randomized study was the SHOCK trial, which showed that early revascularization decreased mortality compared with medical management alone.[1] In this trial, 302 patients were randomized to receive early revascularization (PCI or CABG) versus medical management with an intraaortic balloon pump (IABP). Sixty-four percent of patients in the early-intervention arm received PCI versus 36% in the CABG arm. Although the 30-day mortality rate was lower in the early intervention group, the difference did not reach statistical significance. However, in a 6-year followup, overall survival was markedly higher in the early intervention group (32% versus 19%), and the difference was statistically significant.[14] Of the survivors at 1 year, 83% met the characteristics of heart failure functional class 1 or 2 of the New York Heart Association.[15] Both PCI and CABG are class I recommendations for STEMI patients under 75 years of age who develop cardiogenic shock within 36 hours after infarction.[12,16] Early revascularization did not yield any benefit in patients older than 75 in the SHOCK trial (on the contrary, there was evidence of increased mor-

TABLE 8-4.

Vasoactive agents used in cardiogenic shock

Drug	Dose	Use
Dopamine	Initial dose: 5 mcg/kg/min	First-line agent (vasopressor/ inotrope) to use if SBP <90 mm Hg
	Titrate by 5–10 mcg/kg/min	
	Maximum dose: 20 mcg/kg/min	
Dobutamine	Initial dose: 2.5 mcg/kg/min	First-line inotropic agent to use if SBP >90 mm Hg
	Titrate by 2.5 mcg/kg/min	
	Maximum dose: 20 mcg/kg/min	
Norepinephrine	Initial dose: 0.5–1 mcg/min	Second-line agent added to dopamine if SBP remains <90 mm Hg
	Titrate by 1–2 mcg/min	
	Maximum dose: 30 mcg/min	

TABLE 8-3.

ECG abnormalities in cardiogenic shock

STEMI: ST-segment elevation or new left bundle-branch block

ACS: hyperacute or inverted T waves +/- ST-segment depression

tality), but it was associated with improved outcomes in that patient population in the SHOCK registry and other trials.[17] Therefore, a selective approach of offering revascularization to previously high-functioning individuals with good physiologic reserve is justified.[13]

Additionally, the SHOCK registry demonstrated greater mortality benefit from revascularization with PCI/CABG than with the use of fibrinolytics.[18] In the GUSTO-1 trial, with 2,972 patients in cardiogenic shock, patients who received thrombolytics had a short-term, 30-day mortality rate of 62%; those receiving PCI had a 38% mortality rate.[19,20] The reduced benefits of fibrinolytics in cardiogenic shock have been hypothesized to be due to several factors, including reduced penetration of the fibrinolytic to the occluded vessel in hypotensive patients and a higher rate of reocclusion of the infarcted vessel after thrombolysis administration.[21–23] The ACC/AHA issued a class I recommendation that thrombolytics be used in STEMI patients in cardiogenic shock who do not qualify for revascularization or if transporting the patient to a catheterization laboratory would cause significant delays.[12] PCI is preferred for revascularization if it is available.

PEARL

The mortality rate for patients in cardiogenic shock who undergo revascularization (PCI/CAGB) is lower than that for patients who receive fibrinolytics.

Patients are more likely to be referred for primary CABG versus PCI if they are found to have left main coronary artery disease or severe triple-vessel disease on cardiac catheterization. Mortality rates associated with emergent CABG have ranged from 25% to 60%.[24] In the SHOCK trial, the 30-day mortality rate was equivalent for the CABG and PCI groups (42% versus 45%), and the trial authors recommend emergent CABG for the indications named above.[7] Cardiogenic shock patients with AMI are more likely to have severe three-vessel disease or left main coronary artery disease than their hemodynamically stable counterparts[5] and therefore have a higher need for CABG. Unfortunately, there have been no randomized head-to-head trials comparing outcomes for PCI versus CABG. In patients with moderate triple-vessel disease, it is reasonable to perform PCI on the infarct-related artery and to defer CABG of the other diseased vessels.[13] In patients with severe triple-vessel or left main coronary artery disease, emergent CABG is recommended.

The timing of reperfusion is simple: the faster a patient can get to PCI or CABG, the lower the mortality rate. This was demonstrated in a German Registry (ALKK) trial and the SHOCK trial.[25,26] In the SHOCK trial, mortality rates in-

creased as time to revascularization increased from 0 to 8 hours. A survival benefit of revascularization was still noted up to 18 hours after the onset of shock.[26]

KEY POINTS

Reperfusion therapy is the mainstay treatment in most cardiogenic shock patients.

- PCI is preferred over fibrinolytic therapy.
- Fibrinolytics are indicated in patients who are not candidates for revascularization and in those who would experience significant delays in getting to the catheterization lab.
- CABG is the preferred method of revascularization if coronary angiography reveals severe triple-vessel disease or left main coronary artery disease.
- "Time is muscle"— the faster the revascularization, the lower the mortality risk to the patient.

Mechanical Support Devices

Patients in cardiogenic shock who require mechanical support are at the most critically ill spectrum of disease severity. These are patients who remain hemodynamically unstable despite aggressive supportive care and vasopressor therapy. Initiation of mechanical support is often a key therapeutic step toward definitive therapy, whether it is revascularization or surgical repair (Table 8-5).

Intraaortic Balloon Pump Counterpulsation

IABP counterpulsation can be lifesaving in patients with hemodynamic instability requiring vasopressors to maintain perfusion (Table 8-6). The pump is typically placed by an interventional cardiologist. Balloon pumps improve diastolic coronary flow by as much as 30% by increasing diastolic blood pressure.[27] They also decrease afterload (which lowers myocardial oxygen consumption) and improve subendocardial blood flow. Balloon pumps should be placed as early as possible, ideally before definitive revascularization, especially if the patient requires transfer to another facility for PCI.[6] Not every patient shows hemodynamic improvement with IABP counterpulsation, but a response predicts a better outcome.[28]

IABP counterpulsation is also beneficial in patients with structural causes of cardiogenic shock such as mitral regurgitation or ventricular septal rupture.[7] Studies have shown that balloon pumps improve survival after thrombolytic therapy in

---

TABLE 8-5.

Mechanical support devices used in cardiogenic shock

Intraaortic balloon pump counterpulsation

Ventricular assist devices

Extracorporeal life support

TABLE 8-6

Class I ACC/AHA recommendations for use of intraaortic balloon pump[12]

For cardiogenic shock not reversed with pressors prior to angiography and revascularization

For acute mitral regurgitation and ventricular septal rupture complicating AMI prior to angiography and surgical repair

For refractory post-MI angina as a bridge to angiography and revascularization

patients in cardiogenic shock.[29–31] However, the use of balloon pumps without revascularization has not been shown to reduce mortality.[32] Complications of IABP counterpulsation occur in about 10% to 30% of cases.[7,33,34] Contraindications and complications related to the placement of balloon pumps are listed in Table 8-7.

Ventricular Assist Devices

Ventricular assist devices are used in selected patients who remain unstable despite supportive care, IABP counterpulsation, and revascularization. These patients usually have very low cardiac outputs (<1.2 L/min/m^2).[23] A small trial comparing IABP counterpulsation with percutaneous ventricular assist devices in patients undergoing PCI for cardiogenic shock secondary to AMI found no difference in 30-day mortality but higher complication rates after use of a ventricular assist device.[35] These devices are either inserted percutaneously or implanted surgically. They can assist the left ventricle, the right ventricle, or both.

Percutaneous ventricular assist devices can be inserted rapidly but they cannot be left in place for a long time. The procedure is done in the catheterization lab by an interventional cardiologist. For example, in the TandemHeart percutaneous ventricular assist device (Cardiac Assist, Inc., Pittsburgh, PA), a 21F femoral catheter is placed transseptally across the interatrial septum into the left atrium, which unloads the left atrium and ventricle.[36] Blood is then pumped back to the patient via a 15F to 17F catheter inserted into the femoral artery. Flows of 3.5 to 4 L/min have been reported.[36] In a case series, Kar et al[37] described 11 patients in cardiogenic shock from AMI refractory to IABP counterpulsation and pressors who received percutaneous ventricular assist devices. These patients were supported for an average of 89 hours and had mean cardiac indices of 2.6 L/min/m^2. The authors concluded that a percutaneous ventricular assist device is useful as a bridge to an implantable ventricular assist device or to more definitive therapies such as revascularization, CABG, or cardiac transplantation.

Implantable ventricular assist devices are placed by a cardiothoracic surgeon in the operating room and can support patients for longer periods of time. Tayara and associates[38] supported 49 patients with cardiogenic shock following AMI for an average of 56 days until cardiac transplantation. The use of ventricular assist devices on a long-term basis as definitive therapy is appealing, given the limited supply of donor hearts. More research into this possibility is needed.[39,40]

The resources needed to place percutaneous and implantable ventricular assist devices are not widely available. Therefore, patients in whom IABP counterpulsation and revascularization fail must be transported to a tertiary care center that has the equipment and personnel needed to perform these specialized procedures.

Extracorporeal Life Support

Two types of extracorporeal life support (ECLS) are used in patients in cardiogenic shock: cardiopulmonary bypass and extracorporeal membrane oxygenation (ECMO). Percutaneous cardiopulmonary bypass can be instituted rapidly at the bedside, using the femoral artery and vein to provide nonpulsatile flow of 3 to 5 L/min. This type of support can be used only short term (hours) because of red blood cell destruction.[41] A report from the University of Michigan ECLS program, based on the largest series of ECLS cases at the time, documented a 33% rate of survival to discharge among 31 adults.[42] Both types of ECLS require specialized teams and equipment, so many patients who require this type of intervention must be transported to tertiary care hospitals.

PEARL

Consider ventricular assist devices and extracorporeal life support in patients who remain in shock despite aggressive supportive care, IABP counterpulsation, and revascularization.

TABLE 8-8.

Structural causes of cardiogenic shock[7]

Three structural causes account for 12% of cases of cardiogenic shock:
- Papillary muscle rupture
- Left ventricular free wall rupture
- Ventricular septal rupture

All are associated with very high mortality rates if they are not surgically repaired; therefore, early diagnosis is imperative.

Echocardiography has a vital role in diagnosing/excluding structural causes:
- Severe mitral regurgitation and/or papillary muscle rupture suggests papillary muscle rupture.
- A large pericardial effusion in a patient with an acute anterior wall MI suggests left ventricular free wall rupture.
- Left-to-right shunt across the ventricular septum with acute right ventricular dilatation suggests acute ventricular septal rupture.

TABLE 8-7.

Contraindications to and complications associated with intraaortic balloon pumps

---

Contraindications
- Aortic regurgitation
- Aortic dissection
- Severe peripheral vascular disease

Complications
- Hemorrhage
- Limb ischemia
- Femoral artery laceration
- Aortic dissection
- Infection
- Hemolysis
- Thrombocytopenia
- Thrombosis
- Embolism

Novel Therapy: N^G-Monomethyl-L-Arginine

N^G-monomethyl-L-arginine (L-NMMA) is a nitric oxide inhibitor that is thought to improve outcomes by competitively blocking nitric oxide in patients with shock. High levels of nitric oxide have been associated with decreased contractility. A small trial of 11 patients with severe cardiogenic shock (on mechanical ventilator, IABP, and pressors) demonstrated improvement in hemodynamic measurements (raised mean arterial pressure and lowered wedge pressure) after treatment with L-NMMA. Ten of the 11 patients were weaned off the ventilator and 7 were alive at 1 month.[43] The subsequent TRIUMPH trial did not reveal any benefit of L-NMMA.[44] The SHOCK-2 trial showed improvement in hemodynamic markers but no improvement in survival.[45]

Structural Causes of Cardiogenic Shock

Although LV failure from MI is the most common cause of cardiogenic shock, it is essential to rule out structural causes. These include papillary muscle rupture, LV free wall rupture, and ventricular septal rupture (Table 8-8).[6] Together, these three conditions account for 12% of causes of cardiogenic shock.[46] When any of these complications develops, the patient requires cardiac surgical repair, not just referral to the cardiac catheterization lab. These complications should be suspected in patients presenting in shock after a non-anterior MI, especially if it is their first event. Echocardiography is the imaging modality of choice to detect these complications.[6]

Papillary Muscle Rupture

Papillary muscle rupture occurs when MI produces ischemia at the head of the papillary muscle. Severe mitral regurgitation usually precedes the rupture. It is a relatively uncommon condition, being reported in the SHOCK trial registry in association with 7% of patients in cardiogenic shock.[46,47] It is more likely to occur in patients with acute inferior or posterior MIs and usually occurs within the first 24 hours after the onset of AMI. Risk factors include female sex and age greater than 65 years.[48] Patients present with acute pulmonary edema and often have a loud pansystolic cardiac murmur. Urgent formal echocardiography should be ordered when the diagnosis is suspected. Surgical repair is listed as a class I recommendation by the ACC/AHA. Without surgical repair, these patients have a very high mortality rate (71% in the SHOCK trial registry). Even with surgery, the mortality rate is still approximately 40%.[47] Temporary afterload reduction can improve cardiac output while the patient awaits surgery,[49] although this is difficult to accomplish when patients are already hypotensive. In that case, a combination of vasopressor (for blood pressure support) plus afterload reducer is needed.

Left Ventricular Free Wall Rupture

LV free wall rupture is a rare but lethal complication of acute anterior MI. A substantial majority of patients die immediately from pulseless electrical activity arrest, but a small proportion develop a contained hemorrhagic cardiac tamponade and may be salvageable. This diagnosis has decreased in incidence from 6% to 1% in the revascularization era.[46] Rupture occurs in the first 24 hours after AMI in about half the cases and within 1 week in the remainder.[50] Patients develop nonspecific symptoms such as refractory or recurrent chest pain, nausea, vomiting, syncope, and paradoxic bradycardia.[51] Echocardiography is required to make the diagnosis and will show a significant pericardial effusion. In the SHOCK registry trial, 28 patients (1.4% of the study group) in cardiogenic shock had free wall rupture. Twenty-one of the 28 had surgery to repair the rupture, with a 62% mortality rate. Six patients had pericardiocentesis without surgical repair, and only 3 of them survived.[52]

Ventricular Septal Rupture

Rupture of the intraventricular septum is a very rare complication of AMI and cardiogenic shock. In the GUSTO-I study, it occurred in less than 1% of patients with a STEMI and usually developed within 24 hours after infarction.[12,13] Among patients in cardiogenic shock in the SHOCK registry trial, ventricular septal rupture occurred in 4% of all cases. Patients usually present with acute pulmonary edema and a loud pansystolic murmur. An urgent echocardiogram is required to make the diagnosis; right ventricular overload is seen, with left-to-right shunting of blood though the rupture.[31] Urgent surgical repair is a class I recommendation by the ACC/AHA, but even with surgery, the mortality rate is in excess of 80%.[13]

Conclusion

Cardiogenic shock, a complication of AMI, requires timely diagnosis and resuscitation. A sound knowledge of the various options for aggressive supportive treatment can make the difference between life and death. Early referral for revascularization or cardiac surgical repair in selected cases is often necessary for survival.

References

1. Hochman JS, Sleeper LA, Webb JG, et al. Early revascularization in acute myocardial infarction complicated by cardiogenic shock. SHOCK Investigators. Should we emergently revascularize occluded coronaries for cardiogenic shock? *N Engl J Med.* 1999;341:625-634.

2. Nieminen MS, Bohm C, Cowie MR, et al. Executive summary of the guidelines on the diagnosis and treatment of acute heart failure: the Task Force on Acute Heart Failure of the European Society of Cardiology. *Eur Heart J.* 2005;26:384-416.

3. Goldberg RJ, Samad NA, Yarzdbska J, et al. Temporal trends in cardiogenic shock complicating acute myocardial infarction. *N Engl J Med.* 1999;340:1162-1168.

4. Holmes DR Jr, Berger PB, Hochman JS, et al. Cardiogenic shock in patients with acute ischemic syndromes with and without ST-segment elevation. *Circulation.* 1999;100:2067-2073.

5. Jacobs AK, French JK, Col J, et al. Cardiogenic shock with non-ST-segment elevation myocardial infarction: a report from the SHOCK Trial Registry. Should we emergently revascularize occluded coronaries for cardiogenic shock? *J Am Coll Cardiol.* 2000;36:1091-1096.

6. Reynolds HR, Hochman JS. Cardiogenic shock: current concepts and improving outcomes. *Circulation.* 2008;117:686-697.

7. Gurm HS, Bates ER. Cardiogenic shock complicating myocardial infarction. *Crit Care Clin.* 2007;23:759-777.

8. Lindholm MG, Kober L, Boesgaard S, et al. Cardiogenic shock complicating acute myocardial infarction. *Eur Heart J.* 2003;24:258-265.

9. Sanborn TA, Sleeper LA, Bates ER, et al. Impact of thrombolysis, intra-aortic balloon pump counterpulsation, and their combination in cardiogenic shock complicating acute myocardial infarction: a report from the SHOCK trial registry. *J Am Coll Cardiol.* 2000;36:1123-1129.

10. Niendorff DF, Rassias AJ, Palac R, et al. Rapid cardiac ultrasound of inpatients suffering PEA arrest performed by nonexpert sonographers. *Resuscitation.* 2005;67:81-87.

11. Randazzo MR, Snoey ER, Levitt MA, et al. Accuracy of emergency physician assessment of left ventricular ejection fraction and central venous pressure using echocardiography. *Acad Emerg Med.* 2003;10:973-977.

12. Antman EM, Anbe DT, Armstrong PW, et al. ACC/AHA guidelines for the management of patients with ST-elevation myocardial infarction: a report of the American College of Cardiology/American Heart Association Task Force on Practice Guidelines (Committee to Revise the 1999 Guidelines for the Management of Patients with Acute Myocardial Infarction). *J Am Coll Cardiol.* 2004;44:E1-E211.

13. Menon V, Hochman JS. Management of cardiogenic shock complicating acute myocardial infarction. *Heart.* 2003;88:531-537.

14. Ohman EM, Chang PP. Improving the quality of life after cardiogenic shock: do more revascularization. *J Am Coll Cardiol.* 2005;46:274-276.

15. Menon V, Webb JC, Hillis LD, et al. Outcome and profile of ventricular septal rupture with cardiogenic shock after myocardial infarction: a report from the SHOCK registry trial. *J Am Coll Cardiol.* 2000;36:1110-1116.

16. Eagle KA, Guyton RA, Davidoff R, et al. ACC/AHA 2004 guideline update for coronary artery bypass graft surgery. A report of the American College of Cardiology/American Heart Association Task Force on Practice Guidelines (Committee to Revise the 1999 Guidelines for Coronary Artery Bypass Surgery). *Circulation.* 2004;100:e340-e437.

17. Dzavik V, Sleeper LA, Cocke TP, et al. Early revascularization is associated with improved survival in elderly patients with acute myocardial infarction complicated by cardiogenic shock: a report from the SHOCK trial registry. *Eur Heart J.* 2003;24:828-837.

18. Sanborn TA, Feldman T. Management strategies for cardiogenic shock. *Curr Opin Cardiol.* 2004;19:608-612.

19. Naples RM, Harris JW, Ghaemmahami CA. Critical care aspects in the management of patients with acute coronary syndromes. *Emerg Med Clin North Am.* 2008;26:685-702.

20. Holmes DR Jr, Bates ER, Kleiman NS, et al. Contemporary reperfusion therapy for cardiogenic shock: the GUSTO-I Investigators Global Utilization of Streptokinase and Tissue Plasminogen Activator for Occluded Coronary Arteries. *J Am Coll Cardiology.* 1995;26:668-674.

21. Hollenberg SM, Kavinsky CJ, Parillo JE. Cardiogenic shock. *Ann Intern Med.* 1999;131:47-59.

22. Ellis TC, Lev E, Yasbek NF, et al. Therapeutic strategies for cardiogenic shock, 2006. *Current Treat Options Cardiovasc Med.* 2006;8:79-94.

23. Duvernoy CS, Bates ER. Management of cardiogenic shock attributable to acute myocardial infarction in the reperfusion era. *J Intensive Care Med.* 2005;4:188-198.

24. Bates ER, Moscussi M. Postmyocardial infarction cardiogenic shock. In: Brown DL, ed. *Cardiac Intensive Care.* Philadelphia, PA: WB Saunders; 1998:215-227.

25. Zeymer U, Neuhaus KL. Predictors of in-hospital mortality in 1333 patients with acute myocardial infarction complicated by cardiogenic shock treated with primary percutaneous coronary intervention (PCI): results of the primary PCI registry of the Arbeitsgemeinschaft Leitende Kardiologische Krankenhausarzte (ALKK). *Eur Heart J.* 2004;25:322-328.

26. Hochman JS, Sleeper LA, Webb JG, et al. Early revascularization and long-term survival in cardiogenic shock complicating acute myocardial infarction. *JAMA.* 2006;295:2511-2515.

27. Scheidt S, Wilner G, Mueller H, et al. Intra-aortic balloon counterpulsation in cardiogenic shock: report of a co-operative clinical trial. *N Engl J Med.* 1973;288:979-984.

28. Ramanathan K, Cosmi J, Harkness SM, et al. Reversal of systemic hypoperfusion following intra aortic balloon pumping is associated with improved 30-day survival independent of early revascularization in cardiogenic shock complicating an acute myocardial infarction. *Circulation.* 2003;108(suppl 1):I-672.

29. Anderson RD, Ohman EM, Holmes DR, et al. Use of intra-aortic balloon counterpulsation in patients presenting with cardiogenic shock: observations from the GUSTO-I study. *J Am Coll Cardiol.* 1997;30:708-715.

30. Webb JG. Interventional management of cardiogenic shock. *Can J Cardiol.* 1998;14:233-244.

31. Hochman JS, Sleeper LA, White HD, et al. One-year survival following early revascularization for cardiogenic shock. *JAMA.* 2001;285:190-192.

32. Hudson MP, Ohman EM. Intra-aortic balloon counterpulsation for cardiogenic shock complicating acute myocardial infarction. In: Hollenberg SM, Bates ER, eds. *Cardiogenic Shock.* Armonk, NY: Futura; 2002:81-102.

33. Trost JC, Hillis LD. Intra-aortic balloon counterpulsation. *Am J Cardiol.* 2006;97:J391-J398.

34. Stone GW, Ohman EM, Miller MF, et al. Contemporary utilization and outcomes of intra aortic balloon counterpulsation in acute myocardial infarction: the benchmark registry. *J Am Coll Cardiol.* 2003;41:1940-1945.

35. Thiele H, Sick P, Boudriot E, et al. Randomized comparison of intra-aortic balloon support with a percutaneous left ventricular assist device in patients with revascularized acute myocardial infarction complicated by cardiogenic shock. *Eur Heart J.* 2005;26:1276-1283.

36. Topalian S, Ginsberg F, Parrilo J. Cardiogenic shock. *Crit Care Med.* 2008;36(suppl):S66-S74.

37. Kar B, Adkins LE, Civitello AB, et al. Clinical experience with the TandemHeart percutaneous ventricular assist device. *Tex Heart Inst J.* 2006;33:111-115.

38. Tayara W, Starling RC, Yamani MH, et al. Improved survival after acute myocardial infarction complicated by cardiogenic shock with circulatory support and transplantation: comparing aggressive intervention with conservative treatment. *J Heart Lung Transplant.* 2006;25:504-509.

39. Burkoff D, O'Neill W, Brunckhorst C, et al. Feasbility study of the use of the TandemHeart percutaneous ventricular assist device for the treatment of cardiogenic shock. *Catheter Cardiovasc Interv.* 2006;68:211-217.

40. Meyns B, Dens J, Sergeant P, et al. Initial experience with the Impella device in patients with cardiogenic shock: Impella support for cardiogenic shock. *Thorac Cardiovasc Surg.* 2003;51:312-317.

41. Nichol G, Karmy-Jones R, Salerno C, et al. Systematic review of percutaneous cardiopulmonary bypass for cardiac arrest or cardiogenic shock states. *Resuscitation.* 2006;70:381-394.

42. Bartlett RH, Roloff DW, Custer JR, et al. Extracorporeal life support: the University of Michigan experience. *JAMA.* 2000;283:904-908.

43. Cotter G, Kaluski E, Blatt A, et al. L-NMMA (a nitric oxide synthase inhibitor) is effective in the treatment of cardiogenic shock. *Circulation.* 2000;101:1358-1361.

44. TRIUMPH investigators, Alexander JH, Reynolds HR, et al. Effect of tilarginine acetate in patients with acute myocardial infarction and cardiogenic shock: the TRIUMPH randomized controlled trial. *JAMA.* 2007;297:1657-1666.

45. Dzavik V, Cotter G, Reynolds HR, et al. Effect of nitric oxide synthase inhibition on hemodynamics and outcome of patients with persistent cardiogenic shock complicating acute myocardial infarction: a phase II dose-ranging study. *Eur Heart J.* 2007;28:1009-1016.

46. Hochman JS, Buller CE, Sleeper LA, et al. Cardiogenic shock complicating acute myocardial infarction–etiologies, management and outcome: a report from the SHOCK registry trial. *J Am Coll Cardiol.* 2000;36:1063-1070.

47. Thompson CR, Buller CE, Sleeper LA, et al. Cardiogenic shock due to acute severe mitral regurgitation complicating acute myocardial infarction: a report from the SHOCK trial registry. *J Am Coll Cardiol.* 2000;36:1104-1109.

48. Bates ER, Topol EJ. Limitations of thrombolytic therapy for acute myocardial infarction complicated by congestive heart failure and cardiogenic shock. *J Am Coll Cardiol.* 1991;18:1077-1084.

49. Aronson D, Goldsher N, Zukermann R, et al. Ischemic mitral regurgitation and risk of heart failure after myocardial infarction. *Arch Intern Med.* 2006;166:2362-2368.

50. Wehrens XH, Doevendans PA. Cardiac rupture complicating myocardial infarction. *Int J Cardiol.* 2004;95:285-292.

51. Birnbaum Y, Wagner GS, Gates KB, et al. Clinical and electrocardiographic variables associated with increased risk of ventricular septal defect in acute anterior myocardial infarction. *Am J Cardiol.* 2000;86:830-834.

52. Slater J, Brown RJ, Antonelli TA, et al. Cardiogenic shock due to cardiac free wall rupture or tamponade after acute myocardial infarction: a report from the SHOCK trial registry. *J Am Coll Cardiol.* 2000;36:1117-1122.

CHAPTER 9

Aortic Catastrophes

George C. Willis and Robert L. Rogers

Introduction

Thoracic aortic dissection and abdominal aortic aneurysm (AAA) are two deadly conditions that may mimic many other conditions in emergency medicine and critical care, leading to misdiagnosis with resultant increased morbidity and mortality. Frequently, the diagnosis is missed in the emergency department because it is never considered. When the diagnosis is made, the work for the emergency physician has only begun. Most patients with aortic emergencies are critically ill and must be transported to either an operating room or intensive care unit (ICU) after initial resuscitation. With hospital overcrowding, these patients can remain in the emergency department for an indeterminate amount of time. Any complications that emerge can result in detrimental outcomes. This chapter focuses on the care of the critically ill patient with two specific aortic emergencies: thoracic aortic dissection and AAA.

Thoracic Aortic Dissection

Thoracic aortic dissection is one of the most deadly causes of chest pain. This acute aortic condition arises when a tear occurs in the intima of the aorta, allowing blood to enter the defect and travel within the wall of the aorta. This creates a flap of intima that can freely occlude vital vessels that branch off of the aorta. It is a fairly common condition, occurring in 6,000 to 10,000 patients in the United States each year.[1-3] It is the most common catastrophic condition affecting the aorta, occurring three times more frequently than ruptured AAA.[4]

KEY POINT

Thoracic aortic dissection is three times as prevalent as ruptured AAA.

Several classification schemes for thoracic aortic dissection have been developed. Most management options are based on the Stanford system (Figure 9-1). Stanford type A dissections involve either the aortic arch alone or the aortic arch along with the descending aorta (Figure 9-2). Stanford type B dissections involve only the descending aorta.

Patients with thoracic aortic dissection present with a myriad of complaints. Acute severe chest pain is the most common chief complaint in all patient populations.[5-8] Most patients who present with Stanford type A dissections present with anterior chest pain that radiates to the neck or through to the back, especially if the descending aorta is involved.[8,9] Patients with Stanford type B dissections frequently complain of back and abdominal pain.[8,9] Unfortunately, these so-called classic presentations are found infrequently. Some patients have resolution of their pain or experience no pain whatsoever, making the diagnosis elusive.[9–12] High clinical suspicion is key in determining the diagnosis. However, once the diagnosis is established, the path to survival and recovery remains difficult. As many as 40% of patients die immediately, and 20% to 25% die during or after surgery.[13–15] In addition, for every hour the diagnosis of aortic dissection is delayed, the mortality rate increases 1% to 2%.[5,13,14,16] Early and aggressive diagnosis and management of dissection provide the best chance for better outcomes.

KEY POINTS

Forty percent of patients with thoracic aortic dissection die immediately, and 20% to 25% of patients die in the hospital, even with appropriate management.

Delaying the diagnosis increases the mortality rate 1% to 2% per hour after the initial event.

Stable Aortic Dissections

Stable patients should be managed in a stepwise fashion. All patients with aortic dissection, regardless of classification, should be placed on a cardiac monitor for detection of life-threatening arrhythmias and heart rate. Two large-bore intravenous lines should be placed for purposes of resuscitation. Blood pressure and heart rate monitoring become paramount in the management of dissection. Most patients present with a severely elevated blood pressure, often with a systolic blood pressure (SBP) higher than 200 mm Hg and a diastolic pressure greater than 100 mm Hg; others present normotensive or hypotensive for a number of reasons.[15] Blood pressure should be measured in both arms, and an arterial line should be placed into the radial artery in the arm that measures the highest blood pressure. Invasive blood pressure monitoring with an arterial catheter is necessary, providing the most accurate blood pressure.

Patients should have standard shock screening laboratory

samples sent for analysis. A type and screen will allow preparation of the blood products that will be needed if circulatory collapse occurs. A complete blood count will assess for significant anemia. A basic metabolic panel should be obtained to evaluate for any electrolyte abnormalities, most importantly for renal dysfunction. A lactate level will screen for mesenteric compromise. A coagulation panel will reveal any coagulopathies that are present, and any patients on warfarin will need intravenous vitamin K and fresh frozen plasma to correct the coagulopathy. Patients with thoracic aortic dissection need to be reassessed frequently for evidence of dissection extension, organ malperfusion (Table 9-1), pulse deficits, and new heart murmurs, all of which portend poorer outcomes.

The goals of management are to decrease the shear stress on the aortic wall, accomplished by decreasing the change in pressure over time. The blood pressure target is an SBP of 100 to 110 mm Hg and a heart rate less than 60 beats/min.

PEARL

In the management of aortic dissection, the target SBP is <110 mm Hg and the target heart rate is <60 beats/min.

These goals are most commonly accomplished by administration of easily titratable intravenous antihypertensive agents with a short half-life. The purpose is to make the blood pressure much lower than would be acceptable in other hypertensive emergencies (>25% of mean arterial pressure [MAP] in the first few hours). The most commonly used medications and their dosing regimens are listed in Table 9-2. Initial treatment is usually with intravenous β-blockers, which will primarily decrease the heart rate below 60 beats/min but will also have a moderate effect on lowering the blood pressure. If the patient has a history of asthma or intolerance to β-blockers, the non-dihydropyridine calcium channel blockers may be used. These agents

FIGURE 9-1.

The Stanford classification scheme for aortic dissection. Stanford type A dissections involve either the ascending aorta alone (i) or the ascending aorta as well as the descending aorta (ii). Stanford type B dissections involve the descending aorta alone (iii). Image courtesy of Miya Hunter-Willis.

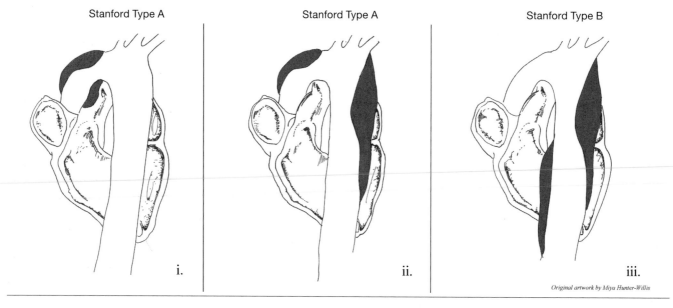

Stanford Type A   Stanford Type A   Stanford Type B

i.   ii.   iii.

Original artwork by Miya Hunter-Willis

have negative inotropic effects and do not produce the reflex tachycardia associated with the dihydropyridine calcium channel blockers. If further blood pressure management is necessary, the use of afterload-reducing agents is usually next-line therapy. These agents should not be used without β-blockade or calcium channel blockade because the decrease in blood pressure will likely result in reflex tachycardia.

KEY POINTS

In hypertensive patients with suspected or confirmed aortic dissection, the blood pressure must be reduced rapidly in the emergency department. The main rule followed in treating hypertensive emergencies, that is, not dropping the blood pressure too rapidly, does not apply to the management of acute aortic disease.

Avoid the use of afterload-reducing agents such as nitroprusside without β-blockers (or calcium channel blockers) to avoid reflex tachycardia.

Pain should be controlled with intravenous narcotic medications. This will decrease the adrenergic response to pain and provide some mild vasodilation to assist with blood pressure control.

Uncomplicated Type A Dissections

Patients who present with type A dissections should be treated as surgical emergencies. These patients have a very high mortality rate, as high as 1% to 2% per hour after symptom onset.[5,13,14,16] Risk factors that portend a poor prognosis are listed in Table 9-3.

Uncomplicated type A dissections, defined simply as not associated with any of the aforementioned complications listed in Table 9-1, are still associated with a high mortality rate. In addition to receiving aggressive blood pressure and heart rate

control, these patients should be monitored and frequently re-evaluated for signs of complications. A thoracic surgeon should be consulted for emergent operative intervention very early in the emergency department course. If a thoracic surgeon is not available, then preparations for transfer to the nearest tertiary care center should be made, once the patient has been stabilized and the heart rate and blood pressure have been optimized to prevent further complications.

Complicated Type A Dissections

Most complications arising from type A dissections are from retrograde extension of the dissection. This occurs when the dissection, which normally extends in an anterograde fashion, extends retrograde toward more proximal structures. Some of the more common and more fatal complications include coronary artery malperfusion, aortic valve insufficiency, and cardiac tamponade. Management of these complications requires an aggressive approach because of the associated high mortality rate.

Cardiac Complications

Coronary artery malperfusion, leading to acute myocardial ischemia or infarction, is one of the most challenging complications of acute aortic dissection. This complication is caused by an intimal flap overlying the lumen of the vessel or a dissection of the coronary vessel. The right coronary artery is most commonly affected, leading to inferior ST-segment elevation myocardial infarction (MI). Patients presenting with chest pain are often thought of as having an MI until proved otherwise. Patients with coronary artery malperfusion can have diagnostic ECGs or elevated troponin levels that lead the physician to a misdiagnosis of an isolated MI.[17] The dilemma arises when a cardiac catheterization suite is not available. When patients with MI caused by aortic dissection receive thrombolytic ther-

FIGURE 9-2.

Computed tomography (CT) scan of a Stanford type A aortic dissection

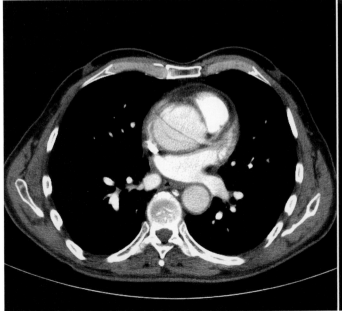
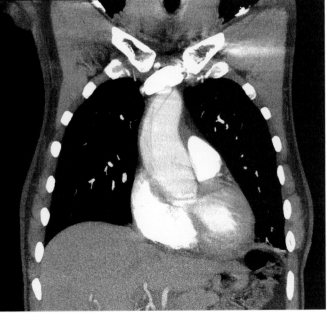

apy for an assumed acute MI, the outcome tends to be poor.[18] Patients who are diagnosed with coronary malperfusion are at higher risk for postoperative complications if the ischemic myocardium is not revascularized on an urgent basis. The bottom line is that all emergency physicians should consider the diagnosis of aortic dissection in every case of acute MI. This is especially true for patients who present with chest and back pain. Any patient with a diagnostic ECG and a low risk for aortic dissection should be managed as presumed acute coronary syndrome (ACS). If there is an increased risk of aortic dissection by history or risk factor analysis, the patient should have diagnostic imaging of the aorta before any antiplatelet therapy or anticoagulation is initiated.

KEY POINT

Aortic dissection most commonly involves the right coronary ostium, leading to right coronary artery occlusion and inferior ST-segment elevation MI. The physician must be on guard for patients with chest and back pain who present with what looks like an isolated acute MI.

TABLE 9-1.

Findings suggestive of organ malperfusion

Mesenteric malperfusion	Abdominal pain, distention, or acute abdomen
	Elevated lactate level
	Signs of ischemic bowel on CT scan (eg, thickened bowel wall, pneumatosis intestinalis, perforation)
Renal malperfusion	Urine output <0.5 mL/kg/hr
	Elevated serum creatinine
	Signs of decreased kidney perfusion on CT scan
Carotid/vertebral malperfusion	Transient ischemic attack or stroke symptoms
	Altered mental status
	Paraplegia
Iliac malperfusion	Pulse deficits
	Leg discomfort
	Paresthesias
Coronary malperfusion	ECG changes
	Troponin elevation
	Coronary artery occlusion on angiogram

Acute aortic regurgitation occurs in 41% to 76% of patients with type A dissections.[7,19–22] This complication is caused by aortic root dilatation or protrusion of the false lumen into the aortic root, not allowing the leaflets to close. Patients can present with a broad spectrum of signs and symptoms, ranging from a hemodynamically insignificant diastolic murmur to frank cardiogenic shock.[23] Acute management of patients with acute aortic regurgitation centers around aggressive afterload reduction with intravenous vasodilators until operative repair can be initiated.

A common practice in the evaluation of the "rule out ACS" chest pain patient is obtaining a portable chest radiograph to rule out aortic dissection by looking for a widened mediastinum. However, a widened mediastinum on the chest radiograph is present in only 60% of patients with confirmed dissection and should not be relied on alone for ruling out the diagnosis.[5,15,24–26] Consultation with a cardiothoracic surgeon

TABLE 9-2.

Antihypertensive agents recommended for use in hypertensive patients with thoracic aortic dissection

β-Blockers	
Esmolol	Load: 500 mcg/kg IV over 1 min
	Maintenance: 50 mcg/kg/min IV and titrate up to 200 mcg/kg/min IV
Labetalol	Bolus: 20 mg IV with repeat boluses of 40–80 mg up to 300 mg total
	Infusion: 2 mg/min IV and titrate to effect
Propranolol	Load: 1–5 mg IV
	Maintenance: 3 mg/hr IV
Metoprolol	2.5–5 mg IV every 5 min up to 15 mg IV every 15 min
Calcium channel blockers	
Diltiazem	5 mg/hr IV and titrate up to 15 mg/hr IV
Verapamil	2.5–5 mg IV then 5–10 mg IV 30 min later
Afterload-reducing agents	
Nitroprusside	0.25-0.5 mcg/kg/min IV and titrate to effect up to a maximum dose of 10 mcg/kg/min (cyanide toxicity is associated with rates higher than 4 mcg/kg/min)
Enalapril	1.25 mg IV every 6 hr

for early operative management is the next step, as emergent coronary revascularization in most cases must precede the dissection repair to preserve myocardium. Consulting interventional cardiology in concert with cardiothoracic surgery often expedites the process. Most surgeons prefer a preoperative angiogram to visualize the anatomy and evaluate which vessels are compromised, although there has been a recent shift toward intraoperative angiograms.[18,27] On patient stabilization, if a cardiothoracic surgeon is not available, transfer to a tertiary care center is the most favorable disposition.

KEY POINT

A chest radiograph is not sensitive enough to rule out aortic dissection.

Neurologic Complications

Central nervous system complications of acute aortic dissection are common and generally occur as a result of carotid artery occlusion. Classic stroke-like symptoms constitute a well-known presentation of proximal aortic dissection. Neurologic manifestations originate from malperfusion of the affected artery secondary to direct occlusion or decreased perfusion from hypotension. Patients with carotid compromise can present with any number of neurologic manifestations, ranging from transient ischemic attack or stroke symptoms to altered mental status or coma. Patients can present with neurologic symptoms without chest pain. All of these patients have a dismal prognosis, as the neurologic manifestations remain or worsen, or they die despite operative intervention.[28,29] These patients require emergent revascularization of compromised tissue. Unfortunately, other than urgent operative intervention, therapeutic interventions are rarely available to assist with revasculariza-

TABLE 9-3.

Risk factors associated with poor prognosis in patients with thoracic aortic dissection

Age >70 years
Abrupt onset of chest pain
Hypotension, shock, or tamponade at presentation
Renal failure at presentation and before surgery
Pulse deficit
Previous aortic valve replacement
Abnormal ECG, particularly ST-segment elevation
Prior MI
Renal and/or visceral ischemia
Underlying pulmonary disease
Preoperative neurologic impairment
Massive blood transfusion

tion. Management of these patients with early consultation by a cardiothoracic surgeon and neurologist or neurosurgeon improves the chance of full neurologic recovery.[30] Reducing time between initial presentation and intervention improves patient outcomes.

Patients with acute aortic dissection, Stanford type A or B, can present with spinal cord ischemia. This is brought about by a dissection flap occluding the ostia to the greater radicular artery, a large branch off the aorta that supplies blood flow to a large portion of the spinal cord.

Unstable Type A Dissections

Most unstable patients presenting with type A dissections have cardiac tamponade. The pathophysiology involves one of two mechanisms: either the false lumen extends into the pericardium and the hypertensive forces bring about a transudative pericardial effusion or, less commonly, the dissection ruptures into the pericardium.[31-33] Tamponade is the leading cause of death in patients with type A dissections.[1,7] The differential diagnoses for an unstable aortic dissection patient should include cardiac tamponade, MI, rupture, and cardiogenic shock from aortic valve insufficiency. Hypotensive patients with a proximal (type A) dissection should be assumed to have pericardial tamponade until proved otherwise.

KEY POINT

Differential diagnoses for unstable type A dissection:

- Pericardial tamponade
- MI
- Aortic rupture
- Aortic insufficiency leading to cardiogenic shock

Unstable patients who present with aortic dissection should be intubated for airway protection and adequate oxygenation and ventilation. Induction agents that have a safe and well-established hemodynamic profile such as etomidate are preferred. After the airway is secured, the next step is to rule out cardiac tamponade. Using bedside ultrasonography, an emergency physician can evaluate for a pericardial effusion. The subxiphoid view is adequate in most cases. Absence of an effusion on bedside ultrasonography rules out tamponade and should trigger the consideration of other causes. If an effusion is present, it must be relieved, but not by traditional means. In most cases of acute cardiac tamponade, pericardiocentesis is warranted; however, this procedure is contraindicated in the setting of aortic dissection, unless the patient is acutely decompensating or in arrest. This procedure has been associated with rebleeding and increased mortality.[34] Pericardiocentesis should be a last resort and used only as a temporizing measure in patients with proximal aortic dissection complicated by rupture to offer stability while an operating room is being prepared. These patients need definitive emergent operative intervention.

Cardiac arrest in patients with type A dissections is usually secondary to life-threatening arrhythmias or pulseless electrical activity secondary to cardiac tamponade, cardiogenic shock secondary to acute aortic insufficiency, or hypovolemia from rupture and exsanguination. These patients are very difficult to resuscitate without operative intervention. Early consultation with a cardiothoracic surgeon is directly linked with survival. Determination of the cause of the cardiac arrest is paramount in the selection of resuscitative measures. The survival rates for patients who present in a hypotensive state or after cardiac arrest are abysmal.

Patients should be placed on a monitor, and defibrillator pads should be placed. Intravenous access should be established, preferably with a central venous line. Advanced cardiovascular life support (ACLS) algorithms should be instituted early for arrhythmias such as ventricular fibrillation and pulseless ventricular tachycardia, and appropriate interventions should be used. As the algorithms are being implemented, the cause of the arrest should be considered. Bedside ultrasonography can be a handy way to determine if a pericardial effusion is present and can be performed at the time of resuscitation. Pericardiocentesis should be considered if tamponade is present because it offers an opportunity for return of spontaneous circulation while en route to an operating room.

Fluid resuscitation and vasopressor administration are mainstays of therapy regardless of the cause of shock. This seems counterintuitive to the purpose of decreasing the stress on the aortic wall; however, hemodynamic compromise will decrease overall organ perfusion and potentially worsen outcomes. If the murmur of aortic regurgitation is present or if cardiogenic shock is suspected, the addition of inotropes can be required to augment cardiac contractility. Examples of vasopressors and inotropes and their dosing are presented in Table 9-4. If rupture is suspected, packed red blood cells (RBCs) should be the resuscitative fluid of choice. The use of untyped, uncrossmatched blood products is encouraged in this patient population. Once spontaneous circulation has returned, the emergency physician must maintain adequate blood pressure through careful titration of medications that likely counteract each other. The ultimate goal at this point should be to expeditiously transfer these patients to the nearest operating room, whether it is in the presenting hospital or a tertiary care facility.

Uncomplicated Type B Dissections

Stanford type B aortic dissection is less likely to extend up the aortic arch and involve the cardiac structures. Patients with this condition are at significantly higher risk for organ malperfusion caused by dissection into or occlusion of a branch vessel leading to other organs (discussed below). Uncomplicated type B dissection is most commonly managed medically with blood pressure and heart rate control. Primary surgical management of type B dissections is associated with a mortality rate as high as 35%, whereas the mortality rate associated with medical management is approximately 10%.[35] Indications for operative intervention of type B dissections are listed in Table 9-5.

Samples for baseline laboratory tests should be drawn. These tests include a comprehensive metabolic panel for baseline liver function along with measurement of creatinine for renal function and lactate to assess for mesenteric compromise. These laboratory studies must be repeated if any suggestion of organ malperfusion arises (see Table 9-1). A Foley catheter should be placed to evaluate for decreased urine output as a sign of renal

malperfusion. Neurovascular checks should be performed on all extremities to evaluate for pulse deficits and neurovascular compromise every 1 or 2 hours. Finally, after the patient has been stabilized and the blood pressure and heart rate have been optimized, monitoring in an ICU setting is necessary to ensure frequent reevaluation for the complications that often arise with type B dissections.

Complicated Type B Dissections

Type B aortic dissections complicated with organ malperfusion are difficult to manage. The organ malperfusion syndromes that occur in patients with proximal (type A) aortic dissection are also possible in association with type B dissections. The mesenteric, renal, and iliac arteries are most often compromised by dissection. The intimal flap overlies the branch artery off of the aorta, which places the false lumen in line with the vessel lumen, compromising blood flow to the branch vessel's target organ. Rarely, the vessel also dissects, compromising blood flow. This is the origin of the phrase "symptoms above and below the diaphragm," as patients can experience chest or upper back pain and symptoms secondary to malperfusion.

Management of organ malperfusion syndromes often involves operative intervention. Patients with organ malperfusion have a higher mortality rate than those without; the mortality rate for these patients approaches that of patients with uncomplicated type A dissection. This is especially true in patients with mesenteric and renal malperfusion, who have a mortality rate between 30% and 50%.[29,30,36] Mesenteric malperfusion is the leading cause of death in type B dissections.[8] Patients who

TABLE 9-4.

Vasopressors and inotropes for patients with unstable thoracic aortic dissection

Vasopressors	
Dopamine	Initial dose: 5 mcg/kg/min
	Titrate by 5-10 mcg/kg/min
	Maximum dose: 20 mcg/kg/min
Norepinephrine	Initial dose: 0.5–1 mcg/min
	Titrate by 1–2 mcg/min
	Maximum dose: 30 mcg/min
Epinephrine	Initial dose: 1 mcg/min
	Titrate by 1 mcg/min
	Maximum dose: 10 mcg/min

Inotropes	
Dobutamine	Initial dose: 2.5 mcg/kg/min
	Titrate by 2.5 mcg/kg/min
	Maximum dose: 20 mcg/kg/min

present with organ malperfusion require urgent revascularization to salvage devitalized tissue. Many cardiothoracic surgeons will not operate on a patient with acute aortic dissection complicated by organ malperfusion until the specific organ malperfusion has been addressed or corrected. The mortality rate for these patients is very high unless the arterial obstruction is corrected surgically.

KEY POINT

Acute aortic dissection complicated by organ malperfusion carries a very high mortality rate. Cardiothoracic surgeons, in general, will not operate until the specific malperfusion syndrome has been corrected.

In addition to aggressive blood pressure and heart rate control, patients also require frequent monitoring for signs of worsening organ malperfusion. Serial blood samples for creatinine levels should be obtained if renal malperfusion is suspected. Urine output below 0.5 mL/kg/hr is an ominous sign, regardless of the serum creatinine level, because it is a sign of inadequate volume status or impending renal failure from malperfusion. In patients with abdominal pain or diarrhea associated with aortic dissection, mesenteric ischemia should be suspected. Serial lactate measurements should be obtained to assess for the possibility of mesenteric ischemia. Liver function tests and amylase measurement, allowing assessment for pancreatic compromise, should be obtained as well. Bowel ischemia has the highest mortality rate of the malperfusion syndromes. Any complaint of leg discomfort or signs of ischemic compromise of a lower limb should raise suspicion of iliac artery malperfusion. Neurovascular checks should be performed every 1 to 2 hours to assess for pulse deficits.

Open aortic repair and revascularization used to be the gold standard of care for patients with malperfusion. In more recent years, surgical intervention for these syndromes has been associated with a higher mortality rate; patients died not as a result of the dissection but as a consequence of malperfusion. Management with endovascular procedures such as aortic fenestration performed by interventional radiology or cardiology is being used more often, with promising results. Aortic fenestration is a procedure in which an angiogram is obtained to determine where the artery is compromised. Then several "fenestrations" are created in the dissection flap (the connection between the true and false lumens) using an endovascular device. This al-

lows blood flow through the fenestration and into the malperfused artery and subsequent target organ(s). The interventional radiologist can also place a stent in the artery to maintain patency, especially in the circumstance of branch vessel dissection. These techniques are associated with a much lower mortality rate than open surgical repair of the aorta (12% versus 28%).[29,37,38] Also, patients who underwent branch vessel intervention had a much lower complication rate than patients who underwent open repair alone, who were more likely to require bowel resections for ischemic gut or permanent hemodialysis for renal insufficiency.[29] Surgeons are now performing delayed surgery for aortic repair, even on type A dissections, allowing an average of 4 days for reperfusion and resolution of symptoms.[39]

KEY POINT

Patients with type A acute aortic dissection complicated by organ malperfusion need an aortic fenestration procedure (open or closed) before or at the time of corrective proximal aortic repair. The emergency physician should consult interventional radiology and vascular surgery in addition to cardiothoracic surgery. If these resources are not available, the patient should be transferred rapidly to a facility that can provide them.

Unstable Type B Dissections

In type B dissections, the causes of unstable vital signs are few, the most common and deadly being aortic rupture. Some patients present in cardiac arrest from hypovolemia. The primary goal is recognition of aortic rupture followed closely by hemodynamic stabilization. All unstable patients must be intubated for airway protection and to maintain adequate oxygenation. Large-bore intravenous access or central catheter placement for large-volume resuscitation is required. Crystalloid can be infused initially, but a rapid switch to packed RBCs to replace lost blood volume is encouraged. Any acute, life-threatening arrhythmias should be managed according to ACLS algorithms. After spontaneous circulation has returned, the patient should be transferred to an operating room for definitive operative intervention. Repair is the only definitive treatment for aortic rupture. The interventional techniques discussed earlier are also being used for rupture; however, the decision to use these techniques should be made in concert with the cardiovascular surgeon.[37,40]

Abdominal Aortic Aneurysm

AAAs occur in 2% to 4% of the US population. Most are diagnosed incidentally on radiographic studies obtained for other reasons. They are most commonly caused by atherosclerosis of the aorta, leading to degenerative changes in the elastic properties of the aorta. This allows the aorta to stretch and enlarge, leading to the development of the aneurysm. Risk factors for development of AAA are age over 60, hypertension, hyperlipidemia, and peripheral vascular disease. Most patients have no symptoms associated with their aneurysms and may be observed by a vascular surgeon every 6 to 12 months. The dilemma occurs when patients present with symptoms, because their presentations often lead to misdiagnosis. Presentations can

TABLE 9-5.

Indications for surgical management of type B dissections

Rapid progression or decompensation

Intractable chest or back pain

Refractory hypertension

Aortic branch vessel involvement with compromised perfusion to vital organs

Impending aortic rupture

vary widely from colicky abdominal or flank pain suggestive of renal colic to altered mental status from hypotension secondary to rupture of the aneurysm. Rupture is infrequent but still occurs in 15,000 patients per year and is the 13th leading cause of death in the United States. The mortality rate associated with AAA rupture is 90%.[41-43] Recognition and emergent management of these presentations are vital to maximize patient benefit.

The goal in managing stable patients with an AAA that is not ruptured is to determine if operative intervention is needed. Patients who present with a history of AAA and complain of abdominal or flank pain need an aorta-imaging study. The diagnosis should be considered in patients with no history of AAA but with any of the risk factors described in the preceding paragraph. Ultrasonography is an adequate screening tool for AAA and is excellent at measuring the diameter of the aortic lumen, but it cannot evaluate for rupture in the retroperitoneal space. Computed tomography (CT) scan with intravenous contrast can evaluate the retroperitoneal space for rupture and measure the diameter of the aortic lumen. Any AAA diameter greater than 5 to 5.5 cm requires operative intervention, and any ruptured AAA requires repair, regardless of the aortic caliber. As the diameter increases beyond 5 cm, the risk of rupture increases significantly to between 4% and 11%; past 6 cm, the risk increases to 7% to 26%.[44-46] Other indications for operative intervention are listed in Table 9-6. Once the diagnosis is established, consultation with a vascular surgeon to discuss surgical or medical management is warranted.

One of the most important issues in the management of a diagnosed AAA is whether the patient is truly stable. Patients can present with stable vital signs and still have a ruptured AAA. The most common pathophysiology behind this presentation is that the rupture has occurred posteriorly, into the retroperitoneum. Since it is a confined potential space, it fills with blood and then the blood loss abates secondary to tamponade in the retroperitoneal space, allowing the vital signs to restabilize. The patient experiences a sudden onset of abdominal or back pain that gradually eases but never resolves completely. Therefore, it should never be assumed that a rupture has not occurred simply because the vital signs are stable.

KEY POINT
Patients with ruptured AAA can have stable vital signs secondary to rupture into the retroperitoneal space and resultant tamponade.

Patients with a suspected ruptured AAA should be placed on a cardiac monitor to evaluate heart rate as well as arrhythmias that can arise from circulatory compromise secondary to hypovolemia. Two large-bore intravenous lines should be placed for access because blood products will likely be needed. Supplemental oxygen should be administered because most of these patients have lost a significant amount of blood into their retroperitoneal space and their hemoglobin should be saturated for adequate oxygen delivery.

If a patient presents with unstable vital signs and a history of AAA, the assumption must be that there is a rupture until it is proven otherwise, even if there are no symptoms. The possibility of ruptured AAA must be considered in patients in cardiac arrest, even in those without a history of AAA. Patients who have unstable vital signs and in whom ruptured AAA is being considered should be intubated for protection of the airway and maximization of oxygenation. The use of induction agents that maintain hemodynamics is preferred because any circulatory compromise can be detrimental.

Laboratory studies, including a complete blood count to evaluate for anemia and an initial hematocrit, should be obtained. A basic metabolic panel should be obtained to evaluate for renal insufficiency, which can develop if the renal artery is compromised. The lactate level should be measured initially as a baseline and serially every 4 to 6 hours. A type and crossmatch for at least 2 units of packed RBCs should be obtained because subsequent units may be needed. A coagulation panel will document any coagulopathies that require correction. If a patient is taking warfarin, presumptive therapy with intravenous vitamin K and fresh frozen plasma should be administered to correct the INR, even before the return of laboratory results.

Once intravenous access has been established, volume resuscitation and stabilization are required. The use of crystalloid is first-line therapy, and at least 2 liters of normal saline or lactated Ringer solution should be given to maintain intravascular volume. Once the crystalloid has been infused, the next volume replacement should be with packed RBCs. This will give the patient some oxygen storage capacity and replace the blood that was lost during the rupture. To monitor the patient's blood pressure, an invasive arterial catheter should be placed to provide the most accurate reading. The targets are an SBP of 100 to 120 mm Hg and a MAP of 60 to 65 mm Hg. Increased blood pressure can exacerbate ongoing blood loss or turn a contained rupture into a free rupture.[47]

Patients can present with hypertension, which is usually attributed to renal artery compromise. The amount of stress on the aortic wall makes the free wall less stable, creating a predisposition toward rupture. These patients must have their blood pressure lowered to the same management goal as those presenting with hypotension (ie, 100 to 120 mm Hg). This is achieved with intravenous antihypertensive medications (see Table 9-2), the most common being β-blockers. Calcium channel blockers and afterload-reducing agents can be used if a patient is intoler-

TABLE 9-6.
Indications for surgical management of abdominal aortic aneurysm

Aortic diameter >5.5 cm in asymptomatic patients

Interval increase of aortic diameter of 0.5 cm in 6 months in asymptomatic patients

Symptomatic patients

Renal malperfusion

Impending or completed rupture

ant to β-blockers. There is no conclusive evidence that lowering the blood pressure in the setting of hypertension and coexisting AAA has any beneficial effect.

PEARL

When AAA rupture is suspected, stabilization maneuvers include lowering the SBP to 100 to 120 mm Hg and the MAP to 60 to 65 mm Hg.

Patients presenting in cardiac arrest and with suspected ruptured aortic aneurysm are likely in arrest due to hypovolemia from exsanguination. These patients should be placed on a monitor, with defibrillator pads in place. Intravenous access should be obtained; a central venous catheter with a percutaneous sheath introducer is excellent for large-volume resuscitation. For patients with ruptured AAA, the most common presenting rhythm on the monitor is pulseless electrical activity, resulting from inadequate blood volume for the heart to produce a palpable pulse. ACLS algorithms should be followed for all other rhythms. Chest compressions should start once arrest is recognized, and adequate volume resuscitation should be performed. Crystalloids can be used, but the best volume resuscitation product is packed RBCs. Waiting for a type and crossmatch to be performed will be detrimental to the patient, so the use of untyped, uncrossmatched blood products is encouraged in this situation until the typed and crossmatched blood arrives. If spontaneous circulation returns, the aforementioned protocols of blood pressure management and hemodynamic maintenance are sufficient to stabilize the patient in preparation for the operating room.

What if spontaneous circulation does not return and the patient is still crashing? Case reports have described patients in the setting of cardiac arrest secondary to ruptured AAA undergoing open thoracotomy and aortic cross-clamping to stop the exsanguination. This preferentially shunts blood to the brain and coronary arteries and away from the rupture to allow enough time for sufficient volume to be infused. This would allow temporary stability for transport to the operating room and definitive repair. The costs and benefits of a thoracotomy need to be weighed. It should be reserved as a last resort for patients in whom cardiac arrest occurred very early after the emergence of symptoms and for those whose cardiac arrest was witnessed. Patients who have undergone prolonged resuscitative efforts without return of spontaneous circulation should not be considered for this procedure.

A vascular surgeon should be consulted early regarding the management of any patient presenting with a ruptured AAA, regardless of stability. Management options include open repair versus endovascular repair. Endovascular repair has proved to have a lower mortality rate.[48,49] Most vascular surgeons will be willing to proceed even without imaging in an unstable patient with a history of AAA. If a vascular surgeon is not available, the patient should be transported to a tertiary care center after being stabilized.

KEY POINT

If the patient is unstable and has a history of AAA, a vascular surgeon should be consulted early (ie, before imaging) to avoid delays in surgical management.

Conclusion

Aortic aneurysms, dissections, and ruptures are difficult to diagnose and treat. Associated complications further complicate the assessment process and therapeutic strategy. Early, aggressive management focusing on blood pressure control can improve outcomes for these critically ill patients. This group of disorders requires an early team approach, calling on the expertise of multiple medical and surgical specialties.

References

1. Meszaros I, Morocz J, Szlavi J, et al. Epidemiology and clinicopathology of aortic dissection. *Chest.* 2000;117:1271-1278.
2. Bickerstaff LK, Pairolero PC, Hollier LH, et al. Thoracic aortic aneurysms: a population-based study. *Surgery.* 1982;92:1103-1108.
3. Clouse WD, Hallett JW Jr, Schaff HV, et al. Acute aortic dissection: population-based incidence compared with degenerative aortic aneurysm rupture. *Mayo Clin Proc.* 2004;79:176-180.
4. Coady MA, Rizzo JA, Goldstein LJ, et al. Natural history, pathogenesis, and etiology of thoracic aortic aneurysms and dissections. *Cardiol Clin.* 1999;17:615-635.
5. Hiratzka L, Bakris G, Beckman J, et al. 2010 CCF/AHA/AATS/ACR/ASA/SCA/SCAI/SIR/STS/SVM Guidelines for the Diagnosis and Management of Patients With Thoracic Aortic Disease. A Report of the American College of Cardiology Foundation/American Heart Association Task Force on Practice Guidelines, American Association for Thoracic Surgery, American College of Radiology, American Stroke Association, Society of Cardiovascular Anesthesiologists, Society for Cardiovascular Angiography and Interventions, Society of Interventional Radiology, Society of Thoracic Surgeons, and Society for Vascular Medicine. *Circulation.* 2010;121:e266-e369.
6. Jex RK, Schaff HV, Piehler JM, et al. Repair of ascending aortic dissection: influence of associated aortic valve insufficiency on early and late results. *J Thorac Cardiovasc Surg.* 1987;93:375-384.
7. Fann JI, Smith JA, Miller DC, et al. Surgical management of aortic dissection during a 30-year period. *Circulation.* 1995;92:II113-II121.
8. Miller DC, Stinson EB, Oyer PE, et al. Operative treatment of aortic dissections: experience with 125 patients over a sixteen-year period. *J Thorac Cardiovasc Surg.* 1979;78:365-382.
9. Moon M. Approach to the treatment of aortic dissection. *Surg Clin North Am.* 2009;89:869-893.
10. Baydin A, Nargis C, Nural MS, et al. Painless, acute aortic dissection presenting as an acute stroke. *Mt Sinai J Med.* 2006;73:1129-1131.
11. Ayrik C, Cece H, Aslan O, et al. Seeing the invisible: painless aortic dissection in the emergency setting. *Emerg Med J.* 2006;23:e24.
12. Young J, Herd AM. Painless acute aortic dissection and rupture presenting as syncope. *J Emerg Med.* 2002;22:171-174.
13. Anagnostopoulos CE, Prabhakar MJ, Kittle CF. Aortic dissections and dissecting aneurysms. *Am J Cardiol.* 1972;30:263-273.
14. Masuda Y, Yamada Z, Morooka N, et al. Prognosis of patients with medically treated aortic dissections. *Circulation.* 1991;84:III7–III13.
15. Trimarchi S, Nienaber C, Rampoldi V, et al. Contemporary results of surgery in acute type A aortic dissection: the International Registry of Acute Aortic Dissection experience. *J Thorac Cardiovasc Surg.* 2005;129:112-122.
16. Hirst AE Jr, Johns VJ Jr, Kime SW Jr. Dissecting aneurysm of the aorta: a review of 505 cases. *Medicine.* 1958;37:217-279.
17. Hansen MS, Nogareda GJ, Hutchison SJ. Frequency of and inappropriate treatment of misdiagnosis of acute aortic dissection. *Am J Cardiol.* 2007;99:852-856.
18. Kawahito K, Adachi H, Murata S, et al. Coronary malperfusion due to type A aortic dissection: mechanism and surgical management. *Ann Thorac Surg.* 2003;76:1471-1476.
19. Mazzucotelli JP, Deleuze PH, Baufreton C, et al. Preservation of the aortic valve in acute aortic dissection: long-term echocardiographic assessment and clinical outcome. *Ann Thorac Surg.* 1993;55:1513-1517.
20. Von Segesser LK, Lorenzetti E, Lachat M, et al. Aortic valve preservation in acute type A dissection: is it sound? *J Thorac Cardiovasc Surg.* 1996;111:381-390.
21. Massimo CG, Presenti LF, Marranci P, et al. Extended and total aortic resection in the surgical treatment of acute type A aortic dissection: experience with 54 patients. *Ann Thorac Surg.* 1998;46:420-424.

22. Movsowitz HD, Levine RA, Hilgenberg AD, et al. Transesophageal echocardiographic description of the mechanisms of aortic regurgitation in acute type A aortic dissection: implications for aortic valve repair. *J Am Coll Cardiol.* 2000;36:884-890.

23. Januzzi JL, Eagle KA, Cooper JV, et al. Acute aortic dissection presenting with congestive heart failure: results from the International Registry of Acute Aortic Dissection. *J Am Coll Cardiol.* 2005;46:733-735.

24. von Kodolitsch Y, Nienaber C, Dieckmann C, et al. Chest radiography for the diagnosis of acute aortic syndrome. *Am J Med.* 2004;116:73-77.

25. Klompas M. Does this patient have an acute thoracic aortic dissection? *JAMA.* 2002;287:2262-2272.

26. Hagan PG, Nienaber CA, Isselbacher EM, et al. The International Registry of Acute Aortic Dissection (IRAD): new insights into an old disease. *JAMA.* 2000;283:897-903.

27. Neri E, Toscano T, Papalia U, et al. Proximal aortic dissection with coronary malperfusion: presentation, management, and outcomes. *J Thorac Cardiovasc Surg.* 2001;121:552-560.

28. Geirsson A, Szeto W, Pochettino A, et al. Significance of malperfusion syndromes prior to contemporary surgical repair for acute type A dissection: outcomes and need for additional revascularizations. *Eur J Cardiothorac Surg.* 2007;32:255-262.

29. Lauterbach S, Cambria R, Brewster D, et al. Contemporary management of aortic branch compromise resulting from acute aortic dissection. *J Vasc Surg.* 2001;33:1185-1192.

30. Girardi L, Krieger K, Lee L, et al. Management strategies for type A dissection complicated by peripheral vascular malperfusion. *Ann Thorac Surg.* 2004;77:1309-1314.

31. Garcia-Jimenez A, Peraza TA, Martinez LG, et al. Cardiac tamponade by aortic dissection in a hospital without cardiothoracic surgery. *Chest.* 1993;104:290-291.

32. Pretre R, Von Segesser LK. Aortic dissection. *Lancet.* 1997;349:1461-1464.

33. Armstrong WF, Bach DS, Carey LM, et al. Clinical and echocardiographic findings in patients with suspected acute aortic dissection. *Am Heart J.* 1998;136:1051-1060.

34. Isselbacher EM, Cigarroa JE, Eagle KA. Cardiac tamponade complicating proximal aortic dissection: is pericardiocentesis harmful? *Circulation.* 1994;90:2375-2378.

35. Umana JP, Lai DT, Mitchell RS, et al. Is medical therapy still the optimal treatment strategy for patients with acute type B aortic dissections? *J Thorac Cardiovasc Surg.* 2002;124:896-910.

36. Shiiya N, Matsuzaki K, Kunihara T, et al. Management of vital organ malperfusion in acute aortic dissection: proposal of a mechanism-specific approach. *Gen Thorac Cardiovasc Surg.* 2007;55:85-90.

37. Cambria R, Crawford R, Cho J, et al. A multicenter clinical trial of endovascular stent graft repair of acute catastrophes of the descending thoracic aorta. *J Vasc Surg.* 2009;50:1255-1264.

38. Patel H, Williams D, Meekov M, et al. Long-term results of percutaneous management of malperfusion in acute type B aortic dissection: implications for thoracic aortic endovascular repair. *J Thorac Cardiovasc Surg.* 2009;138:300-308.

39. Patel H, Williams D, Dasika N, et al. Operative delay for peripheral malperfusion syndrome in acute type A aortic dissection: a long-term analysis. *J Thorac Cardiovasc Surg.* 2008;135:1288-1296.

40. Patel H, Williams D, Upchurch G, et al. A comparative analysis of open and endovascular repair for the ruptured descending thoracic aorta. *J Vasc Surg.* 2009;50:1265-1270.

41. Mealy K, Salman A. The true incidence of ruptured abdominal aortic aneurysms. *Eur J Vasc Surg.* 1988;2:405-408.

42. Heikkinen M, Salenius J, Zeitlin R, et al. The fate of AAA patients referred electively to vascular surgical unit. *Scand J Surg.* 2002;91:345-352.

43. Johansen K, Kohler TR, Nicholls SC, et al. Ruptured abdominal aortic aneurysm: the Harborview experience. *J Vasc Surg.* 1991;13:240-245.

44. Brown LC, Powell JT. Risk factors for rupture in patients kept under ultrasound surveillance: the UK Small Aneurysm Trial Participants. *Ann Surg.* 1999;230:289-297.

45. Reed WW, Hallett JW Jr, Damiano MA, Ballard DJ. Learning from the last ultrasound: a population-based study of patients with abdominal aortic aneurysm. *Arch Intern Med.* 1997;157:2064-2068.

46. Brewster D, Cronenwett J, Hallett J, et al. Guidelines for the treatment of abdominal aortic aneurysms: report of a subcommittee of the Joint Council of the American Association for Vascular Surgery and Society for Vascular Surgery. *J Vasc Surg.* 2003;37:1106-1117.

47. Arthurs Z, Sohn V, Starnes B. Ruptured abdominal aortic aneurysms: remote aortic occlusion for the general surgeon. *Surg Clin North Am.* 2007;87:1035-1045.

48. Eliason J, Clouse W. Current management of infrarenal abdominal aortic aneurysms. *Surg Clin North Am.* 2007;87:1017-1033.

49. Hirsch AT, Haskal ZJ, Hertzer NR, et al. ACC/AHA 2005 guidelines for the management of patients with peripheral arterial disease (lower extremity, renal, mesenteric, and abdominal aortic): executive summary. A collaborative report from the American Association for Vascular Surgery/Society for Vascular Surgery, Society for Cardiovascular Angiography and Interventions, Society for Vascular Medicine and Biology, Society of Interventional Radiology, and the ACC/AHA Task Force on Practice Guidelines (Writing Committee to Develop Guidelines for the Management of Patients With Peripheral Arterial Disease) endorsed by the American Association of Cardiovascular and Pulmonary Rehabilitation; National Heart, Lung, and Blood Institute; Society for Vascular Nursing; TransAtlantic Inter-Society Consensus; and Vascular Disease Foundation. *J Am Coll Cardiol.* 2006;47:1239-1312.

CHAPTER 10

The Unstable Patient with Pulmonary Embolism

Timothy J. Ellender, Ryan G.K. Mihata, and J. C. Skinner

IN THIS CHAPTER

Pathophysiology of pulmonary insufficiency and right ventricular dysfunction

Identification of unstable patients with pulmonary embolism

Intravenous fluids, ventilation, vasopressors, and inotropes

Anticoagulation and thrombolysis: indications, contraindications, and applications

Alternative therapies: interventional and surgical approaches

Introduction

Pulmonary embolism (PE) is a common cardiovascular and cardiopulmonary illness with an incidence that exceeds 1 in 1,000 and a mortality rate that exceeds 15% in the first 3 months after diagnosis.[1-5] The hemodynamic collapse that follows a large PE can be one of the more anxiety-provoking encounters of an emergency physician's career. Massive PE is marked by abrupt hemodynamic instability caused by acute right ventricular (RV) dysfunction (cor pulmonale), which is caused by a sequence of pulmonary arterial vasoconstriction and obstruction that directly increases pulmonary vascular resistance and RV afterload.[6]

The emergency department diagnosis and treatment of PE can be challenging. Primary presentations in PE share common features with other commonly encountered emergencies (acute myocardial infarction, sepsis, heart failure). PE can progress to cause moderate or profound RV dysfunction with decreased cardiac output and eventually cardiac arrest, which heralds increased mortality.[7] Thus, making the correct diagnosis and distinguishing massive from submassive PE are important steps in the therapeutic algorithm.[7] Goldhaber described six syndromes of acute PE. The first two, massive PE and moderate to large PE, apply to patients with significant pulmonary perfusion de-

fects and RV dyskinesis.[6] These two syndromes can be distinguished from one another by a transition from relatively normal systemic pressures (moderate to large PE: 30% perfusion obstruction) to persistent systemic arterial hypotension (massive PE: >50% obstruction).[6] A "massive" PE can be distinguished from a "submassive" one on the basis of hemodynamic stability; this distinction becomes part of an overall strategy for risk stratification and treatment.[8] Biomarker assays combined with measurements of ventricular chamber size by computed tomography (CT) and echocardiography aid not only in the differentiation of shock states but also in the determination of patient acuity and the assignment of risk.

Patients with massive PE, hemodynamic instability, and/or cardiogenic shock (identified by a systolic blood pressure [SBP] <90 mm Hg without other explanation) have increased mortality rates and can benefit from immediate time-dependent therapy.[1,6,9-16] Much of the emergency literature focuses on stratifying patients for risk of PE or on identifying PE as a differential cause of pathology using various tests and algorithms. Surprisingly, there is a paucity of data to support a single approach to resuscitating the unstable patient with PE.

Although optimal management of massive PE requires multidisciplinary input, it is imperative that emergency physicians be knowledgeable in the acute management of patients with

FIGURE 10-1.

Algorithm for the treatment of unstable patients with pulmonary embolism

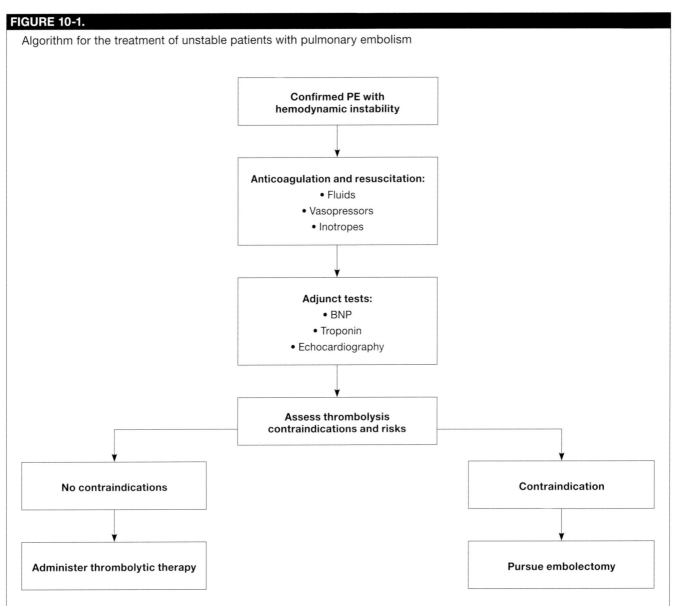

- Massive PE with shock is the clearest indication for thrombolysis. To many clinicians, hypotension in the setting of acute PE marks hemodynamic instability and is an indication for thrombolytic therapy.

- In unstable patients, fluids should be administered and vasopressor therapy initiated when indicated.

- Severe RV enlargement and dysfunction portend a worse prognosis and help identify patients who could most benefit from resuscitation and thrombolysis. Although the presence of positive biomarkers should be considered together with other criteria, these tests have not allowed stratification of groups who will benefit from thrombolysis.

- In extremely unstable patients, thrombolysis should not be delayed for additional assays or confirmatory testing.

massive PE since most deaths occur in the first 1 to 2 hours of care.[17] Optimal care orchestrates rapid differentiation of massive from submassive PE, implementation of evidence-based resuscitation, and early initiation of time-sensitive anticoagulant and thrombolytic therapy (Figure 10-1).

KEY POINTS

The mortality rate for PE exceeds 15% during the first 3 months of treatment.

Most deaths caused by PE occur in the first 1 or 2 hours of care.

Pathophysiology

Pulmonary Insufficiency

In massive PE, the increased vascular resistance caused primarily by thrombosis obstruction and secondarily by vasoconstrictive triggers (thromboxanes/serotonin) leads to decreased pulmonary vascular flow.[18-20] Low-flow perfusion defects increase alveolar dead space and subsequently impair gas exchange, which manifests as hypoxemia.[19,20] Hypoxemia in conjunction with irritant receptor stimulation leads to alveolar hyperventilation, which drives hypocapnia and respiratory alkalosis.[21] These acid–base shifts combined with an augmentation in sympathetic tone, increase in platelet activation, and escalation of inflammatory cascades can trigger bronchospasm and further vasoconstriction.[21,22] Finally, hydrostatic and oncotic imbalance drives the formation of pulmonary edema, which further dilutes alveolar surfactant and lowers pulmonary compliance.[18]

Right Ventricular Dysfunction

RV dysfunction can be classified as impaired RV contractility, RV pressure overload, and RV volume overload.[23] Many PE patients with acutely decompensated RV function have a combination of these three entities.[6,23] Compared with the left ventricle, the right ventricle is better suited to volume overload than pressure overload.[24] Unless conditioned over time (hypertrophied) to gradual increases in pulmonary vascular resistance, the thin-walled, compliant right ventricle does not have the myocardial bulk and contractility to overcome an elevated afterload.[25] Acutely increased end-diastolic pressure causes a shift in the normal contour of the interventricular septum toward the left ventricle and increases intrapericardial pressures, which limit both RV and left ventricular (LV) filling (Figure 10-2).[26] In time, RV pressure overload, secondary to pulmonary artery obstruction and pulmonary hypertension, leads to increased RV wall tension, RV chamber dilation, and impaired diastolic and systolic function.[1] Increased ventricular wall tension and decreasing cardiac output contribute to decreased coronary perfusion. This decreased oxygen supply comes at a time of increased myocardial oxygen consumption, which can lead to RV ischemia or infarction.[27]

As RV dysfunction progresses, a decreasing RV cardiac output alters LV preload, which affects LV cardiac output. Pressure imbalances created by a failing pump further exacerbate interventricular septum dyskinesis, affecting LV chamber size

and preload, which leads to systemic hypotension. As systemic hypotension in turn lowers coronary perfusion pressure, a vicious cycle termed *auto-aggravation* continues to worsen RV dysfunction.[28-30]

Identification of Unstable Patients with Pulmonary Embolism

Clinical Presentation

Hemodynamic collapse can be initiated by a multitude of disease processes, the clinical presentation of which can be nonspecific and overlapping. Therefore, a thorough history and physical examination along with rapid bedside diagnostic testing (Table 10-1) can aid in identifying PE as the cause and selecting further management.

Patients with PE can present with dyspnea, lightheadedness, fatigue, and/or chest discomfort. Severe dyspnea, significant tachypnea, hypoxemia (SpO$_2$ <90), cyanosis, and syncope are suggestive of a massive PE. Clinical criteria for massive PE are hypotension (SBP <90 mm Hg or a drop of 40 mm Hg from a baseline systolic arterial pressure) and cardiogenic shock.[7,31] Common physical examination findings in massive PE include hypotension, tachycardia, tachypnea, elevated jugular venous pressure in the presence of clear lung fields, parasternal heave, tricuspid regurgitation, a right-sided S$_3$ gallop, and accentuated pulmonic valve closure (loud S$_2$).[1]

Diagnostic Testing

High clinical suspicion for massive PE should be maintained in an unstable patient with clinical evidence of RV dysfunction. In a patient with evidence of shock or hypotension, a focused bedside echocardiogram should be performed urgently. Evidence of RV dilation or dysfunction in the setting of high clinical concern for PE should prompt the clinician to initiate treatment prior to performing other confirmatory tests.

The literature lists multiple diagnostic options for further evaluation and confirmation, including electrocardiogram (ECG), cardiac biomarkers, chest radiography (plain, CT, and cardiac magnetic resonance imaging [MRI]), echocardiography, and right-heart catheterization. Not all of these tests are feasible, available, or necessary given the specific clinical scenario. However, familiarity with these tests and their individual and combined diagnostic accuracy is useful in the setting of RV decompensation. These diagnostic investigations facilitate rapid diagnosis and delineation of the cause of RV failure and aid in the interpretation of volume status and cardiac output.

Electrocardiogram

Electrocardiographic findings are nonspecific in massive PE. Sinus tachycardia is by far the most common abnormality noted. Rhythm disturbances, axis deviations, right bundle-branch blocks, nonspecific ST-segment changes, evidence of RV strain (precordial T-wave inversions), and an S$_1$Q$_3$T$_3$ pattern (seen in only 15%–20% of patients with PE) can all be seen.[32] However, in 10% to 25% of patients with PE, the ECG is normal.[33]

PEARL

The most useful role of the ECG in the unstable patient is to differentiate massive PE from acute myocardial infarction as the primary cause of cardiogenic shock.

Cardiac Biomarkers

Cardiac biomarkers, which often rise over a 6-hour window, have limited utility in the hemodynamically unstable patient who presents with an abrupt onset of symptoms. Although D-dimer ELISA and cardiac biomarker testing might aid in risk stratification, these tests are often redundant in the critically ill and should not delay therapeutic optimization. Brain natriuretic peptide (BNP) and pro-natriuretic peptide (proBNP) are re-

leased during myocardial wall stress and ischemia and can help predict the seriousness of PE.[23] A BNP level less than 500 pg/mL is a good prognostic indicator, whereas higher levels mark increased risk for inhospital adverse events (OR, 6.8; 95% CI, 4.4–10) and 30-day mortality (OR, 7.6; 95% CI, 3.4–17).[34,35] Similar studies with troponins have shown that elevated levels herald RV compromise and reflect a higher level of morbidity

TABLE 10-1.

Clinical and diagnostic findings in massive PE

Clinical signs and symptoms

Dyspnea

Tachycardia

Tachypnea

Cyanosis

Anxiety

Pleuritic pain

Hemoptysis

Arterial hypotension

Distended neck veins

Right parasternal heave

Accentuated valve closure, P_2

Tricuspid regurgitant murmur

Right-sided S_3 gallop

Diagnostic findings

Sinus tachycardia on ECG

$S_1Q_3T_3$ pattern on ECG

T-wave inversions in V_1 or V_4

Qr (pseudo-infarction) in V_1

Incomplete or complete right bundle-branch block

BNP >50 pg/mL

Troponin I >0.04 ng/mL

Troponin T >0.01 ng/mL

D-Dimer ELISA >1,500 ng/mL^{-1}

Westermark sign on chest film

Hampton hump on chest film

RV dilation >25 mm on CT scan

RV:LV ratio >1.5

FIGURE 10-2.

Cardiac hemodynamic relationships in massive pulmonary embolism. 1, Pulmonary vascular resistance and pulmonary pressures increase. 2, RV afterload and end-diastolic pressures increase. 3, RV chamber dilates (limited by pericardium). 4, RV wall tension increases (increases oxygen demand). 5, Interventricular septum shifts leftward. 6, LV ejection fraction is impaired by decreased LV chamber size and preload volume. From: Creative Commons, Creative Commons Attribution 2.5 License 2006. Patrick J. Lynch, Medical Illustrator. http://upload.wikimedia.org/wikipedia/commons/4/4f/Heart_anterior_large.jpg.

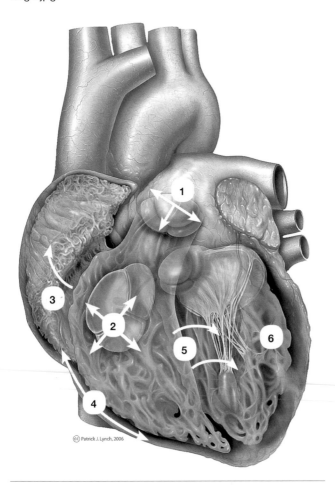

(OR, 5.2; 95% CI, 3.3–8.4) and mortality (OR, 7.0; 95% CI, 2.4–20.4).[1,6,11,13,31,36-38]

Chest Radiography

No specific finding on plain chest radiographs is diagnostic of PE, but the film will be abnormal in 76% to 90% of cases.[39] Findings include enlargement of the pulmonary artery, elevation of the diaphragm, and right heart enlargement. A Westermark sign (oligemia or lack of vascular markings) and Hampton hump (wedge-based opacification) are present in less than 20% of cases.[39] Ventilation-perfusion scintigraphy (V/Q scan) can be useful in the stable patient. A normal perfusion scan can safely exclude PE; a high-probability V/Q scan in the right context establishes the diagnosis. Although this might be a safe alternative in the stable patient, V/Q imaging is typically impractical in assessing massive PE because of the associated time delays and transport logistics.

Spiral CT and CT angiography have become the diagnostic modalities of choice. The overall sensitivity of the test varies according to a number of factors, including technical aspects, selection bias, interpretation of the test, and the quality of the CT scanner.[40] Two advantages of CT are its ability to detect an alternative diagnosis and the relative speed with which the scan can be obtained in most emergency departments.

Bedside Transthoracic Echocardiogram

A bedside transthoracic echocardiogram or goal-directed ultrasonography should be performed as soon as possible (Table 10-2). This helps confirm RV dysfunction and dilation as well as excludes alternative causes of shock (eg, pericardial tamponade).[41] In the setting of shock or hypotension, the absence of echocardiographic signs of RV dysfunction can help exclude PE as the cause.[13] In massive PE, regional RV wall dysfunction with hypokinesis that spares the apex is specific for PE.[13,27,43] The right ventricle can be dilated to the point that it causes poor filling of the left ventricle, which can be observed in real time. Other signs of massive PE seen on transthoracic echocardiogram include paradoxical septal motion toward the left ventricle, tricuspid regurgitation, right atrial enlargement, and a lack of inferior vena cava inspiratory variation (Figure 10-3).

TABLE 10-2.

Ultrasonography findings in PE

RV dilation (best seen in parasternal long-axis view)
    Normal RV diameter: 21±1 mm
    Abnormal: >25–30 mm

Leftward septal deviation/shift (apical four-chamber view)

Septal flattening (parasternal short-axis view)

RV hypokinesis with wall thinning (parasternal short-axis view)

Tricuspid regurgitation

Right atrial dilation

Dilated inferior vena cava with loss of respiratory variability

---

Resuscitation and Supportive Care

The treatment of the cardiopulmonary derangements of massive PE is aimed at disrupting the auto-aggravation cycle triggered by pulmonary vascular obstruction. The specific clinical scenario requires prioritized stabilization with minimal to aggressive support and the use of thrombolysis or possible percutaneous or surgical interventions (Figure 10-1). Therapeutic strategies proposed for hemodynamic support of acute circulatory failure caused by massive PE include volume expansion, inotropes, and vasopressors.[3,13,23,31,43,47] Very few clinical studies have evaluated these treatments. Worse yet, most of the knowledge about the effectiveness of supportive measures in PE comes from experimental studies that are difficult to extrapolate into clinical practice.[47]

Intravenous Fluids

Because most deaths from massive PE occur within the first hour after symptom onset, thrombolytic therapy or pulmonary embolectomy alone is insufficient.[31,48] Fluid loading, the initial therapy used in various types of shock, remains controversial in massive PE. Most authors recommend cautious use of fluids in the initial phase of resuscitation and caution against aggressive volume expansion.[9,13,43,48] Human and animal data are conflicting as to the effectiveness of fluid loading in massive PE.[28,31,46,47,49-55] Mercat and colleagues[47] showed that a 500-mL loading volume was relatively safe and improved ventricular performance and cardiac output. Based on these findings and other human data, a moderate volume challenge (250–500 mL) is an acceptable strategy in PE resuscitation.[9,13,44,45,47,48,56] Low central venous pressures (<13 mm Hg), smaller RV chamber size, and lower RV end-diastolic volume make success and an increase in cardiac output more likely with this strategy.[47,56,57]

Determining if volume is needed in the setting of PE and RV failure can be difficult. Tools such as echocardiography and right heart catheterization can help assess right atrial filling pressures to indicate whether RV pressures are elevated.[25,47,52,58-60] In patients with moderate or severe PE, plasma volume expansion can have a negative effect on RV performance. If the right ventricle has reached a state of optimal stretch to allow maximal pressure generation, further volume could be detrimental because of overstretch, which would decrease RV ejection fraction. When RV afterload rises, RV function worsens with the addition of volume because of the pericardial constraint on RV expansion.[52] Cardiac overload can decrease RV coronary perfusion pressure (to <30 mm Hg), which exacerbates RV myocardial ischemia and acute RV failure.[47] This can lead to a downward spiral resulting in RV infarction, circulatory arrest, and death.

KEY POINTS

Use caution with volume administration.

Attempt to estimate right-sided pressures.

Avoid fluid loading if pressures are elevated, as indicated by the following:

Marked jugular venous distention

Central venous pressure >12 mm Hg

Marked RV dilation on sonography

Lack of inferior vena cava collapse on sonography

A 500-mL fluid challenge may be attempted when right-sided pressures are normal or minimally elevated and may be repeated as tolerated.

KEY POINT

Avoid aggressive fluid resuscitation in patients with PE, as it can overdistend the ventricle and worsen RV failure.

Respiratory Support and Mechanical Ventilation

Supplemental oxygen is practical in all patients with massive PE. Oxygen debt and respiratory distress often necessitate more advanced ventilatory support. Physiologically, full ventilatory support in patients with massive PE would seem logical because

FIGURE 10-3.

Two-dimensional, parasternal long-axis view of the heart in a 45-year-old man with massive PE and hemodynamic instability. Note the shift in septal wall positioning (A) with aortic outflow tract obstruction by the posterior mitral valve leaflet (B) and the increased chamber size (distance lines: RV size [1]>LV size [2]).

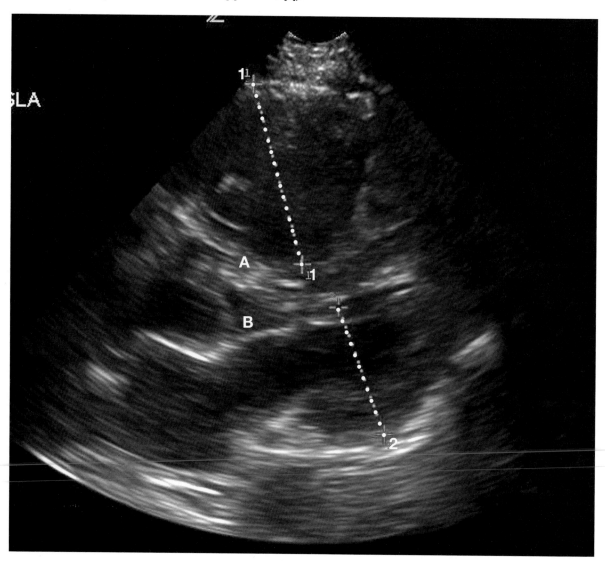

as much as 20% of cardiac output can be recruited by reducing the work of breathing.[20,61] However, negative interactions between the heart and lungs can destabilize an already unstable situation. Thus, emergency physicians must approach respiratory support of these patients with some degree of caution and preparation (Table 10-3).

Patients with massive PE frequently require intubation and mechanical ventilation because of progressive hypoxia; however, these procedures should be undertaken cautiously. Intubation can be complicated by cardiovascular collapse for several reasons. As in most shock states, sedatives can blunt catecholamine-driven peripheral vasoconstriction and central pulmonary vasodilation, resulting in further compromise of biventricular filling (preload). Lung overinflation can decrease venous return and increase pulmonary vascular resistance, which further worsens left heart filling. Thus, for patients with massive PE, emergency physicians should consider rapid-sequence intubation using sedative agents that preserve hemodynamic function (ie, etomidate and ketamine) and ventilator settings that limit overinflation.

PEARL

Prepare for worsened hypotension in association with intubation and ventilation. Have vasopressors immediately available or already infusing.

Although mechanical ventilation is often a necessary adjunct in the management of patients with massive PE, positive-pressure ventilation can lead to elevated airway pressures, increased transpulmonary pressures, decreased venous return, limited RV diastolic filling, and increased RV afterload, which impede RV systolic function.[62,63] Limiting tidal volumes (6–8 mL/kg) and positive-end expiratory pressure (PEEP) (5 cm H_2O) can decrease airway pressures and minimize RV dysfunction. This low-volume, low-pressure ventilation strategy can worsen hypercarbia and hypoxemia, which can exacerbate pulmonary

TABLE 10-3.

Key elements in respiratory management for patients with massive PE

Limit reflex responses to airway manipulation
   Plan for rapid sequence intubation
   Use hemodynamically neutral induction agents
      Etomidate: 0.15–0.3 mg/kg IV
      Ketamine: 1–2 mg/kg IV

Initial ventilator settings
   Mode: Assist control
   Tidal volume: 8 mL/kg of *ideal body weight*
   Respiratory rate: 14–18 bpm
   PEEP: 5 cm H_2O
   F_{IO_2}: 100%

Maintain pH >7.15

Maintain plateau pressures <30 cm H_2O

Maintain $PaCO_2$ between 35 and 45 mm Hg

vasoconstriction and hypertension if adequate ventilation and oxygenation are not maintained. Oxygenation can be improved by manipulating PEEP and expiratory times to optimize recruitment and limit gas trapping. The tidal volume and respiratory rate should be set to minimize hypercarbia. Each of these settings might require repeated fine-tuning to minimize the effect of ventilation on ventricular hemodynamics.[13,19,62]

PEARL

Avoid lung hyperinflation, because it can worsen hemodynamic compromise.

Vasopressors and Inotropes

Norepinephrine, epinephrine, phenylephrine, dopamine, and vasopressin may be used to offset the systemic hypotension that occurs with RV failure in patients with massive PE (Table 10-4). Although vasoconstriction seems counterintuitive in massive PE, it is important to realize that the right ventricle is perfused in both diastole and systole.[30,65] Therefore, in the setting of increased myocardial oxygen demand, maintaining a mean arterial pressure can increase RV myocardial perfusion. In massive PE, the ideal agent would increase systemic vasoconstriction without increasing pulmonary vascular resistance, but no such agent exists.

Data extrapolated from animal models suggest that norepinephrine is the vasopressor of choice for shock secondary to massive PE.[13,46,53,57,65,66] It appears to improve survival by maintaining mean arterial pressure and adequate coronary flow to the stressed right ventricle. It appears that norepinephrine improves function through alpha vasoconstriction, which improves arterial pressures. Additionally, norepinephrine's β_1-mediated inotropic properties enhance RV function.[46] Norepinephrine may be used as monotherapy, but it is more often mixed with inotropic medication to correct shock in patients with massive PE. Epinephrine has been advocated as a second-line agent in case-based literature for treatment of refractory shock complicating PE.[67] Vasopressin has also been used in low doses to treat inotrope-induced hypotension without detriment to cardiac output or pulmonary artery pressures.[68] Despite the promise of these small studies, there are no outcome data to support one agent over another for hypotension in the setting of RV failure in massive PE.

Vasoconstriction alone is often inadequate for hemodynamic support of patients with massive PE.[46] Although dopamine, dobutamine, milrinone, and amrinone have historically been used in patients with cardiogenic shock with LV dysfunction, limited studies have specifically evaluated their use in isolated RV failure.[69] Isoproterenol, amrinone, and milrinone have been investigated in animal models of acute PE with mixed results.[53,55,68,70-75] Of the available agents, dobutamine has the best available data and is considered the first-line inotropic agent for the treatment of PE-related cardiac failure. This drug is a β-adrenergic agonist with positive inotropic and pulmonary vasodilating properties that lead to increased RV contractility and decreased pulmonary vascular resistance. In patients with massive PE with hemodynamic compromise, a dobutamine infusion (5–10 mcg/kg/min) is associated with an increase in cardiac index and a reduction in right atrial pressure, pulmonary vascular resistance, and systemic vascular resistance.[46,76,77]

KEY POINT

Titrate vasopressors and inotropes to maintain a mean arterial pressure of 70 to 80 mm Hg.

Vasodilators

Vasodilators might be used to reduce pulmonary vasoconstriction and unload the right ventricle, but they have limited applicability in the emergency department. Systemic vasodilators such as nitroglycerin, sodium nitroprusside, sildenafil, glyceryl trinitrate, nesiritide, and hydralazine all reduce pulmonary vascular resistance, but they also cause systemic hypotension, which can decrease coronary perfusion and worsen RV dysfunction. Therefore, their use in the setting of acute RV failure is not advocated.[78]

Inhaled vasodilators such as prostaglandin I and E act on vascular endothelial smooth muscle via nitric oxide release, which leads to pulmonary vasodilation. Inhaled prostaglandins

are relatively inexpensive and can be nebulized, not requiring a special delivery system. Inhalation results in pulmonary vasodilation and limits the amount that is systemically delivered; however, particle size cannot be controlled easily, risking potential systemic spillover and hypotension.[79] Inhaled nitric oxide acts on the vascular smooth muscle via cyclic guanosine monophosphate, leading to pulmonary vasodilation. Nitric oxide requires a special delivery system, which limits its use in emergency medicine.

KEY POINTS

Data extrapolated from animal models suggest that norepinephrine is the vasopressor of choice for shock secondary to massive PE.

Norepinephrine improves survival by maintaining mean arterial pressure and adequate coronary flow to the stressed right ventricle.

In patients with massive PE and hemodynamic compromise, dobutamine infusion is associated with an increase in cardiac index and a reduction in right atrial pressure, pulmonary vascular resistance, and systemic vascular resistance.

Anticoagulation and Thrombolysis

Anticoagulation with heparin should be initiated immediately to halt further clot propagation. Low-molecular-weight heparins appear to be as effective as unfractionated heparin in

TABLE 10-4.

Vasopressors and inotropes used for hemodynamic support in massive PE

Vasopressors

Drug	Dosing Regimen
Norepinephrine (first-line agent)	Initial dose: 1 mcg/min
	Titrate by 1–2 mcg/min
	Maximum dose: 50 mcg/min
Epinephrine	Initial dose: 1 mcg/min
	Titrate by 1–2 mcg/min
	Maximum dose: 10 mcg/min
Phenylephrine	Initial dose: 5 mcg/kg/min
	Titrate by 1–2 mcg/kg/min
	Maximum dose: 20 mcg/kg/min
Vasopressin	Initial dose: 0.01 units/min
	Titrate by 0.01 units/min
	Maximum dose: 0.04 units/min

Inotropes

Drug	Dosing Regimen
Dobutamine (first-line agent)	Initial dose: 2.5 mcg/kg/min
	Titrate by 2.5 mcg/kg/min
	Maximum dose: 20 mcg/kg/min

TABLE 10-5.

Guidelines for antithrombotic therapy[82]

All PE patients should undergo rapid risk stratification (grade 1C).

For patients with hemodynamic compromise, we recommend use of thrombolytic therapy unless there are major contraindications owing to bleeding risk (grade 1B).
Thrombolysis in these patients should not be delayed because irreversible cardiogenic shock may ensue.

The decision to use thrombolytic therapy depends on the clinician's assessment of PE severity, prognosis, and risk of bleeding.

In patients with acute PE, when a thrombolytic agent is used, we recommend that treatment be administered via a peripheral vein rather than through a pulmonary artery catheter (grade 1B).

In selected highly compromised patients who are unable to receive thrombolytic therapy because of bleeding risk, or whose critical status does not allow sufficient time for systemic thrombolytic therapy to be effective, we suggest use of interventional catheterization techniques if appropriate expertise is available (grade 2C).

Grade 1 = strong recommendation; Grade 2 = weak recommendation; A = high-quality evidence; B = moderate-quality evidence; C = low-quality or very low-quality evidence.

the prevention of recurrence of submassive PE.[80] However, patients with massive PE should receive unfractionated heparin, which can be bolused, infused, titrated, and paused as other therapies are arranged.[80] Heparin should be administered as an 80-units/kg bolus, followed by an 18-units/kg/hr continuous infusion, and titrated to maintain an activated partial thromboplastin time (aPTT) two times the normal control value. Heparin should be discontinued as soon as the decision to administer thrombolytics is made, but it should be restarted after thrombolytic infusion. An aPTT should be obtained after thrombolytic infusion, and intravenous heparin should be restarted if the aPTT is less than 80 seconds.

The use of thrombolytics in hemodynamically stable patients with PE and RV dysfunction remains controversial, but the use of thrombolytics in the hemodynamically unstable patient is well guided (Table 10-5). The administration of thrombolytics to patients with life-threatening massive PE decreases the size of the obstructing clot burden and results in more rapid hemodynamic improvement. Anticoagulation with heparins only prevents clot extension; thrombolytics selectively dissolve and remove clot.

TABLE 10-6.

Contraindications to thrombolytic therapy in massive PE

Absolute contraindications

History of intracranial hemorrhage

Active internal bleeding

Relative contraindications

Known intracranial neoplasm, arteriovenous malformation, or aneurysm

Significant head trauma within the past 15 days

Intracranial or intraspinal surgery within the past 3 months

Cerebrovascular accident within the past 2 months

Recent surgery or organ biopsy

Recent trauma (within the past 15 days)

Venipuncture at a noncompressible site

Uncontrolled hypertension (SBP >180 mm Hg, DBP >110 mm Hg)

Recent gastrointestinal or internal bleeding (within the past 10 days)

Known bleeding diathesis

Significant hepatic or renal impairment

Pregnancy

There are few absolute contraindications to fibrinolysis in massive PE.

PEARL

Consider early thrombolytic therapy in the hemodynamically unstable patient with suspected massive PE.

A metaanalysis and recent Cochrane review strongly endorse the use of rapid fibrinolytic therapy versus the use of heparin alone as a means of reducing recurrence (OR, 0.63; 95% CI, 0.33–1.20) and death (OR, 0.89; 95% CI, 0.45–1.78).[16] Rapid fibrinolytic therapy is less invasive and is the primary method of treatment for hemodynamically unstable PE patients in the emergency department who lack contraindications to systemic therapy (Table 10-6).

Three thrombolytic agents have been approved by the US Food and Drug Administration for use in patients with acute PE: streptokinase, urokinase, and alteplase (Table 10-7). A 2005 metaanalysis designed to compare thrombolytic regimens failed to demonstrate any statistically significant differences in efficacy.[81] Despite the lack of data proving superiority, guidelines published by the American College of Chest Physicians (ACCP) suggest using the thrombolytic regimen with the shortest infusion time (alteplase).[82]

In patients with acute PE, thrombolytic therapy should be given via a peripheral intravenous line as standard practice.[17] The ACCP recommends that right-heart catheterization techniques be reserved for highly compromised patients who are unable to receive systemic thrombolytic therapy (a grade 2C recommendation) (Table 10-5).[82] If a central venous catheter is required for additional access or medications, it should be placed in a compressible site (internal jugular or femoral vein) using ultrasound guidance to minimize iatrogenic arterial puncture and bleeding risk.

KEY POINTS

Low-molecular-weight heparins are not recommended for the treatment of massive PE since they cannot be immediately discontinued or reversed if other interventions need to be initiated (ie, thrombolytics).

Heparin should be paused during the infusion of thrombolytics and resumed when the infusion is completed.

Alteplase is the recommended thrombolytic because it has the shortest infusion time (2 hours).

TABLE 10-7.

Thrombolytic regimens for acute PE

Drug	Dosing Regimen
Streptokinase	Initial dose: 250,000 units over 30 min, then
	Infusion: 100,000 units/hr over 24 hr
Urokinase	Initial dose: 4,400 units/kg over 10 min, then
	Infusion: 4,400 units/kg/hr over 12 hr
Alteplase	Initial dose: 10 mg bolus, then
	Infusion: 90 mg over 2 hr

Alternative Therapies

Interventional therapy is another option in the emergency management of PE. Potential candidates for interventional procedures include hemodynamically unstable patients with contraindications to systemic thrombolytics, PE-positive patients who fail fibrinolytic therapy, and patients who remain hemodynamically unstable despite resuscitation. The methods of interventional PE therapy include percutaneous embolectomy, catheter-directed thrombolysis, and percutaneous fragmentation techniques. Surgical embolectomy has the same indications as interventional therapy. The practical use of these therapies in the emergency department is limited by local hospital resources and expertise.

Conclusion

PE with acute RV dysfunction leading to hypotension requires rapid evaluation, diagnosis, and management. The clinician with an understanding of the pathophysiology of RV dysfunction in PE is better prepared to guide therapy based on clinical acumen. Beginning fluid resuscitation and escalating to inotropic and vasopressor support while initiating definitive therapy are the mainstays of resuscitation. Support for a specific volume strategy or choice of medication is lacking. Heparinization and thrombolytic therapy are essential in the successful treatment of patients with massive PE. Emergency physicians armed with a standardized approach to the treatment of massive PE can help limit the morbidity and mortality associated with this devastating condition.

References

1. Goldhaber SZ, Elliott CG. Acute pulmonary embolism: part I: epidemiology, pathophysiology, and diagnosis. *Circulation*. 2003;108:2726-2729.
2. Goldhaber SZ, Visani L, De Rosa M. Acute pulmonary embolism: clinical outcomes in the International Cooperative Pulmonary Embolism Registry (ICOPER). *Lancet*. 1999;353:1386-1389.
3. Kasper W, Konstantinides S, Geibel A, et al. Management strategies and determinants of outcome in acute major pulmonary embolism: results of a multicenter registry. *J Am Coll Cardiol*. 1997;30:1165-1171.
4. Anderson FA Jr, Wheeler HB, Goldberg RJ, et al. A population-based perspective of the hospital incidence and case-fatality rates of deep vein thrombosis and pulmonary embolism. The Worcester DVT Study. *Arch Intern Med*. 1991;151:933-938.
5. Silverstein MD, Heit JA, Mohr DN, Petterson TM, O'Fallon WM, Melton LJ 3rd. Trends in the incidence of deep vein thrombosis and pulmonary embolism: a 25-year population-based study. *Arch Intern Med*. 1998;158:585-593.
6. Lualdi JC, Goldhaber SZ. Right ventricular dysfunction after acute pulmonary embolism: pathophysiologic factors, detection, and therapeutic implications. *Am Heart J*. 1995;130:1276-1282.
7. Kucher N, Goldhaber SZ. Management of massive pulmonary embolism. *Circulation*. 2005;112:e28-e32.
8. Fengler BT, Brady WJ. Fibrinolytic therapy in pulmonary embolism: an evidence-based treatment algorithm. *Am J Emerg Med*. 2009;27:84-95.
9. Goldhaber SZ. Advanced treatment strategies for acute pulmonary embolism, including thrombolysis and embolectomy. *J Thromb Haemost*. 2009;7:322-327.
10. Goldhaber SZ, Haire WD, Feldstein ML, et al. Alteplase versus heparin in acute pulmonary embolism: randomised trial assessing right-ventricular function and pulmonary perfusion. *Lancet*. 1993;341:507-511.
11. Kline JA, Zeitouni R, Marchick MR, Hernandez-Nino J, Rose GA. Comparison of 8 biomarkers for prediction of right ventricular hypokinesis 6 months after submassive pulmonary embolism. *Am Heart J*. 2008;156:308-314.
12. Come PC, Kim D, Parker JA, et al. Early reversal of right ventricular dysfunction in patients with acute pulmonary embolism after treatment with intravenous tissue plasminogen activator. *J Am Coll Cardiol*. 1987;10:971-978.
13. Torbicki A, Perrier A, Konstantinides S, et al. Guidelines on the diagnosis and management of acute pulmonary embolism. *Eur Heart J*. 2008;29:2276-2315.
14. Kline JA, Steuerwald MT, Marchick MR, et al. Prospective evaluation of right ventricular function and functional status 6 months after acute submassive pulmonary embolism: frequency of persistent or subsequent elevation in estimated pulmonary artery pressure. *Chest*. 2009;136:1202-1210.
15. Nass N, McConnell MV, Goldhaber SZ, et al. Recovery of regional right ventricular function after thrombolysis for pulmonary embolism. *Am J Cardiol*. 1999;83:804-806, A10.
16. Wan S, Quinlan DJ, Agnelli G, Eikelboom JW. Thrombolysis compared with heparin for the initial treatment of pulmonary embolism: a meta-analysis of the randomized controlled trials. *Circulation*. 2004;110:744-749.
17. Tapson VF. Acute pulmonary embolism. *N Engl J Med*. 2008;358:1037-1052.
18. Stein M, Levy SE. Reflex and humoral responses to pulmonary embolism. *Prog Cardiovasc Dis*. 1974;17:167-174.
19. Smulders YM. Pathophysiology and treatment of haemodynamic instability in acute pulmonary embolism: the pivotal role of pulmonary vasoconstriction. *Cardiovasc Res*. 2000;48:23-33.
20. Elliott CG. Pulmonary physiology during pulmonary embolism. *Chest*. 1992;101:163S-171S.
21. Wilson JE 3rd, Pierce AK, Johnson RL Jr, et al. Hypoxemia in pulmonary embolism, a clinical study. *J Clin Invest*. 1971;50:481-491.
22. Tapson VF. Acute pulmonary embolism. *Cardiol Clin*. 2004;22:353-365.
23. Piazza G, Goldhaber SZ. The acutely decompensated right ventricle: pathways for diagnosis and management. *Chest*. 2005;128:1836-1852.
24. Brieke A, DeNofrio D. Right ventricular dysfunction in chronic dilated cardiomyopathy and heart failure. *Coron Artery Dis*. 2005;16:5-11.
25. Cecconi M, Johnston E, Rhodes A. What role does the right side of the heart play in circulation? *Crit Care*. 2006;10(suppl 3):S5.
26. Goldstein JA. Pathophysiology and management of right heart ischemia. *J Am Coll Cardiol*. 2002;40:841-853.
27. Vieillard-Baron A, Page B, Augarde R, et al. Acute cor pulmonale in massive pulmonary embolism: incidence, echocardiographic pattern, clinical implications and recovery rate. *Intensive Care Med*. 2001;27:1481-1486.
28. Louie EK, Lin SS, Reynertson SI, et al. Pressure and volume loading of the right ventricle have opposite effects on left ventricular ejection fraction. *Circulation*. 1995;92:819-824.
29. Budev MM, Arroliga AC, Wiedemann HP, Matthay RA. Cor pulmonale: an overview. *Semin Respir Crit Care Med*. 2003;24:233-244.
30. Mebazaa A, Karpati P, Renaud E, Algotsson L. Acute right ventricular failure—from pathophysiology to new treatments. *Intensive Care Med*. 2004;30:185-196.
31. Kucher N, Rossi E, De Rosa M, Goldhaber SZ. Massive pulmonary embolism. *Circulation*. 2006;113:577-582.
32. Daniel KR, Courtney DM, Kline JA. Assessment of cardiac stress from massive pulmonary embolism with 12-lead ECG. *Chest*. 2001;120:474-481.
33. Rogers RL, Winters M, Mayo P. Pulmonary embolism: remember that patient you saw last night? *Emerg Med Pract*. 2004;6:1-18.
34. Klok FA, Mos IC, Huisman MV. Brain-type natriuretic peptide levels in the prediction of adverse outcome in patients with pulmonary embolism: a systematic review and meta-analysis. *Am J Respir Crit Care Med*. 2008;178:425-430.
35. Sanchez O, Trinquart L, Colombet I, et al. Prognostic value of right ventricular dysfunction in patients with haemodynamically stable pulmonary embolism: a systematic review. *Eur Heart J*. 2008;29:1569-1577.
36. Tapson VF. Diagnosing and managing acute pulmonary embolism: role of cardiac troponins. *Am Heart J*. 2003;145:751-753.
37. Scridon T, Scridon C, Skali H, et al. Prognostic significance of troponin elevation and right ventricular enlargement in acute pulmonary embolism. *Am J Cardiol*. 2005;96:303-305.
38. Becattini C, Vedovati MC, Agnelli G. Prognostic value of troponins in acute pulmonary embolism: a meta-analysis. *Circulation*. 2007;116:427-433.
39. Elliott CG, Goldhaber SZ, Visani L, DeRosa M. Chest radiographs in acute pulmonary embolism: results from the International Cooperative Pulmonary Embolism Registry. *Chest*. 2000;118:33-38.
40. Roy PM, Colombet I, Durieux P, Chatellier G, Sors H, Meyer G. Systematic review and meta-analysis of strategies for the diagnosis of suspected pulmonary embolism. *BMJ*. 2005;331:259.
41. Jones AE, Tayal VS, Sullivan DM, Kline JA. Randomized, controlled trial of immediate versus delayed goal-directed ultrasound to identify the cause of nontraumatic hypotension in emergency department patients. *Crit Care Med*. 2004;32:1703-1708.
42. Jardin F, Dubourg O, Bourdarias JP. Echocardiographic pattern of acute cor pulmonale. *Chest*. 1997;111:209-217.
43. Konstantinides S. Acute pulmonary embolism. *N Engl J Med*. 2008;359:2804-2813.
44. Otero R, Trujillo-Santos J, Cayuela A, et al. Haemodynamically unstable pulmonary embolism in the RIETE Registry: systolic blood pressure or shock index? *Eur Respir J*. 2007;30:1111-1116.
45. Sanchez O, Planquette B, Meyer G. Update on acute pulmonary embolism. *Eur Respir Rev*. 2009;18:137-147.
46. Layish DT, Tapson VF. Pharmacologic hemodynamic support in massive pulmonary embolism. *Chest*. 1997;111:218-224.
47. Mercat A, Diehl JL, Meyer G, Teboul JL, Sors H. Hemodynamic effects of fluid loading in acute massive pulmonary embolism. *Crit Care Med*. 1999;27:540-544.
48. Pastores SM. Management of venous thromboembolism in the intensive care unit. *J Crit Care*. 2009;24:185-191.

49. Ghignone M, Girling L, Prewitt RM. Volume expansion versus norepinephrine in treatment of a low cardiac output complicating an acute increase in right ventricular afterload in dogs. *Anesthesiology.* 1984;60:132-135.

50. Hauser CJ, Shoemaker WC. Volume loading in massive acute pulmonary embolus. *Crit Care Med.* 1979;7:304-306.

51. Belenkie I, Dani R, Smith ER, Tyberg JV. Effects of volume loading during experimental acute pulmonary embolism. *Circulation.* 1989;80:178-188.

52. Belenkie I, Dani R, Smith ER, Tyberg JV. The importance of pericardial constraint in experimental pulmonary embolism and volume loading. *Am Heart J.* 1992;123:733-742.

53. Molloy WD, Lee KY, Girling L, et al. Treatment of shock in a canine model of pulmonary embolism. *Am Rev Respir Dis.* 1984;130:870-874.

54. Mathru M, Venus B, Smith RA, et al. Treatment of low cardiac output complicating acute pulmonary hypertension in normovolemic goats. *Crit Care Med.* 1986;14:120-124.

55. Tanaka H, Tajimi K, Matsumoto A, Kobayashi K. Vasodilatory effects of milrinone on pulmonary vasculature in dogs with pulmonary hypertension due to pulmonary embolism: a comparison with those of dopamine and dobutamine. *Clin Exp Pharmacol Physiol.* 1990;17:681-690.

56. Wood KE. Major pulmonary embolism. *Chest.* 2002;121:877-905.

57. deBoisblanc BP. Treatment of massive pulmonary embolism. *Clin Pulm Med.* 1995;2:353-358.

58. Michard F, Reuter DA. Assessing cardiac preload or fluid responsiveness? It depends on the question we want to answer. *Intensive Care Med.* 2003;29:1396.

59. Bendjelid K, Romand JA. Fluid responsiveness in mechanically ventilated patients: a review of indices used in intensive care. *Intensive Care Med.* 2003;29:352-360.

60. Michard F, Teboul JL. Predicting fluid responsiveness in ICU patients: a critical analysis of the evidence. *Chest.* 2002;121:2000-2008.

61. Viires N, Sillye G, Aubier M, Rassidakis A, Roussos C. Regional blood flow distribution in dog during induced hypotension and low cardiac output. Spontaneous breathing versus artificial ventilation. *J Clin Invest.* 1983;72:935-947.

62. Jardin F, Vieillard-Baron A. Right ventricular function and positive pressure ventilation in clinical practice: from hemodynamic subsets to respirator settings. *Intensive Care Med.* 2003;29:1426-1434.

63. Haddad F, Couture P, Tousignant C, Denault AY. The right ventricle in cardiac surgery, a perioperative perspective: I. Anatomy, physiology, and assessment. *Anesth Analg.* 2009;108:407-421.

64. Lee FA. Hemodynamics of the right ventricle in normal and disease states. *Cardiol Clin.* 1992;10:59-67.

65. Angle MR, Molloy DW, Penner B, et al. The cardiopulmonary and renal hemodynamic effects of norepinephrine in canine pulmonary embolism. *Chest.* 1989;95:1333-1337.

66. Hirsch LJ, Rooney MW, Wat SS, et al. Norepinephrine and phenylephrine effects on right ventricular function in experimental canine pulmonary embolism. *Chest.* 1991;100:796-801.

67. Boulain T, Lanotte R, Legras A, Perrotin D. Efficacy of epinephrine therapy in shock complicating pulmonary embolism. *Chest.* 1993;104:300-302.

68. Gold J, Cullinane S, Chen J, et al. Vasopressin in the treatment of milrinone-induced hypotension in severe heart failure. *Am J Cardiol.* 2000;85:506-508.

69. Ellender TJ, Skinner JC. The use of vasopressors and inotropes in the emergency medical treatment of shock. *Emerg Med Clin North Am.* 2008;26:759-786.

70. Halmagyi DF, Colebatch HJ, Starzecki B, et al. Effect of isoproterenol in "severe" experimental lung embolism with and without postembolic collapse. *Am Heart J.* 1963;65:208-219.

71. Molloy DW, Lee KY, Jones D, et al. Effects of noradrenaline and isoproterenol on cardiopulmonary function in a canine model of acute pulmonary hypertension. *Chest.* 1985;88:432-435.

72. Wolfe MW, Saad RM, Spence TH. Hemodynamic effects of amrinone in a canine model of massive pulmonary embolism. *Chest.* 1992;102:274-278.

73. Rosenberg JC, Hussain R, Lenaghan R. Isoproterenol and norepinephrine therapy for pulmonary embolism shock. *J Thorac Cardiovasc Surg.* 1971;62:144-150.

74. Spence TH, Newton WD. Pulmonary embolism: improvement in hemodynamic function with amrinone therapy. *South Med J.* 1989;82:1267-1268.

75. Ducas J, Duval D, Dasilva H, et al. Treatment of canine pulmonary hypertension: effects of norepinephrine and isoproterenol on pulmonary vascular pressure-flow characteristics. *Circulation.* 1987;75:235-242.

76. Jardin F, Genevray B, Brun-Ney D, Margairaz A. Dobutamine: a hemodynamic evaluation in pulmonary embolism shock. *Crit Care Med.* 1985;13:1009-1012.

77. Prewitt RM. Hemodynamic management in pulmonary embolism and acute hypoxemic respiratory failure. *Crit Care Med.* 1990;18:S61-S69.

78. Woods J, Monteiro P, Rhodes A. Right ventricular dysfunction. *Curr Opin Crit Care.* 2007;13:532-540.

79. Fattouch K, Sbraga F, Bianco G, et al. Inhaled prostacyclin, nitric oxide, and nitroprusside in pulmonary hypertension after mitral valve replacement. *J Card Surg.* 2005;20:171-176.

80. Quinlan DJ, McQuillan A, Eikelboom JW. Low-molecular-weight heparin compared with intravenous unfractionated heparin for treatment of pulmonary embolism: a meta-analysis of randomized, controlled trials. *Ann Intern Med.* 2004;140:175-183.

81. Capstick T, Henry MT. Efficacy of thrombolytic agents in the treatment of pulmonary embolism. *Eur Respir J.* 2005;26:864-874.

82. Kearon C, Kahn SR, Agnelli G, et al. Antithrombotic therapy for venous thromboembolic disease: American College of Chest Physicians Evidence-Based Clinical Practice Guidelines (8th edition). *Chest.* 2008;133:454S-545S.

CHAPTER 11

The Unstable Patient with Gastrointestinal Hemorrhage

Eduardo Borquez and Stuart P. Swadron

IN THIS CHAPTER

General approach to the unstable patient with gastrointestinal hemorrhage

Intubation, mechanical ventilation, and circulatory resuscitation of the unstable patient

Indications for endoscopy, angiography, and surgical intervention

Balloon tamponade

Introduction

An unstable patient with gastrointestinal (GI) hemorrhage is rarely simple to manage (Figure 11-1). Multiple factors complicate the resuscitation, including occult, often sporadic, blood loss that is difficult to predict, localize, and control. Additionally, many patients have underlying comorbidities that can mask changes in vital signs, thereby masking true hemodynamic instability and delaying resuscitation. Several consultants may be necessary in the management of a patient. The emergency physician is a critical link in the chain of survival for unstable patients with GI bleeding. The physician must diagnose and resuscitate the patient in parallel with mobilizing subspecialists and arranging definitive care, often with incomplete information.

Approach to the Patient

Definitions of severe GI bleeding vary. Objective criteria include a marked decrease in hematocrit, vital sign changes consistent with hemorrhagic shock, and copious amounts of hematemesis and hematochezia. These objective measures can be foreshadowed by a toxic appearance and changes in mental status. Although GI bleeding is usually clinically obvious, occasionally, epistaxis and hemoptysis, which both can result in bloody discharge from the nose and mouth, mimic GI bleeding.

The most common sources of GI bleeding are summarized in Table 11-1. GI hemorrhage is typically divided anatomically into upper GI bleeding, originating proximal to the ligament of Treitz in the distal duodenum, and lower GI bleeding, distal to the ligament of Treitz. It is important to differentiate upper from lower GI bleeding as early as possible.[1] Although patients with massive hematemesis clearly have an upper GI source, patients who present with only rectal bleeding could have either an upper or lower source. When upper GI bleeding is particularly brisk, the cathartic effect of its expulsion decreases transport time, resulting in the production of blood that is bright red, not melenic.

Thus, when assessing a patient who is hemodynamically unstable, it is safest to first consider an upper GI source of bleeding. An upper source is responsible for 76% to 90% of all GI bleeds,[2,3] and patients with upper GI bleeding have a poorer prognosis and a higher mortality rate than those with lower GI bleeding. Three of four patients who die from GI bleeding have an upper source.[4,5] Peptic ulcers (duodenal and gastric) represent the source of more than half of upper GI bleeds,[2] and 60% of patients who die from GI bleeding do so from varices or peptic ulcers.[4] In contrast, the overall mortality rate for lower GI bleeding is comparatively low, at 4%.[6] Treatment options for upper GI bleeding are more readily available and feasible in the

FIGURE 11-1.

Approach to the unstable patient with suspected GI bleeding

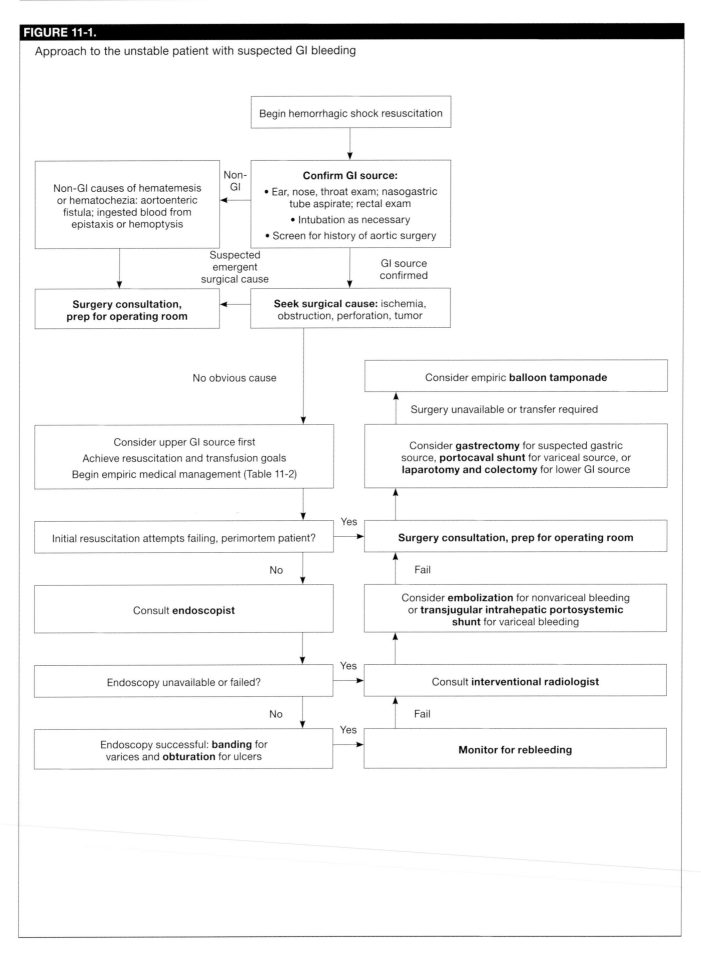

emergency department. Empiric therapeutic interventions immediately available to emergency physicians are geared toward upper GI bleeding in general and gastroesophageal varices in particular. Moreover, endoscopy of the upper tract, unlike that of the lower tract, is possible without any special bowel preparation and can be performed by a qualified operator, if necessary, in the emergency department.

PEARLS
General approach and resuscitation

- Even in cases of seemingly "clear-cut" lower GI bleeding with frank hematochezia, more than 10% of patients have an upper source of the bleeding.[7]

- In patients suspected of end-stage liver disease, empiric and aggressive use of plasma is indicated simultaneously with packed red blood cells (RBCs). Vitamin K supplementation is also indicated.

- A negative nasogastric tube aspirate does not exclude an upper GI source.

- Even in patients with a history and obvious physical signs of cirrhosis with portal hypertension, ulcerative bleeding is extremely common.

KEY POINTS
General approach

- The emergency physician must diagnose and treat GI hemorrhage in parallel with mobilizing subspecialists, often with incomplete data.

- Upper sources are the most common and deadly causes of GI bleeding. They are also the most amenable to empiric treatment by emergency physicians prior to definitive diagnostic testing.

TABLE 11-1.

Most common causes of GI hemorrhage[2]

Upper	
Duodenal ulcer	28%
Gastric ulcer	25.7%
Gastritis erosions	12.9%
Esophageal and gastric varices	11.8%
Esophagitis	7.7%
Lower	
Diverticula	29.7%
Arteriovenous malformations	10.3%
Polyps	9%
Cancer	7.6%
Ulcerative colitis	7.6%

Resuscitation
Airway and Breathing

Early endotracheal intubation in the unstable patient with GI bleeding has several advantages and allows the physician to take control of one of the most critical variables in the resuscitation. Intubation serves a diagnostic purpose when the source of the bleeding is still in question. In some cases, it can be difficult to differentiate among massive hematemesis, hemoptysis, epistaxis, and oropharyngeal sources of bleeding. Although endotracheal intubation will be complicated by the presence of blood, it will immediately differentiate between pulmonary and GI sources as well as facilitate examination of the oropharynx and nasopharynx. Moreover, it can prevent massive aspiration in a patient with altered mental status, and it provides better control of the airway and therefore breathing during endoscopy than procedural sedation alone. A sudden burst of hematemesis in the sedated patient who is not intubated can have catastrophic consequences. Despite these theoretical advantages, studies have not demonstrated improved patient outcomes with early intubation.[8] Such studies have been retrospective and may not inform practice in the most critically ill subset of patients. Thus, in hemodynamically unstable patients with GI bleeding, we nevertheless recommend intubation before endoscopic or other invasive procedures.

The preoxygenation step in rapid sequence intubation (RSI) should be emphasized. In patients with upper GI bleeding, oxygen desaturation during intubation attempts that necessitate bag-valve-mask ventilation leads to abdominal distention and increases the risk of aspiration. With respect to the sedative used for RSI, hemodynamically neutral agents such as etomidate are preferred. Similarly, agents with neutral or positive hemodynamic profiles such as ketamine are a good option for postintubation sedation until blood pressures stabilize.

KEY POINTS
RSI in the unstable patient with GI bleeding

- Intubation before endoscopic procedures is recommended for unstable GI bleeding patients.

- In the conscious patient, eight vital capacity breaths using a well-fitted nonrebreathing mask will maximize the time to desaturation. If the patient is unable to cooperate, at least 3 minutes of normal breathing on a nonrebreathing mask will serve a similar purpose.

- Use etomidate or ketamine for induction of patients in hemorrhagic shock.

- Be prepared to suction copious hematemesis that could obscure direct laryngoscopy.

- Use short-acting and hemodynamically neutral sedatives while these patients are on mechanical ventilation.

Circulation

Several features of the patient with GI bleeding that can impede the initial recognition of a shock state should be highlighted. Like all patients with hemorrhagic shock, patients with GI bleeding may fail to mount a tachycardia. In fact, patients with GI bleeding can present with paradoxic bradycardia.[8,9] Patients with known varices are often receiving primary or secondary prophylaxis with β-blocker therapy or nitrates,[10] which will invariably blunt a normal tachycardic response to acute shock and lower baseline blood pressures. Patients with cirrhosis and portal hypertension often have low baseline blood pressures[11,12] in the absence of treatment. This can delay the diagnosis of shock if the low blood pressures are not recognized as pathologic.

At least two large-bore intravenous catheters are necessary to provide large-volume resuscitation. Although resuscitation may begin with crystalloids, blood must be transfused as quickly as possible. Type O blood may be used initially until type-specific and then fully cross-matched blood is available. In patients in whom end-stage liver disease is suspected, empiric and aggressive use of plasma is indicated simultaneously with packed RBCs. Although colloid solutions have been advocated by some to restore circulating volume in patients with end-stage liver disease, the volume of plasma required to restore function to the deficient coagulation cascade is substantial (20–30 mL/kg). Very little evidence supports the use of colloids over crystalloids.[13] Platelets should be administered to patients with severe thrombocytopenia. Desmopressin should be used in patients with end-stage renal disease, and it may be of value in patients receiving therapy with antiplatelet agents.

PEARL
Desmopressin should be used in patients with end-stage renal disease, and it may be of value in patients receiving therapy with antiplatelet agents.

There is currently no consensus and there are few data to recommend any particular blood pressure targets in the setting of hemorrhagic shock resulting from GI bleeding. Although some authors have suggested that overzealous resuscitation can worsen GI bleeding, the data to support this opinion are retrospective.[14] A reasonable goal for resuscitation is evidence of adequate perfusion of vital organs (eg, mental status and urine output) rather than a particular blood pressure.

KEY POINTS
Resuscitation goals

- Circulatory resuscitation in patients with severe GI bleeding focuses on achieving hemodynamic stability, tissue perfusion, and the correction of anemia and coagulopathy.[15]

- Keep hemoglobin above 10 g/dL in critically ill patients, older patients (age >55 years), and those with multiple comorbidities or cardiac disease.[15-17]

- Keep the platelet count above 50,000/mm³.[18]

- Keep the INR below 1.8.[15]

Emergency physicians should watch for any evidence of end organ dysfunction, which can develop as a consequence of hemorrhagic shock and complicate management. An electrocardiogram can reveal cardiac ischemia; decreasing urine output and elevated blood urea nitrogen and creatinine could indicate

renal failure; and decreasing oxygen saturation can represent acute respiratory distress syndrome, which often results from aspiration. Although control of GI bleeding ultimately lies at the heart of managing all of these complications, awareness of them could influence other treatment decisions and possibly the choice of venue for ongoing resuscitative efforts (eg, operating room, intensive care unit, interventional radiology suite).

The utility of routine nasogastric tube (NGT) aspiration in patients with GI bleeding has come into question. Although traditionally used as a diagnostic tool to distinguish upper from lower GI bleeding in patients without hematemesis, it has poor sensitivity for the detection of upper GI bleeding in this subset of patients.[19] In the sickest patients, however, the pretest probability of having an active upper GI bleeding source is much higher. One major disadvantage of NGT aspiration, patient discomfort, is of less concern in intubated and sedated patients. In patients at risk for concomitant hepatic encephalopathy or hepatorenal syndrome, aspirating blood decreases the absorbed protein load that exacerbates these conditions. Finally, NGT aspirate in patients with severe ongoing losses can essentially serve as an additional very sensitive vital sign, foreshadowing changes in blood pressure, pulse, and hemoglobin measurements. Thus, in an unstable patient with GI bleeding, ongoing losses of large quantities of blood via NGT suction can be one important predictor of impending circulatory collapse.

TABLE 11-2.
Medical treatment strategies for GI bleeding

Drug	Dose	Note
Octreotide	50-mcg bolus followed by 50-mcg/hr infusion	Of benefit in **both variceal and nonvariceal** upper GI bleeding Consider empiric administration until a diagnosis is made, given its low side-effect profile.
Pantoprazole	80-mg bolus followed by 8-mg/hr infusion	Of benefit in **peptic ulcer disease** Consider empiric administration until a diagnosis is made, given its low side-effect profile.
Omeprazole	80-mg bolus followed by 8-mg/hr infusion	
Vasopressin	20 units IV over 20 min, then 0.2–0.4 units/min infusion	Of benefit in **variceal bleeding** Given its high side-effect profile, consider giving empirically if other options have been exhausted.
Antibiotics	Ceftriaxone, 1 g/day	Mortality benefit in patients with **cirrhosis and GI bleeding**[34]

Treatment Strategies

Medical Treatment

The administration of proton pump inhibitors (PPIs) to patients with gastric and peptic ulcer disease is recommended.[20,21] There is no evidence that PPIs acutely stop hemorrhage, but they may have a role in decreasing the incidence of rebleeding, transfusion requirements, the need for surgery, and hospital length of stay.[22,23] Because of their low side-effect profile and the fact that it is difficult to distinguish between ulcerative and variceal disease prior to endoscopy, some authors advocate empiric administration of PPIs to patients with undifferentiated upper GI bleeding while awaiting definitive diagnosis.[24]

Somatostatin and its synthetic analogue octreotide decrease splanchnic blood flow and have been used to arrest variceal[25–27] and nonvariceal[28–30] bleeding (Table 11-2), although evidence of their efficacy in the latter group is weak. The argument for early liberal use of octreotide is similar to that for PPIs: it rests on its low side-effect profile, the high prevalence of variceal hemorrhage in critically ill patients with upper GI bleeding, and the imperfect ability of noninvasive techniques (eg, physical examination, laboratory tests, and ultrasonography) to predict the presence of esophageal varices[31–33] (with sensitivity ranging from 75% to 93% and specificity from 37% to 76%).

Vasopressin and its analogue terlipressin are vasoconstrictors that can be used systemically (intravenously) or selectively (intraarterially) through angiography. When used intravenously, serious side effects such as arrhythmias and systemic vasoconstriction causing cerebral, cardiac, intestinal, and extremity ischemia necessitate discontinuation of these agents in 10% of cases.[28] Therefore, vasopressin is typically used only when other medical treatments are exhausted and there is a high suspicion of variceal bleeding (Table 11-2).

Antibiotics are routinely administered to patients with suspected variceal bleeding, given the high incidence of comorbid infections such as spontaneous bacterial peritonitis and as prophylaxis for invasive endoscopic procedures.[34]

Endoscopic Treatment

Endoscopy is a first-line intervention for the definitive diagnosis and treatment of both variceal and nonvariceal upper GI bleeding (Table 11-3).[20,35,36] It should be performed emergently in those with life-threatening GI bleeding, even if the bleeding has been controlled temporarily by medical therapy, to establish the diagnosis and prevent rebleeding. The preferred treatment for esophageal variceal bleeding is banding, whereas the use of tissue adhesives (obturation) is favored for gastric varices.[37] Treatment options for nonvariceal bleeding include cautery, injection, and coagulation. If upper GI tract endoscopy fails to identify a source of bleeding, lower GI bleeding sources should be sought. Although colonoscopy may be considered a first-line strategy for definitive diagnosis and treatment of lower GI bleeding, without bowel preparation it is technically difficult.[38]

Angiographic and Interventional Radiologic Treatment

Angiography should be used when endoscopy is unavailable, unsuccessful, or contraindicated (Table 11-4). Like endoscopy, angiography offers both diagnostic and therapeutic capability. It is also considered first-line treatment in patients with suspected biliary or pancreatic bleeding.[36]

Sclerotherapy via angiography involves selective infusion of either intraarterial vasopressin or embolizing agents. Lesions particularly amenable to this treatment include gastric ulcers and Mallory-Weiss tears. In patients with variceal hemorrhage in whom endoscopic banding has failed, a transjugular intrahepatic portosystemic shunt (TIPS) can be created by passing a catheter through the internal jugular vein to the hepatic vein, and then creating a shunt from the hepatic vein to the portal vein (through the liver parenchyma), thereby lowering

---

TABLE 11-3.

Indications for emergent endoscopy[3,21]

Massive bleeding

Active bleeding with unstable vital signs

TABLE 11-4.

Indications for angiography for nonvariceal upper GI bleeding[36]

Failure of endoscopy

Poor surgical candidates

Transcatheter arteriography and intervention are best for treating hemorrhage in the biliary or pancreatic vessels.

TABLE 11-5.

Indications for surgical consultation[1,21,46]

Surgical abdomen: suspected perforation, obstruction, malignancy, peritonitis, mesenteric ischemia, recent surgery

Massive bleeding (half the patient's volume in 24 hr) or bleeding that is recurrent or requires massive transfusion

Failure or high risk of failure of medical, endoscopic, or angiographic therapy

---

TABLE 11-6.

Indications for surgical treatment of peptic ulcer disease[1,45]

Failure of resuscitative measures and persistent severe hemorrhage

Failure or unavailability of endoscopic and angiographic techniques

Concurrent or causative surgical emergency such as bowel ischemia, perforation, obstruction, or malignancy

portal pressure. In cases of lower GI bleeding, angiography is typically considered second-line therapy, but it is an important alternative when colonoscopy is unavailable or fails. Computed tomography (CT) angiography is emerging as a potential modality in severe GI bleeding. Given its availability and ability to diagnose other surgical pathology, it may have a role, particularly when upper GI bleeding has been ruled out and another source is being sought.[39–42]

Surgery

In the past, surgery had a major role in the management of GI bleeding. Advances in endoscopic and angiographic techniques have reduced this role, but surgery continues to have a place in the definitive management of approximately 10% of patients with GI bleeding.[2,43] Modern surgeons are reluctant to operate without definitive diagnosis and localization of the bleeding. Because endoscopic and angiographic techniques are often diagnostic and therapeutic, success with these techniques usually obviates the need for surgery. In many cases of lower GI bleeding, surgery can still be necessary as definitive therapy, after bleeding is stopped with less invasive techniques (Table 11-5).[1,21,44]

The indications for surgical intervention in peptic ulcer hemorrhage are summarized in Table 11-6. They range from excision of the gastric ulcer or ligation of the duodenal ulcer to partial or total gastrectomy.[1] Emergent surgical intervention for variceal hemorrhage is rare and occurs only after failure of nonoperative techniques, including ligation and TIPS. Surgical procedures for varices are typically divided into operative creation of portocaval shunts and devascularization of the distal esophagus.[1] Additional surgical procedures can be performed for less common causes of upper GI bleeding such as angiodysplasia, Dieulafoy lesion, pancreatic pseudoaneurysm, malignancy, and aortoenteric fistula. The underlying theme for all surgical interventions is that they are typically done only after endoscopy or angiography has localized the lesion, after other treatment options have failed, or as a desperation maneuver in patients who are persistently unstable despite resuscitative efforts. The exception to this rule is aortoenteric fistula, which should be suspected in anyone with a history of aortic surgery or an aortic graft and acute GI bleeding. In such cases, immediate vascular surgery consultation is warranted for consideration of emergent exploratory laparotomy. In cases of lower GI bleeding, surgery is typically reserved for patients in whom a surgical lesion has been diagnosed by colonoscopy, CT, or angiography.

However, exploratory laparotomy can be warranted in a subset of unstable patients.[1]

Balloon Tamponade

Balloon tamponade tubes function by compressing bleeding varices in the stomach and esophagus through inflation of a gastric or esophageal balloon. Hemostatic pressure is applied to the fundus of the stomach (and, by extension, to the left gastric vein, which feeds the esophageal venous plexus) by way of traction with a weight mechanism applied to the balloon. These devices have a variable number of ports that continue to aspirate, irrigate, and quantify bleeding in the esophagus and stomach. Commercially available devices include the Linton-Nachlas, Sengstaken-Blakemore, and Minnesota tubes (Table 11-7). A radiograph of a Linton-Nachlas tube *in situ* is presented as Figure 11-2. Although, theoretically, these adjuncts are to be used only in the setting of known variceal disease, in practice, patients may present with no prior diagnosis of variceal disease, so balloon tamponade may be attempted empirically as a bridge to endoscopy, angiography, surgery, or patient transfer (Table 11-8).

Balloon tamponade has a reported success rate of 60% to 90%[46] and a 50% rate of rebleeding when used alone.[44] Complications are common (14% major, 3%–6% fatal[44,47]), many arising from displacement of the tube, which causes respiratory obstruction or esophageal, tracheal, or duodenal rupture.

The procedure is more appropriately described in detail in a procedural textbook but is outlined here. First, proper position of the gastric balloon must be confirmed, preferably with a radiograph, to avoid inflation in the esophagus, which can cause a catastrophic rupture. Second, depending on the kit, inflation requires 400 to 700 mL of air or contrast-water medium in the gastric balloon; the ports do not come equipped with a one-way valve. Some tubes have an additional esophageal balloon that can be inflated if the gastric balloon fails to stop the bleeding. Therefore, a tube clamp or other securing mechanism must be used to prevent deflation, as the filling syringe will have to be removed several times. Third, traction should be applied with a 1-liter saline bag and may need to be adjusted, based on the clinical results. Last, tube placement should be confirmed initially if possible and intermittently thereafter with radiographs to ensure that migration has not occurred.

TABLE 11-7.

Comparison of common balloon tamponade tubes

Tube	Linton-Nachlas	Sengstaken-Blakemore	Minnesota
Lumens	3	3	4
Balloons	1: gastric only	2: esophageal and gastric	2: esophageal and gastric
Ports for suction and lavage	2: esophageal and gastric	1: gastric only	2: esophageal and gastric

PEARLS
Balloon tamponade

Ideally, balloon tamponade is used only when varices are known, but it can be used in extreme cases despite an inability to confirm this diagnosis.

Confirmation and reconfirmation of placement are critical to avoid catastrophic complications.

This procedure is used as a bridge to endoscopy, angiography, surgery, or transfer, not as definitive management.

Use a clamp to prevent deflation of the balloon between syringes and after filling.

Keep shears at the bedside and deflate the balloon if the patient experiences sudden cardiovascular collapse.

TABLE 11-8.

Indications for balloon tamponade in patients with suspected variceal bleeding

Massive bleeding renders endoscopy futile

Consultants are unavailable and other treatments have been exhausted

As a temporizing measure while the patient is transferred to an interventional radiology suite, an operating room, or a facility providing a higher level of care

FIGURE 11-2.

Radiograph of Linton-Nachlas tube *in situ*.

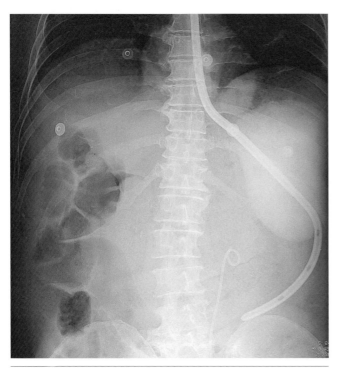

Conclusion

Unstable patients with GI hemorrhage present particular challenges for emergency physicians. The established emergency medicine adage of thinking and treating "worst first" diagnoses will serve the practitioner well in the initial management. An upper GI source, specifically bleeding esophageal varices, should be sought first. Although emergency physicians cannot be expected to perform the myriad procedures that may be necessary to stop the bleeding, a working knowledge of each is important to anticipate what will be required next in the chain of survival. Because there are multiple, typically scarce, subspecialists involved in the definitive management of these patients, parallel approaches are necessary.

References

1. Stabile BE, Stamos MJ. Surgical management of gastrointestinal bleeding. *Gastroenterol Clin North Am.* 2000;29:189-222.
2. Peura DA, Lanza FL, Gostout CJ, et al. The American College of Gastroenterology bleeding registry: preliminary findings. *Am J Gastroenterol.* 1997;92:924-928.
3. Apel D, Riemann JF. Emergency endoscopy. *Can J Gastroenterol.* 2000;14:199-203.
4. Afessa B. Triage of patients with acute gastrointestinal bleeding for intensive care unit admission based on risk factors for poor outcome. *J Clin Gastroenterol.* 2000;30:281-285.
5. Meaden C, Makin AJ. Diagnosis and treatment of patients with gastrointestinal bleeding. *Curr Anaesthes Crit Care.* 2004;15:123-132.
6. Strate LL, Ayanian JZ, Kotler G, et al. Risk factors for mortality in lower intestinal bleeding. *Clin Gastroenterol Hepatol.* 2008;6:1004-1010.
7. Jensen DM, Machicado GA. Diagnosis and treatment of severe hematochezia: the role of urgent colonoscopy after purge. *Gastroenterol Clin North Am.* 1988;95:1569-1574.
8. Rehman A, Iscimen R, Yilmaz M, et al. Prophylactic endotracheal intubation in critically ill patients undergoing endoscopy for upper GI hemorrhage. *Gastrointest Endosc.* 2009;69:e55-e59.
9. Barriot P, Riou B. Hemorrhagic shock with paradoxical bradycardia. *J Intensive Care Med.* 1987;13:203-207.
10. Garcia-Tsao G, Sanyal AJ, Grace ND. Prevention and management of gastroesophageal varices and variceal hemorrhage in cirrhosis. *Hepatology.* 2007;46:922-923.
11. Melo J, Peters J. Low systemic vascular resistance: differential diagnosis and outcome. *Crit Care.* 1999;3:71-77.
12. Newby DE, Hayes PC. Hyperdynamic circulation in liver cirrhosis: not peripheral vasodilatation but 'splanchnic steal.' *QJM.* 2002;95:827-830.
13. Perel P, Roberts I. Colloids versus crystalloids for fluid resuscitation in critically ill patients. *Cochrane Database Syst Rev.* 2007;17(4):CD000567.
14. Ginn JL, Ducharme J. Recurrent bleeding in acute upper gastrointestinal hemorrhage: transfusion confusion. *Can J Emerg Med.* 2001;3:193-198.
15. Baradarian R, Ramdhaney S, Chapalamadugu R, et al. Early intensive resuscitation of patients with upper gastrointestinal bleeding decreases mortality. *Am J Gastroenterol.* 2004;99:619-622.
16. Dallal HJ, Palmer KR. ABC of the upper gastrointestinal tract: upper gastrointestinal haemorrhage. *BMJ.* 2001;323:1115-1117.
17. Hebert PC, Wells G, Blajchman MA, et al. A multicenter, randomized, controlled clinical trial of transfusion requirements in critical care. *N Engl J Med.* 1999;340:409-417.
18. Contreras M. Final statement from the consensus conference on platelet transfusion. *Transfusion.* 1998;38:796-797.
19. Witting MD, Magder L, Heins AE, et al. Usefulness and validity of diagnostic nasogastric aspiration in patients without hematemesis. *Ann Emerg Med.* 2004;43:525-532.
20. Jutabha R, Jensen DM. Management of severe upper gastrointestinal bleeding in the patient with liver disease. *Med Clin North Am.* 1996;80:1035-1068.
21. Kupfer Y, Cappell MS, Tessler S. Acute gastrointestinal bleeding in the intensive care unit: the intensivist's perspective. *Gastroenterol Clin North Am.* 2000;29:275-307.
22. Leontiadis GI, Sharma VK, Howden CW. Systematic review and meta-analysis: proton-pump inhibitor treatment for ulcer bleeding reduces transfusion requirements and hospital stay—results from the Cochrane Collaboration. *Aliment Pharmacol Ther.* 2005;22:169-174.
23. Selby NM, Kubba AK, Hawkey CJ. Acid suppression in peptic ulcer haemorrhage: a 'meta-analysis'. *Aliment Pharmacol Ther.* 2000;14:1119-1126.
24. Barkun A, Bardou M, Marshall JK, et al. Consensus recommendations for managing patients with nonvariceal upper gastrointestinal bleeding. *Ann Intern Med.* 2003;139:843-857.

25. Gøtzsche PC, Gjørup I, Bonnén H, et al. Somatostatin v placebo in bleeding oesophageal varices: randomised trial and meta-analysis. *BMJ.* 1995;310:1495-1498.

26. Planas R, Quer JC, Boix J, et al. A prospective randomized trial comparing somatostatin and sclerotherapy in the treatment of acute variceal bleeding. *Hepatology.* 1994;20:370-375.

27. Sung JJ, Chung SC, Lai CW, et al. Octreotide infusion or emergency sclerotherapy for variceal haemorrhage. *Lancet.* 1993;342:637-641.

28. Imperiale TF, Teran JC, McCullough AJ. A meta-analysis of somatostatin versus vasopressin in the management of acute esophageal variceal hemorrhage. *Gastroenterology.* 1995;109:1289-1294.

29. Junquera F, Saperas E, Videla S, et al. Long-term efficacy of octreotide in the prevention of recurrent bleeding from gastrointestinal angiodysplasia. *Am J Gastroenterol.* 2007;102:254-260.

30. Lin HJ, Perng CL, Wang K, et al. Octreotide for arrest of peptic ulcer hemorrhage—a prospective, randomized controlled trial. *Hepatogastroenterology.* 1995;42:856-860.

31. Berzigotti A, Gilabert R, Abraldes JG, et al. Noninvasive prediction of clinically significant portal hypertension and esophageal varices in patients with compensated liver cirrhosis. *Am J Gastroenterol.* 2008;103:1159-1167.

32. Park SH, Park TE, Kim YM, et al. Non-invasive model predicting clinically-significant portal hypertension in patients with advanced fibrosis. *J Gastroenterol Hepatol.* 2009;24:1289-1293.

33. Prihatini J, Lesmana LA, Manan C. Detection of esophageal varices in liver cirrhosis using non-invasive parameters. *Acta Med Indones.* 2005;37:126-131.

34. Soares-Weiser K, Brezis M, Tur-Kaspa R, et al. Antibiotic prophylaxis for cirrhotic patients with gastrointestinal bleeding. *Cochrane Database Syst Rev.* 2002;(2): CD002907.

35. Adang RP, Vismans JF, Talmon JL, et al. Appropriateness of indications for diagnostic upper gastrointestinal endoscopy: association with relevant endoscopic disease. *Gastrointest Endosc.* 1995;42:390-397.

36. Millward SF. ACR Appropriateness Criteria on treatment of acute nonvariceal gastrointestinal tract bleeding. *J Am Coll Radiol.* 2008;5:550-554.

37. Garcia-Tsao G, Bosch J. Management of varices and variceal hemorrhage in cirrhosis. *N Engl J Med.* 2010;362:823-832.

38. Zuccaro G. Management of the adult patient with acute lower gastrointestinal bleeding. American College of Gastroenterology. Practice Parameters Committee. *Am J Gastroenterol.* 1998;93:1202-1208.

39. Ernst O, Bulois P, Saint-Drenant S, et al. Helical CT in acute lower gastrointestinal bleeding. *Eur J Radiol.* 2003;13:114-117.

40. Laing CF. Acute gastrointestinal bleeding: emerging role of multidetector CT angiography and review of current imaging techniques. *Radiographics.* 2007;27:1055-1070.

41. Scheffel H, Pfammatter T, Wildi S, et al. Acute gastrointestinal bleeding: detection of source and etiology with multi-detector-row CT. *Eur J Radiol.* 2006;17:1555-1565.

42. Yoon W, Jeong YY, Shin SS, et al. Acute massive gastrointestinal bleeding: detection and localization with arterial phase multi-detector row helical CT. *Radiology.* 2006;239:160-167.

43. Rockall TA. Management and outcome of patients undergoing surgery after acute upper gastrointestinal haemorrhage. Steering Group for the National Audit of Acute Upper Gastrointestinal Haemorrhage. *J R Soc Med.* 1988;91:518-523.

44. Haddock G, Garden OJ, McKee RF, et al. Esophageal tamponade in the management of acute variceal hemorrhage. *Dig Dis Sci.* 1989;34:913-918.

45. Stabile BE. Current surgical management of duodenal ulcers. *Surg Clin North Am.* 1992;72:335-356.

46. Feneyrou B, Hanana J, Daures JP, et al. Initial control of bleeding from esophageal varices with the Sengstaken-Blakemore tube: experience in 82 patients. *Am J Surg.* 1988;155:509-511.

47. Henneman PL. Gastrointestinal bleeding. In: Marx J, Hockberger R, Walls R, et al, eds. *Rosen's Emergency Medicine: Concepts and Clinical Practice.* 7th ed. Philadelphia, PA: Mosby Elsevier; 2009:170-174.

CHAPTER 12

Severe Sepsis and Septic Shock

Alan C. Heffner

Introduction

Sepsis is the 10th leading cause of death in the United States and results in 750,000 hospitalizations annually.[1] Statistically, one patient presents to a US emergency department with severe sepsis every minute. The rate of hospitalization for severe sepsis doubled during the past decade and is projected to exceed one million cases per year in the near future.[2,3] Half of these patients are admitted via the emergency department, which highlights the importance of emergency care in acute sepsis management. Of most concern, severe sepsis carries a hospital mortality rate of 25% to 50%, and estimates of age-adjusted mortality rate are increasing.

The Sepsis Syndromes

Infection is classically defined as pathologic microbial invasion of a normally sterile tissue or fluid. In practice, confirmation is rare at initial presentation, and infection is presumed based on clinical observations coupled with laboratory and radiologic findings. Bacteremia defines the presence of viable bacteria in the blood and is confirmed in less than half of severe sepsis cases.[4] Rarely, clinically important manifestations of infection arise from cytopathic or exotoxin effects in the absence of microbial tissue invasion (eg, *Clostridium difficile* colitis, staphylococcal toxic shock syndrome).

Host response has a key role in the pathogenesis of many diseases, including sepsis. The term *systemic inflammatory response syndrome* (SIRS) describes the complex activation of innate immune response manifested as systemic inflammation and endothelial dysfunction.[5] SIRS reflects a generalized (patho-) physiologic response to disease. The cytokine and immunologic storm underlying SIRS holds the potential to damage organs remote from the initial insult.

In practice, the SIRS signs (Figure 12-1) of tachycardia, tachypnea, and abnormal temperature or white blood cell count represent markers to identify patients at risk of progression to more severe disease. SIRS criteria are readily available, easy to identify, reproducible, and associated with prognosis.[6] However, SIRS is not specific to infection.[7–9] The generalized immune reaction represents a conserved response to diverse insults, including tissue injury (eg, burns and trauma) and noninfectious inflammatory and immuno-stimulating diseases. The need for a standardized and practical diagnostic framework for sepsis trials codified use of clinical SIRS criteria in defining clinical sepsis.[10]

Sepsis is the clinical syndrome of systemic response to microbial infection. In patients with known or suspected infection, SIRS constitutes evidence of sepsis. Sepsis encompasses a broad range of disease, from minor self-limited infection to life-threatening conditions. The sepsis syndromes denote a

FIGURE 12-1.

Example of an early severe sepsis and septic shock treatment pathway flowchart

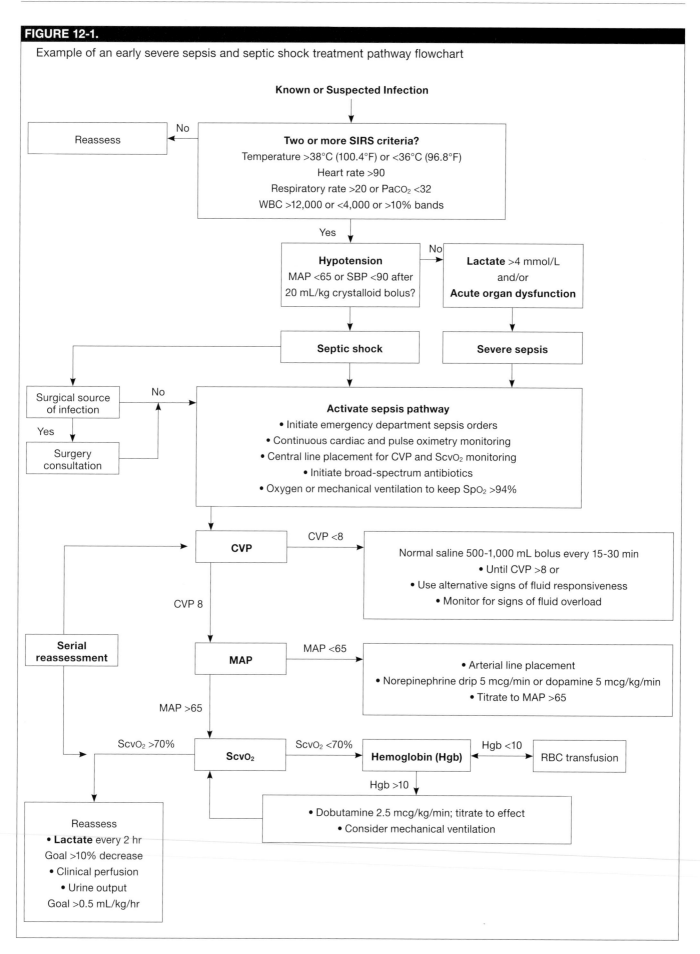

continuum of disease progressing from sepsis (infection with inflammatory response) to severe sepsis (sepsis plus acute organ dysfunction) and septic shock (severe sepsis with cardiovascular failure)[11] (Table 12-1). A minority of patients with clinical sepsis present with or progress to severe disease.[12] This group incurs substantial morbidity and mortality.

Severe Sepsis Identification

Sepsis is a challenging clinical diagnosis. Signs and symptoms of infection are protean and often subtle and nonspecific. There is no pathognomonic sign or single reliable test to diagnose early sepsis. Although the current diagnosis of sepsis is based on physiologic indicators of SIRS in the setting of infection, the clinical presentation and course of infected patients are rarely distinct, as the definitions suggest. In practice, SIRS should prompt consideration and investigation for infection. However, the absence of categorical SIRS (two or more of the four criteria) does not exclude clinically important infection.

PEARL

The two markers considered classic for infection—fever and peripheral leukocytosis (with or without bandemia)—are inconsistent and do not reliably discriminate infectious from noninfectious disease.[4]

Immunocompromised and elderly patients at greatest risk for severe infection exhibit attenuated host response, which also limits bedside detection. Difficult clinical recognition is compounded by the absence of laboratory markers for sepsis. The promise of specific biomarkers to confirm early infection is yet to be realized. Rapid nonculture microbiologic diagnostics such

TABLE 12-1.

The sepsis syndromes

Infection	Microbial invasion of normally sterile host tissue or fluid
SIRS	The systemic inflammatory response to a variety of insults
	Manifested by two or more of the following: 　　Temperature >38°C (100.4°F) or <36°C (96.8°F) 　　Heart rate >90 beats/min 　　Respiratory rate >20 breaths/min or $PaCO_2$ <32 mm Hg 　　WBC count >12,000/mm^3 or <4,000/mm^3, or >10% immature bands
Sepsis	The systemic inflammatory response to infection
	Clinical infection plus SIRS
Severe sepsis	Sepsis with acute organ dysfunction: Acute lung injury: 　　PaO_2/FIO_2 <300 　　Acute respiratory failure Acute kidney injury: 　　Serum creatinine >0.5 mg/dL from baseline 　　Oliguria: urine output <0.5 mL/kg/hr for 2 consecutive hours
	Encephalopathy ranging from confusion or apathy to agitation
	Coagulopathy: 　　Prothrombin time (PT) >16 sec or activated partial thromboplastin time (aPTT) >60 sec
	Thrombocytopenia: 　　Platelet count <100,000/μL
	Hyperbilirubinemia: 　　Serum bilirubin >4 mg/dL
	Blood lactate >2.5 mmol/L
	Clinical malperfusion: 　　Cool extremities, mottling, delayed capillary refill
Septic shock	Sepsis with hypotension refractory to initial fluid resuscitation (20 mL/kg)
	SBP <90 mm Hg or >40 mm Hg drop from baseline
	MAP <65 mm Hg or >25 mm Hg drop from baseline

as polymerase chain reaction and antigen screens may evolve to have clinical utility in the future.

Microbiologic confirmation of infection is rare early in the course of illness, so patients must be treated based on suspected or presumed infection. The source of infection remains unidentified in up to one third of patients with severe sepsis. Occult or unidentified infection is associated with increased death rates, in part due to delays in recognition and treatment.[12] Given the prevalence and morbidity of severe sepsis, constant surveillance and heightened suspicion are warranted. Ill-appearing patients and those presenting with unexplained SIRS or shock warrant consideration of infection and expedited investigation and treatment.

Severe sepsis should be considered in all patients diagnosed with acute infection. Specific sources are more commonly associated with severe disease. Pulmonary and intraabdominal infections account for half of severe sepsis cases. Other common high-risk sources include the urinary tract, skin and soft tissues, and endovascular sites. However, any source or agent, including atypical organisms (eg, virus, spirochete, *Rickettsia*, and yeast), can produce life-threatening disease. The difficulty in clinical identification of sepsis is underscored by the fact that a primary source and site of infection remain unidentified in up to 20% of strongly suspected cases.[4]

PEARL

Pulmonary and intraabdominal infections account for half of severe sepsis cases.

Septic Shock and Severe Sepsis

Shock defines a state of inadequate tissue perfusion in which oxygen delivery does not meet metabolic needs. Contrary to popular use, the term does not reflect perfusion pressure.

KEY POINT

Blood pressure is an unreliable gauge of cardiac output and oxygen delivery.

Hypoperfusion can occur with low, normal, or elevated blood pressure.[13] Up to half of patients with severe sepsis present in compensated shock with normal blood pressure. The difficulty in identifying these patients has spawned the terms *occult shock* and *cryptic shock*. Since blood pressure alone is insufficient to identify infected patients at high risk, it is important to consciously evaluate patients for signs of hypoperfusion, end-organ dysfunction, and metabolic stress.

Septic shock is defined by cardiovascular failure manifesting as hypotension or hypoperfusion following initial fluid resuscitation. *Uncompensated shock* characterized by hypotension defines a late stage of shock that develops when physiologic attempts to maintain normal perfusion pressure are overwhelmed or exhausted. Even if organ blood flow and function are not compromised, their potential to become so should be assumed. Although some patients manifest low blood pressure without apparent distress or hypoperfusion, hypotension is pathologic until proven otherwise.

KEY POINT

A mean arterial pressure (MAP) less than 65 mm Hg, systolic blood pressure (SBP) less than 90 mm Hg, or SBP more than 40 mm Hg below baseline warrants prompt investigation for cause and comparison with the patient's historic baseline.

Transient hypotension often heralds hemodynamic deterioration. Physiologically, nonsustained hypotension represents progressive exhaustion of cardiovascular reserve and is the first sign of uncompensated shock. These episodes are an early warning associated with increased mortality and should not be dismissed as spurious or inconsequential.[14,15]

Severe sepsis is marked by the presence of acute organ dysfunction (Table 12-1). Acute lung and kidney injury are most common, followed by cardiovascular, hematologic, and neurologic dysfunction. Patients with sepsis can be confused, apathetic, or agitated, but the association between infection and delirium is often underappreciated by physicians. Laboratory variables aid in identification, with thrombocytopenia, coagulopathy, hyperbilirubinemia, and elevated lactate being notable evidence of end-organ dysfunction. Mild elevations of serum creatinine (>0.5 mg/dL from baseline), even in the absence of oliguria, represent acute kidney injury, which is associated with increased risk of adverse outcome.[16] Increasing severity of kidney dysfunction is associated with stepwise increases in mortality.[17] Similarly, end-organ dysfunction has an additive effect on mortality, such that failure of three or more organs is associated with mortality rates of more than 60%.

Lactate is a useful biomarker to confirm and risk stratify critical illness, including that associated with sepsis. The admission lactate level grades illness severity and predicts outcome in a variety of critical illnesses.[18–21] Hyperlactatemia is well recognized in the setting of acute infection and has been historically attributed to anaerobic metabolism as a consequence of tissue hypoxia and hypoperfusion. The true source of hyperlactatemia in sepsis is multifactorial, but the contribution of catechol-stimulated aerobic lactate production is more considerable than previously appreciated.[22] This corroborates the clinical observation of hyperlactatemia in hemodynamically stable patients without hypoperfusion. Thus, in many patients, hyperlactatemia is a marker of metabolic stress rather than occult hypoperfusion.

The source of lactate should not distract from its utility in stratifying an individual patient's risk of disease progression and associated outcome. The blood lactate concentration stratifies patients independent of hemodynamics and organ dysfunction.[23,24] Mild supranormal (>2 mmol/L) lactate levels are as-

TABLE 12-2.

Conditions placing patients at high risk for adverse outcome

Septic shock

Severe sepsis with acute organ dysfunction

Sepsis with blood lactate >4 mmol/L

sociated with increased disease severity and mortality. Among patients with suspected infection, a lactate concentration higher than 4 mmol/L carries a one-in-four rate of death, which is 10-fold higher than in patients with a normal lactate level.[24] This mortality figure holds true even among patients with normal blood pressure.[25]

Lactate is a powerful screening biomarker to identify infected patients at high risk, analogous to the use of cardiac markers in suspected acute coronary syndrome. Arterial, venous, and capillary lactate levels are clinically equivalent and unaffected by Ringer lactate infusion.

KEY POINT
Lactate should be measured directly because serum bicarbonate, anion gap, and base excess are insensitive for clinically important hyperlactatemia.

Treatment

Early recognition of severe sepsis is critical but must be coupled with timely and effective therapy in order to influence outcome. The presence of shock, hyperlactatemia (>4 mmol/L), and/or acute organ dysfunction defines a high-risk patient group with hospital mortality rates ranging from 25% to 50% (Table 12-2). Aggressive management of these patients confers short-term and persistent mortality advantage.[26,27]

Bundling evidence-based practices strives to improve outcomes to a level higher than those achieved with individual components of care. The utility of this approach is well recognized in critical care and is particularly valuable for high-risk diseases that have a brief therapeutic window. The Surviving Sepsis Campaign and the Institute for Healthcare Improvement advocate a structured resuscitation bundle to improve process and outcomes of patients with severe sepsis (Table 12-3).[28] Potential benefits of such an approach include consensus, organization, and standardization of care, leading to enhanced patient identification and intervention completion. Bundle compliance generally improves with time.[29,30] The highest survival rates are associated with 100% compliance with all care components.[31,32]

Early Cardiovascular Resuscitation and Hemodynamic Optimization

There is no single cardiovascular abnormality of sepsis. The disease manifests a complex and dynamic cascade of cardiovascular dysfunction, which includes hypovolemia, abnormal vasomotor tone, and primary cardiac dysfunction. These derange-

TABLE 12-3.
Treatment components of the Severe Sepsis Bundle of the Surviving Sepsis Campaign

1) Administer appropriate antibiotics within 3 hours after emergency department admission.

2) Administer early goal-directed therapy, including the following:
   • Fluids to achieve CVP ≥8–12 mm Hg
   • Vasopressors to achieve MAP ≥65 mm Hg
   • Hemodynamic support for goal ScvO$_2$ reading >70%

ments lead to tissue and organ hypoperfusion, which propagate multiorgan dysfunction.[33]

Treatment at proximate stages of care affects outcomes and cannot be delayed. The window to reverse critical organ hypoperfusion is measured in hours and often transpires in the emergency department. Acute structured resuscitation of patients with severe sepsis and septic shock influences longitudinal survival, while equivalent but delayed therapy does not yield the same benefit.[34,35] The opportunity for early therapy to alter the clinical trajectory of severe sepsis is supported by comparison with former sepsis trials focused on patients at later stages of disease.[35]

KEY POINT
The immediate goal of cardiovascular support is to restore and maintain systemic oxygen delivery and end-organ perfusion.

The hemodynamic approach to patients with severe sepsis is similar to the support of patients with other critical illnesses. A systematic goal-oriented strategy aims to rapidly optimize preload, maintain systemic perfusion pressure, and balance oxygen delivery and perfusion to meet metabolic needs (Table 12-4).

Fluid Therapy and Optimization

Vasodilation induced by transcapillary leak and nitric oxide contributes to absolute and relative hypovolemia in sepsis. Vascular refilling in the form of fluid resuscitation is a central component of early cardiovascular support. Initial volume expansion is achieved through rapid fluid administration under direct observation at the bedside. Serial aliquots of crystalloid (10–20 mL/kg) or colloid (5–10 mL/kg) solution should be infused over 15 to 30 minutes, with sequential boluses titrated to perfusion endpoints while monitoring for adverse effects, including pulmonary congestion. Although total volume re-

TABLE 12-4.
Prioritized end points of resuscitation

1) Adequate intravenous access

2) Preload optimization
   a. Serial fluid challenges guided by clinical examination and patient response
   b. CVP ≥8 mm Hg (≥12 mm Hg if mechanically ventilated)
   c. Fluid guided by evidence of volume responsiveness gauged by dynamic hemodynamic variables

3) MAP ≥65 mm Hg

4) Sustain organ perfusion and match oxygen delivery and consumption
   a. Clinical regional markers
      • Cutaneous perfusion
      • Urine output >0.5 mL/kg/hr
      • Mental status
   b. Global markers
      • ScvO$_2$ reading ≥70%
      • Lactate clearance and normalization

quirements are difficult to predict at the onset of resuscitation, empiric crystalloid loading of 50 to 60 mL/kg is generally indicated and well tolerated.

Colloid and crystalloid resuscitation differentially affect a range of physiologic parameters. To date, there is no clear survival benefit with one class or agent.[36,37] In most situations, the clinical endpoint guiding the dose of fluid resuscitation is more important than whether crystalloid or colloid is used. Greater response to a given dose of isotonic colloid is consistent with its expected volume of distribution.[38] As such, a greater volume of crystalloid is required to obtain the same hemodynamic response compared with synthetic and natural colloid. This can influence fluid selection for patients in whom the interstitial edema that follows large-volume crystalloid administration could threaten organ function (eg, hypoxemic lung injury, abdominal ascites, or compartment syndrome).

Persistent hypoperfusion following initial volume loading (>50 mL/kg crystalloid) complicates 50% of severe sepsis cases.[39] Inappropriate continuation of fluid resuscitation to a patient assumed to have stroke volume responsiveness delays appropriate therapy and contributes to unnecessary fluid overload.[40,41] A rational approach to the situation when patients are no longer volume responsive incorporates selection and titration of subsequent therapy under the guidance of objective cardiovascular monitoring.

The primary goal of fluid therapy is stroke volume augmentation. Making an informed prediction of the patient's hemodynamic response to fluid therapy before beginning fluids avoids the administration of ineffective, and potentially deleterious, fluid. Central venous pressure (CVP) is a widely advocated preload measure. In the absence of conflicting data, a target CVP of 8 to 12 mm Hg is recommended to optimize preload.[42] Cardiac filling pressures reflect the net influence of vascular volume, venous tone, cardiac function, and intrathoracic pressure. These myriad influences explain why pressure surrogates of preload (CVP and pulmonary artery occlusion pressure) are poor predictors of fluid response and why there is no consistent threshold of CVP to reliably estimate response to fluid.[40,41]

Fluid responsiveness is best predicted by dynamic indices of preload reserve. Positive-pressure mechanical ventilation induces cyclic alteration in preload, which provides individualized insight into cardiovascular function and status. Observation of respirophasic variation in stroke volume during mechanical ventilation identifies patients capable of augmenting stroke volume in response to fluid administration. It is among the most reliable signs of fluid responsiveness.[41,43] A regular (preferably sinus) rhythm, positive-pressure ventilation with a tidal volume of more than 8 mL/kg, and absence of significant patient interaction with the ventilator are important requirements for interpretation of these data.

Predicting volume responsiveness is more difficult in spontaneously breathing patients.[44] Provocative maneuvers test the cardiovascular system to predict individual response prior to fluid administration. Passive leg raising translocates venous blood from the lower extremities to the thorax.[45] Volume-responsive patients transiently increase stroke volume within 3 minutes of the maneuver. Rapid feedback stroke volume mea-

surement tools are therefore required to identify the transient response. A passive leg-raising maneuver helps gauge volume responsiveness in a wide variety of patients, including ventilated and spontaneously breathing patients and those with irregular cardiac rhythms. Transthoracic echocardiography for assessment of biventricular function and dynamic respiratory vena cava collapse can also aid in titrating fluid and drug therapy.

Vasopressor Support

The abnormal vasomotor tone and impaired vascular reactivity of sepsis manifest as persistent hypotension despite fluid optimization. The goal of vasopressor therapy is to restore blood pressure within organ autoregulatory range. Ideally, fluid optimization is achieved prior to catecholamine support, but severe hemodynamic compromise can require vasopressors early and in the midst of ongoing volume resuscitation. A MAP target of 65 mm Hg is commonly recommended. Titrating vasopressors to higher targets is not associated with consistent benefit in regional perfusion.[46] However, individualized therapy is indicated in the face of concomitant or preexisting comorbid disease. For example, higher perfusion pressure goals can be required to maintain organ blood flow in patients with right-shifted autoregulation associated with chronic hypertension. Invasive arterial measurement is recommended to improve monitoring in patients exhibiting persistent hypotension and requiring catecholamine support.[42]

PEARL

There is no clear evidence that supports a single superior vasopressor agent.

Norepinephrine is generally considered the drug of choice because of its availability, effectiveness, and wide dosing range. Dopamine is also commonly used and has the benefit of cardiac acceleration for patients with bradycardia or cardiomyopathy. There is no role for low-dose "renal" dopamine in an attempt to preserve renal function during vasopressor support.[47] Vasodilatory shock is associated with endogenous vasopressin deficiency and is responsive to vasopressin replacement. Unfortunately, mortality benefit remains uncertain.[48] Vasopressin (0.01–0.04 units/min IV) is typically used as an adjunct for hypotension refractory to typical doses of catecholamine therapy. Dose escalation is not recommended because of its ischemic complications.

End Points of Resuscitation

The ultimate goal of resuscitation is to restore oxygen delivery and tissue perfusion to meet global and regional metabolic needs. The most appropriate endpoint for resuscitation remains controversial. Historically, resuscitation aimed to normalize clinical markers, but a growing body of evidence shows that resuscitation targeting customary markers of blood pressure, pulse, CVP, and urine output does not guarantee normal organ perfusion. We now recognize that macrocirculatory signs provide little insight into the balance of systemic oxygen delivery and utilization.[49] Resuscitation aimed at these targets risks leaving the patient in compensated shock.

Forty percent of patients with severe sepsis suffer deficits in global perfusion despite resuscitation to traditional end points.[34]

Central venous oxygen saturation (ScvO$_2$) and serum lactate measurement have emerged as rapid and reliable markers of global perfusion and physiologic stress. Inadequate oxygen delivery is compensated by enhanced tissue extraction and results in relative desaturation of blood returning to the heart. Mixed (SvO$_2$) and central venous oximetry measure the balance between systemic oxygen delivery and consumption. ScvO$_2$ is a practical bedside measurement based on a sample taken from a catheter (central or peripheral) positioned in the superior vena cava. Physiologic response is rapid such that monitoring provides immediate feedback on resuscitation efforts (and clinical deterioration) to guide the adequacy of therapy.

ScvO$_2$ is the most well studied contemporary resuscitation target in severe sepsis. An ScvO$_2$ reading greater than 70% was a central management variable in the early goal-directed therapy trial.[34] Subsequent integration into institutional protocols and the Surviving Sepsis Campaign corroborate the importance of this endpoint.[26] The maximal ScvO$_2$ measurement achieved during the first 6 hours of care is associated with the risk of death. Patients with persistent venous hypoxia have a mortality rate nearly double that of patients in whom normalization is achieved.[50,51]

The level of lactate clearance is inversely related to mortality.[52] Lactate trends are therefore used to corroborate response to therapy. Clearance of more than 10% of the lactate volume during the first 6 hours of care is associated with improved survival.[53] More significantly, in one trial, targeting lactate clearance as a primary resuscitation endpoint was equivalent to targeting the ScvO$_2$ reading.[54]

There is no single best endpoint of resuscitation for all clinical circumstances. For example, abnormal ScvO$_2$ and lactate measurements should prompt intervention, but normalized values do not guarantee adequate perfusion. A multimodal approach seeking to normalize a combination of global (ScvO$_2$ and lactate) and regional perfusion markers is most prudent. Urine output and clinical perfusion remain legitimate gauges of resuscitation and should be monitored serially. Regional perfusion estimations by measures of tissue capnometry, oximetry, and near-infrared spectroscopy show promise as future endpoints of resuscitation, but their roles remain to be clarified.

Perfusion Optimization

Treatment targets are tied inextricably to resuscitation, as they guide the choice and dose of therapies that influence clinical outcomes. Persistent hypoperfusion despite preload and blood pressure optimization warrants consideration of additional therapy to enhance oxygen delivery or reduce metabolic demand.

Cardiac dysfunction is common in patients with severe sepsis as a consequence of chronic disease or acute sepsis-associated cardiomyopathy.[55,56] Elevated cardiac filling pressures are a clue to primary cardiac dysfunction in patients who fail to meet resuscitation endpoints and can be confirmed by echocardiography. Dobutamine is the preferred inotrope to augment cardiac performance. Low-dose initiation (2.5 mcg/kg/min IV) is recommended to monitor for adverse hypotension or tachycardia, with subsequent titration to clinical effect. Milrinone is an alternative choice for patients with significant tachycardia or previous β-blocker use.

Augmentation of oxygen-carrying capacity via transfusion of red blood cells is an option for patients with persistent oxygen delivery–consumption mismatch despite cardiac performance optimization. There is little evidence to declare the optimal hemoglobin for patients with acute severe infection. A restrictive transfusion strategy targeting hemoglobin of 7 to 9 g/dL is not associated with increased mortality in critically ill patients.[57] However, this strategy has not been investigated in patients undergoing acute resuscitation. Transfusion should be considered for patients with critical anemia, defined by persistent hypoperfusion despite preload and cardiac performance optimization and hemoglobin of less than 10 g/dL.

Serial single-unit transfusions are most appropriately guided by the resuscitation targets rather than an arbitrary hemoglobin level.

Decreasing systemic oxygen consumption is another potential target of therapy. Respiration and pyrexia are two common sources of enhanced oxygen demand in infected patients. The work and metabolic cost of breathing during acute sepsis can be substantial and divert blood flow from other vital organs.[58] Persistent venous hypoxia can be a sign of increased respiratory work. Initiation of mechanical ventilation often normalizes the ScvO$_2$ reading.[59] Noninvasive ventilation is an option for patients with evolving respiratory insufficiency but should be centered on awake and cooperative patients without severe hypoxemia. Rapid sequence intubation and sedation are required

TABLE 12-5.

Priorities of infection control

1) Source identification

2) Culture collection
 • Do not allow culture collection to significantly delay therapy.

3) Antibiotics within 1 hour after recognition of severe sepsis

4) Broad-spectrum antibiotics
 • Dual antibiotic coverage for gram-negative organisms when indicated
 • Consider atypical organisms
 • Choose drug appropriate for host target tissue penetration
 • Use full loading antibiotic dose
 • Consider rapid and simultaneous administration of the first antibiotic doses

5) Decompressive source control when indicated
 • Minimally invasive procedures are preferred when available.

for more severe disease. Following intubation, patients are managed with titrated sedation and analgesia.

PEARL

Long-acting neuromuscular blockade is rarely required and should be avoided because of the downstream consequence of neuromyopathy.[60]

Early Antibiotics and Source Control

Source identification and effective infection control are central goals during the early resuscitation of patients with life-threatening infection. Blood and other culture specimens should be collected prior to the administration of antibiotics, but sampling should not significantly delay therapy. Time to initiation of effective antimicrobial therapy is an important determinant of patient outcome. The recommendation to administer antibiotics within 1 hour after the recognition of severe sepsis is supported by the association of mortality with even brief delays in therapy.[42,61–63] Equally important, empiric coverage should be broad to cover all potential culprit organisms. Inappropriate therapy is associated with a five-fold reduction in survival.[64] Patients with resistant and atypical organisms (eg, methicillin-resistant *Staphylococcus aureus*; vancomycin-resistant enterococci; extended-spectrum, β-lactamase producing gram-negative rods) are more likely to suffer the consequences of inappropriate empiric therapy. The choice of empiric agents should be individualized according to the patient's drug tolerance, local microbe resistance patterns, suspected source, and host tissue involved (Table 12-5).

Anatomic source identification should always be coupled

with consideration for definitive infection control measures (Table 12-6). Common foci of infection that are amenable to intervention include peritonitis, intestinal ischemia, cholangitis, pyelonephritis, empyema, indwelling vascular hardware, necrotizing soft-tissue infection, and other deep space infections. Drainage, débridement, and removal of these sources often require coordinated multidisciplinary effort but are part of resuscitation and should not be delayed for the hope of improved cardiovascular stabilization. Percutaneous drainage is generally preferred over open débridement to minimize additional physiologic insult.

Adjunctive Therapies

A number of adjunctive therapies have potential roles in subsets of patients with severe sepsis (Table 12-7). Inadequate adrenal response in the setting of acute critical illness is called *relative adrenal insufficiency*. Steroid supplementation aims to replace physiologic hormone function in patients with this inadequate reserve. Unfortunately, the ability to diagnose this condition is limited because of inconsistencies in proposed criteria and cortisol immunoassays.[65] Adrenocorticotropic hormone testing is therefore not advised to select infected patients for steroid therapy.

Patients exhibiting vasopressor-refractory shock are candidates for intravenous steroids. Hydrocortisone is the preferred agent and promotes shock reversal, although its mortality benefit remains unclear.[66,67] Stress-dose steroids are also indicated for patients with severe sepsis and known adrenal dysfunction or chronic steroid dependency, even in the absence of shock. Dexamethasone is a suboptimal substitute for hydrocortisone; high-dose corticosteroids are potentially harmful and not indicated in acute infection.

Activated protein C (drotrecogin alfa) exerts anti-inflammatory and anticoagulant properties capable of altering the common pathways of organ dysfunction in severe sepsis. The role of recombinant human activated protein C (rhAPC) was established based on a mortality benefit in adult patients at high risk of death, defined by the presence of multiorgan dysfunction or an APACHE II score of 25 or more.[68,69] The most important risk associated with rhAPC is hemorrhage, and the risk may be higher than initially defined.[70] Current controversies regarding the methodologic quality and potential complications of the initial rhAPC trial[68] may be clarified by an upcoming trial. In the interim, rhAPC should be considered after aggressive hemo-

---

TABLE 12-6.

Common infections warranting consideration for emergency source control

Sources	Control Technique
Infected implant	Device removal
Infected vascular access	
Urinary catheter	
Abscess	Drainage
Cholangitis	
Pyelonephritis with ureteral obstruction	
Septic arthritis	
Thoracic empyema	
Complicated soft-tissue infection	Débridement
Intestinal infarction	
Mediastinitis	
Small-bowel obstruction	

TABLE 12-7.

Adjunctive therapies for severe sepsis

1) Steroid therapy for refractory septic shock
   - Hydrocortisone, 100 mg IV, then 200–300 mg/day in divided doses

2) Activated protein C (drotrecogin alfa)

3) IV immunoglobulin (IVIG)
   - 1 g/kg IV every 24 hr

dynamic optimization followed by an individualized appraisal of disease severity and bleeding risk.

Polyvalent intravenous immunoglobulin (IVIG) theoretically provides a protective effect in sepsis via several immuno-modulating pathways. To date, pooled analyses have failed to provide clear consensus on the role of various IVIG formulations in the management of severe sepsis and septic shock in adults.[71,72] IVIG remains a recommended adjunct in the treatment of streptococcal toxic shock syndrome.[73]

Supportive Therapies

The fragility of critically ill patients mandates detailed attention to routine general care to prevent complications and improve outcomes. Evidence-based support strategies are not specific to the ICU and warrant consideration early in the course of care. The current challenges related to delay in ICU admission because of hospital crowding reinforce the importance of having an understanding of these strategies for implementation in the emergency department (Table 12-8).

Sepsis is the most common cause of acute lung injury (ALI). Many patients with this condition require mechanical ventilation. Volume control is the most common mode of ventilation in the absence of evidence pointing to a clearly superior method of support. Adequate gas exchange and lung protection are the overriding principles of ventilator management. In patients with ALI or acute respiratory distress syndrome, appropriate mechanical ventilation targets are low tidal volume (V_T) (V_T <7 mL/kg ideal body weight) and plateau airway pressure (<30 cm H_2O).[74] Pulmonary shear and strain caused by high V_T contribute to ALI. The same low-V_T management goals are being extrapolated to patients without hypoxemia or abnormal lung compliance.[75]

Derangements of the blood glucose concentration are common during critical illness and are associated with worse outcome.[76] Diabetic complications, including ketoacidosis and severe hyperglycemia, warrant standard therapy during early care. Maintenance of strict normoglycemia during critical illness remains controversial. Current evidence supports setting a target blood sugar level less than 150 to 180 mg/dL via intermittent subcutaneous administration of insulin or an insulin infusion following patient stabilization.[42,77] Patients with severe sepsis are at risk for hypoglycemia even without insulin therapy, so the blood glucose concentration should be monitored serially during resuscitation.

Conclusion

There is perhaps no other critical illness more commonly encountered by emergency physicians than severe sepsis or septic shock. Emergency physicians are uniquely positioned to greatly affect morbidity and mortality in patients with sepsis, unlike those with other medical conditions. It is imperative that emergency physicians rapidly identify and treat any patient with severe sepsis or septic shock. Key components of the emergency department treatment of severe sepsis and septic shock include early administration of antibiotics; source control; and cardiovascular resuscitation, including fluid therapy, vasopressor medications, and possibly inotropic support. The use of adjunctive therapies (eg, initiation of mechanical ventilation, transfusion of packed red blood cells, and administration of corticosteroids or activated protein C) depends on the patient and is based on close monitoring for signs of continued hypoperfusion.

References

1. Angus DC, Linde-Zwirble WT, Lidicker J, Clermont G, Carcillo J, Pinsky MR. Epidemiology of severe sepsis in the United States: analysis of incidence, outcome, and associated costs of care. *Crit Care Med.* 2001;29:1303-1310.
2. Dombrovskiy VY, Martin AA, Sunderram J, Paz HL. Rapid increase in hospitalization and mortality rates for severe sepsis in the United States: a trend analysis from 1993 to 2003. *Crit Care Med.* 2007;35:1244-1250.
3. Martin GS, Mannino DM, Eaton S, Moss M. The epidemiology of sepsis in the United States from 1979 through 2000. *N Engl J Med.* 2003;348:1546-1554.
4. Heffner AC, Horton JM, Marchick MR, Jones AE. Etiology of illness in patients with severe sepsis admitted to the hospital from the emergency department. *Clin Infect Dis.* 2010;50:814-820.
5. Bone RC. Toward an epidemiology and natural history of SIRS (systemic inflammatory response syndrome). *JAMA.* 1992;268:3452-3455.
6. Rangel-Frausto MS, Pittet D, Costigan M, Hwang T, Davis CS, Wenzel RP. The natural history of the systemic inflammatory response syndrome (SIRS): a prospective study. *JAMA.* 1995;273:117-123.
7. Brun-Buisson C. The epidemiology of the systemic inflammatory response. *Intensive Care Med.* 2000;26(suppl 1):S64-S74.
8. Sands KE, Bates DW, Lanken PN, et al. Epidemiology of sepsis syndrome in 8 academic medical centers. *JAMA.* 1997;278:234-240.
9. Vincent JL. Dear SIRS, I'm sorry to say that I don't like you. *Crit Care Med.* 1997;25:372-374.
10. Bone RC, Balk RA, Cerra FB, et al. Definitions for sepsis and organ failure and guidelines for the use of innovative therapies in sepsis. The ACCP/SCCM Consensus Conference Committee. American College of Chest Physicians/Society of Critical Care Medicine. *Chest.* 1992;101:1644-1655.
11. Levy MM, Fink MP, Marshall JC, et al. 2001 SCCM/ESICM/ACCP/ATS/SIS International Sepsis Definitions Conference. *Crit Care Med.* 2003;31:1250-1256.
12. Smith SW, Pheley A, Collier R, Rahmatullah A, Johnson L, Peterson PK. Severe sepsis in the emergency department and its association with a complicated clinical course. *Acad Emerg Med.* 1998;5:1169-1176.
13. Wo CC, Shoemaker WC, Appel PL, Bishop MH, Kram HB, Hardin E. Unreliability of blood pressure and heart rate to evaluate cardiac output in emergency resuscitation and critical illness. *Crit Care Med.* 1993;21:218-223.
14. Jones AE, Yiannibas V, Johnson C, Kline JA. Emergency department hypotension predicts sudden unexpected in-hospital mortality: a prospective cohort study. *Chest.* 2006;130:941-946.
15. Marchick MR, Kline JA, Jones AE. The significance of non-sustained hypotension in emergency department patients with sepsis. *Intensive Care Med.* 2009;35:1261-1264.
16. Bagshaw SM, George C, Bellomo R. Early acute kidney injury and sepsis: a multicentre evaluation. *Crit Care.* 2008;12:R47.
17. Joannidis M, Metnitz B, Bauer P, et al. Acute kidney injury in critically ill patients classified by AKIN versus RIFLE using the SAPS 3 database. *Intensive Care Med.* 2009;35:1692-1702.
18. Smith I, Kumar P, Molloy S, et al. Base excess and lactate as prognostic indicators for patients admitted to intensive care. *Intensive Care Med.* 2001;27:74-83.

TABLE 12-8.

Evidence-based critical care support therapies

---

1) Sterile barrier precautions for all invasive procedures

2) Safe mechanical ventilation
   - Low V_T <7 mL/kg (ideal body weight)
   - Plateau airway pressure <30 cm H_2O
   - Endotracheal tube cuff pressure <25 cm H_2O

3) Aspiration precautions for mechanically ventilated patients
   - Head of bed elevation >30°–45° unless contraindicated
   - Orogastric or nasogastric tube decompression

4) Blood sugar control goal <150–180 mg/dL

5) Prophylaxis
   - Gastrointestinal stress ulcer prophylaxis
   - Deep venous thrombosis prophylaxis

19. Bakker J, Coffernils M, Leon M, Gris P, Vincent JL. Blood lactate levels are superior to oxygen-derived variables in predicting outcome in human septic shock. *Chest.* 1991;99:956-962.

20. Kaplan LJ, Kellum JA. Initial pH, base deficit, lactate, anion gap, strong ion difference, and strong ion gap predict outcome from major vascular injury. *Crit Care Med.* 2004;32:1120-1124.

21. Husain FA, Martin MJ, Mullenix PS, Steele SR, Elliott DC. Serum lactate and base deficit as predictors of mortality and morbidity. *Am J Surg.* 2003;185:485-491.

22. Levy B, Gibot S, Franck P, Cravoisy A, Bollaert PE. Relation between muscle Na⁺K⁺ ATPase activity and raised lactate concentrations in septic shock: a prospective study. *Lancet.* 2005;365(9462):871-875.

23. Trzeciak S, Dellinger RP, Chansky ME, et al. Serum lactate as a predictor of mortality in patients with infection. *Intensive Care Med.* 2007;33:970-977.

24. Howell MD, Donnino M, Clardy P, Talmor D, Shapiro NI. Occult hypoperfusion and mortality in patients with suspected infection. *Intensive Care Med.* 2007;33:1892-1899.

25. Shapiro NI, Howell MD, Talmor D, et al. Serum lactate as a predictor of mortality in emergency department patients with infection. *Ann Emerg Med.* 2005;45:524-528.

26. Rivers EP, Coba V, Whitmill M. Early goal-directed therapy in severe sepsis and septic shock: a contemporary review of the literature. *Curr Opin Anaesthesiol.* 2008;21:128-140.

27. Puskarich MA, Marchick MR, Kline JA, Steuerwald MT, Jones AE. One year mortality of patients treated with an emergency department based early goal directed therapy protocol for severe sepsis and septic shock: a before and after study. *Crit Care.* 2009;13:R167.

28. Dellinger RP, Carlet JM, Masur H, et al. Surviving Sepsis Campaign guidelines for management of severe sepsis and septic shock. *Crit Care Med.* 2004;32:858-873.

29. Levy MM, Dellinger RP, Townsend SR, et al. The Surviving Sepsis Campaign: results of an international guideline-based performance improvement program targeting severe sepsis. *Crit Care Med.* 2010;38:367-374.

30. Barochia AV, Cui X, Vitberg D, et al. Bundled care for septic shock: an analysis of clinical trials. *Crit Care Med.* 2010;38:668-678.

31. Gao F, Melody T, Daniels DF, Giles S, Fox S. The impact of compliance with 6-hour and 24-hour sepsis bundles on hospital mortality in patients with severe sepsis: a prospective observational study. *Crit Care.* 2005;9:R764-R770.

32. Nguyen HB, Corbett SW, Steele R, et al. Implementation of a bundle of quality indicators for the early management of severe sepsis and septic shock is associated with decreased mortality. *Crit Care Med.* 2007;35:1105-1112.

33. Marshall JC, Cook DJ, Christou NV, Bernard GR, Sprung CL, Sibbald WJ. Multiple organ dysfunction score: a reliable descriptor of a complex clinical outcome. *Crit Care Med.* 1995;23:1638-1652.

34. Rivers E, Nguyen B, Havstad S, et al. Early goal-directed therapy in the treatment of severe sepsis and septic shock. *N Engl J Med.* 2001;345:1368-1377.

35. Jones AE, Brown MD, Trzeciak S, et al. The effect of a quantitative resuscitation strategy on mortality in patients with sepsis: a meta-analysis. *Crit Care Med.* 2008;36:2734-2739.

36. Roberts I, Alderson P, Bunn F, Chinnock P, Ker K, Schierhout G. Colloids versus crystalloids for fluid resuscitation in critically ill patients. *Cochrane Database Syst Rev.* 2004;(4):CD000567.

37. Vincent JL, Gerlach H. Fluid resuscitation in severe sepsis and septic shock: an evidence-based review. *Crit Care Med.* 2004;32(11 suppl):S451-S454.

38. Trof RJ, Sukul SP, Twisk JW, Girbes AR, Groeneveld AB. Greater cardiac response of colloid than saline fluid loading in septic and non-septic critically ill patients with clinical hypovolaemia. *Intensive Care Med.* 2010;36:697-701.

39. Hollenberg SM, Ahrens TS, Annane D, et al. Practice parameters for hemodynamic support of sepsis in adult patients: 2004 update. *Crit Care Med.* 2004;32:1928-1948.

40. Michard F, Boussat S, Chemla D, et al. Relation between respiratory changes in arterial pulse pressure and fluid responsiveness in septic patients with acute circulatory failure. *Am J Respir Crit Care Med.* 2000;162:134-138.

41. Michard F, Teboul JL. Predicting fluid responsiveness in ICU patients: a critical analysis of the evidence. *Chest.* 2002;121:2000-2008.

42. Dellinger RP, Levy MM, Carlet JM, et al. Surviving Sepsis Campaign: international guidelines for management of severe sepsis and septic shock: 2008. *Crit Care Med.* 2008;36:296-327.

43. Marik PE, Cavallazzi R, Vasu T, Hirani A. Dynamic changes in arterial waveform derived variables and fluid responsiveness in mechanically ventilated patients: a systematic review of the literature. *Crit Care Med.* 2009;37:2642-2647.

44. Heenen S, De BD, Vincent JL. How can the response to volume expansion in patients with spontaneous respiratory movements be predicted? *Crit Care.* 2006;10:R102.

45. Monnet X, Teboul JL. Passive leg raising. *Intensive Care Med.* 2008;34:659-663.

46. LeDoux D, Astiz ME, Carpati CM, Rackow EC. Effects of perfusion pressure on tissue perfusion in septic shock. *Crit Care Med.* 2000;28:2729-2732.

47. Kellum JA, Decker M. Use of dopamine in acute renal failure: a meta-analysis. *Crit Care Med.* 2001;29:1526-1531.

48. Russell JA, Walley KR, Singer J, et al. Vasopressin versus norepinephrine infusion in patients with septic shock. *N Engl J Med.* 2008;358:877-887.

49. Rady MY, Rivers EP, Nowak RM. Resuscitation of the critically ill in the ED: responses of blood pressure, heart rate, shock index, central venous oxygen saturation, and lactate. *Am J Emerg Med.* 1996;14:218-225.

50. Pope JV, Jones AE, Gaieski DF, Arnold RC, Trzeciak S, Shapiro NI. Multicenter study of central venous oxygen saturation (ScvO₂) as a predictor of mortality in patients with sepsis. *Ann Emerg Med.* 2010;55:40-46.

51. Castellanos-Ortega A, Suberviola B, Garcia-Astudillo LA, et al. Impact of the Surviving Sepsis Campaign protocols on hospital length of stay and mortality in septic shock patients: results of a three-year follow-up quasi-experimental study. *Crit Care Med.* 2010;38:1036-1043.

52. Bakker J, Gris P, Coffernils M, Kahn RJ, Vincent JL. Serial blood lactate levels can predict the development of multiple organ failure following septic shock. *Am J Surg:*1996;171:221-226.

53. Nguyen HB, Rivers EP, Knoblich BP, et al. Early lactate clearance is associated with improved outcome in severe sepsis and septic shock. *Crit Care Med.* 2004;32:1637-1642.

54. Jones AE, Shapiro NI, Trzeciak S, Arnold RC, Claremont HA, Kline JA. Lactate clearance vs central venous oxygen saturation as goals of early sepsis therapy: a randomized clinical trial. *JAMA.* 2010;303:739-746.

55. Parrillo JE, Burch C, Shelhamer JH, Parker MM, Natanson C, Schuette W. A circulating myocardial depressant substance in humans with septic shock: septic shock patients with a reduced ejection fraction have a circulating factor that depresses in vitro myocardial cell performance. *J Clin Invest.* 1985;76:1539-1553.

56. Jardin F, Fourme T, Page B, et al. Persistent preload defect in severe sepsis despite fluid loading: a longitudinal echocardiographic study in patients with septic shock. *Chest.* 1999;116:1354-1359.

57. Hebert PC, Wells G, Blajchman MA, et al. A multicenter, randomized, controlled clinical trial of transfusion requirements in critical care. Transfusion Requirements in Critical Care Investigators, Canadian Critical Care Trials Group. *N Engl J Med.* 1999;340:409-417.

58. Robertson CH Jr, Pagel MA, Johnson RL Jr. The distribution of blood flow, oxygen consumption, and work output among the respiratory muscles during unobstructed hyperventilation. *J Clin Invest.* 1977;59:43-50.

59. Hernandez G, Pena H, Cornejo R, et al. Impact of emergency intubation on central venous oxygen saturation in critically ill patients: a multicenter observational study. *Crit Care.* 2009;13:R63.

60. Freebairn RC, Derrick J, Gomersall CD, Young RJ, Joynt GM. Oxygen delivery, oxygen consumption, and gastric intramucosal pH are not improved by a computer-controlled, closed-loop, vecuronium infusion in severe sepsis and septic shock. *Crit Care Med.* 1997;25:72-77.

61. Gaieski DF, Mikkelsen ME, Band RA, et al. Impact of time to antibiotics on survival in patients with severe sepsis or septic shock in whom early goal-directed therapy was initiated in the emergency department. *Crit Care Med.* 2010;38:1045-1053.

62. Kumar A, Roberts D, Wood KE, et al. Duration of hypotension before initiation of effective antimicrobial therapy is the critical determinant of survival in human septic shock. *Crit Care Med.* 2006;34:1589-1596.

63. Ferrer R, Artigas A, Levy MM, et al. Improvement in process of care and outcome after a multicenter severe sepsis educational program in Spain. *JAMA.* 2008;299:2294-2303.

64. Kumar A, Ellis P, Arabi Y, et al. Initiation of inappropriate antimicrobial therapy results in a fivefold reduction of survival in human septic shock. *Chest.* 2009;136:1237-1248.

65. Briegel J, Sprung CL, Annane D, et al. Multicenter comparison of cortisol as measured by different methods in samples of patients with septic shock. *Intensive Care Med.* 2009;35:2151-2156.

66. Annane D, Sebille V, Charpentier C, et al. Effect of treatment with low doses of hydrocortisone and fludrocortisone on mortality in patients with septic shock. *JAMA.* 2002;288:862-871.

67. Sprung CL, Annane D, Keh D, et al. Hydrocortisone therapy for patients with septic shock. *N Engl J Med.* 2008;358:111-124.

68. Bernard GR, Vincent JL, Laterre PF, et al. Efficacy and safety of recombinant human activated protein C for severe sepsis. *N Engl J Med.* 2001;344:699-709.

69. Abraham E, Laterre PF, Garg R, et al. Drotrecogin alfa (activated) for adults with severe sepsis and a low risk of death. *N Engl J Med.* 2005;353:1332-1341.

70. Bernard GR, Margolis BD, Shanies HM, et al. Extended evaluation of recombinant human activated protein C United States Trial (ENHANCE US): a single-arm, phase 3B, multicenter study of drotrecogin alfa (activated) in severe sepsis. *Chest.* 2004;125:2206-2216.

71. Laupland KB, Kirkpatrick AW, Delaney A. Polyclonal intravenous immunoglobulin for the treatment of severe sepsis and septic shock in critically ill adults: a systematic review and meta-analysis. *Crit Care Med.* 2007;35:2686-2692.

72. Turgeon AF, Hutton B, Fergusson DA, et al. Meta-analysis: intravenous immunoglobulin in critically ill adult patients with sepsis. *Ann Intern Med.* 2007;146:193-203.

73. Norrby-Teglund A, Muller MP, Mcgeer A, et al. Successful management of severe group A streptococcal soft tissue infections using an aggressive medical regimen including intravenous polyspecific immunoglobulin together with a conservative surgical approach. *Scand J Infect Dis.* 2005;37:166-172.

74. Ventilation with lower tidal volumes as compared with traditional tidal volumes for acute lung injury and the acute respiratory distress syndrome. The Acute Respiratory Distress Syndrome Network. *N Engl J Med.* 2000;342:1301-1308.

75. Determann RM, Royakkers A, Wolthuis EK, et al. Ventilation with lower tidal volumes as compared with conventional tidal volumes for patients without acute lung injury: a preventive randomized controlled trial. *Crit Care.* 2010;14:R1.

76. Krinsley JS. Association between hyperglycemia and increased hospital mortality in a heterogeneous population of critically ill patients. *Mayo Clin Proc.* 2003;78:1471-1478.

77. Finfer S, Chittock DR, Su SY, et al. Intensive versus conventional glucose control in critically ill patients. *N Engl J Med.* 2009;360:1283-1297.

The Unstable Patient with Asthma or Chronic Obstructive Pulmonary Disease

Lillian L. Emlet

IN THIS CHAPTER

Clinical characteristics (similarities and differences) of exacerbations of severe acute asthma and chronic obstructive pulmonary disease (COPD)

Noninvasive positive-pressure ventilation in COPD exacerbation

Initiating mechanical ventilation in severe asthma and COPD

Troubleshooting and preventing lung injury of the mechanically ventilated patient with asthma or COPD

Introduction

Asthma afflicts 20 million people in the United States and accounts for one quarter of emergency department visits each year.[1–3] Fortunately, public health initiatives have improved patients' and physicians' understanding of asthma management and critical care has evolved, so that the mortality rate among asthmatics requiring ventilatory support has decreased.[4] Chronic obstructive pulmonary disease (COPD) is the fourth leading cause of death in the United States; despite technological advances, the mortality associated with this disease has increased.[5] There are significant similarities and differences in the spectrum of the clinical presentations of asthma and COPD (Tables 13-1 and 13-2).

Asthma is classically described as a severely reactive, reversible inflammatory process of large and medium-sized airways. The hallmark of asthma is airway hyperresponsiveness. Allergic inflammation mediated by mast cell IgE release activates macrophages, eosinophils, neutrophils, and lymphocytes.[6,7] Activation of cytokines (IL-1 to IL-5), tumor necrosis factor-α, interferon-γ, and granulocyte-macrophage colony-stimulating factor induces further proliferation of inflammatory cells, resulting in chronic inflammatory changes, including basement membrane thickening, bronchial smooth muscle hyperplasia, and loss of airway epithelium. Early asthma is characterized by wheezing and airflow obstruction from bronchial smooth muscle constriction and airway edema caused by mast cell histamine release. Late asthma is characterized by airflow obstruction and prolonged bronchospasm from increased airway mucus production and bronchial smooth muscle spasm caused by persistent cytokine and cellular activation. Chronic inflammation can result in airway remodeling, causing chronic irreversible airflow limitation.[8,9]

COPD is a progressive fixed obstruction with loss of elastic recoil of lung tissue, causing resting and dynamic lung hyperinflation and oxygen diffusion. Airflow limitation in COPD is progressive, not fully reversible, and is associated with an abnormal chronic inflammatory response.[10] Inflammation mediated by neutrophils, lymphocytes, and macrophages activates different mediators, resulting in cellular destruction of lung parenchyma in a centrilobular pattern. Scarring and narrowing occur in large and small airways, and increased goblet cells that secrete mucus contribute to mucus plugging and obstruction. Alveolar destruction results in hypoxia, causing thickened pulmonary vasculature, which results in pulmonary hypertension.

Patients with severe asthma and COPD can present with similar progressive ventilatory failure. Oxygenation usually remains preserved initially until enough alveoli are damaged.

COPD is characterized by neutrophilic infiltration, lack of airway hyperreactivity, lack of bronchodilator response, and lack of steroid response. Asthma is characterized by eosinophilic infiltration, airway hyperreactivity, response to bronchodilators, and response to steroids. Approximately 10% of patients have overlapping disease and are difficult to distinguish structurally, functionally, and clinically; they also have incompletely reversible disease.[11,12]

Clinical Presentation and Initial Treatment

Asthma

Coughing, wheezing, and dyspnea characterize acute asthma exacerbations. Persistently increased work of breathing causes restlessness, agitation, and diaphoresis. In the most severe airway obstruction, wheezing decreases or becomes absent. However, the character and degree of wheezing do not determine asthma severity. Although most patients are tachycardic and tachypneic, respiratory rate also does not determine asthma severity unless it is faster than 40 breaths/min. Peak flow meters allow measurement of the peak expiratory flow rate and estimation of the severity of asthma. These values are useful in determining response to treatment provided in the emergency department and therefore contribute to the decision to admit or discharge. Many critically ill asthmatic patients are unable to comply with testing because their speech is fragmented and their work of breathing is labored. Pulsus paradoxus, altered mental status, and bradypnea are late signs suggestive of impending respiratory failure.[13]

The mainstay in the treatment of acute severe asthma in the emergency department is the reversal of acute airflow obstruction. Although the most common treatment is administration of racemic albuterol, comparative studies of levalbuterol and albuterol suggest that levalbuterol may improve pulmonary function longer and to a greater extent, especially in patients who have maximized home nebulizer treatments with racemic albuterol.[14–18] Either drug can be used in emergent therapy. Side effects of β-agonists include tachycardia, tremor, and a slight decrease in serum potassium. For extremely severe cases refractory to β-agonists, 0.25 mg of terbutaline or 0.3 mL of a 1:1,000 concentration of epinephrine can be administered subcutaneously. Helium blended with oxygen (60%–80% helium with 40%–20% oxygen) can reduce resistance from nonlaminar flow and increases diffusion of carbon dioxide, theoretically reducing the work of breathing until bronchodilation has occurred. However, no published reports suggest that heliox reduces the need for intubation or mortality. Noninvasive positive-pressure ventilation (NPPV) can also be beneficial in selected cases.

Diagnostic tests are of limited utility with severe asthma, but they are often performed. Routine laboratory measurements such as a complete blood count, basic metabolic panel, and electrolytes are not helpful, either. The decision to intubate is based on clinical assessment. Arterial blood gases (ABGs) can be helpful if hypercarbia is suspected, but they usually show normal values or respiratory alkalosis. An elevated lactate level is not predictive of the severity of near-fatal asthma. Chest radiographs can rule out superimposed pneumothorax or pneumomediastinum.

Near-fatal asthma exacerbations are generally of two clinical presentations: slow onset and rapid onset. Slow-onset near-fatal asthma presents as chronic poorly controlled asthma with gradual deterioration over several days. Rapid-onset near-fatal asthma presents as rapidly progressive hypercapnic respiratory failure.[19]

COPD

Worsening dyspnea and increased sputum volume and purulence characterize acute COPD exacerbations. Viral or bacterial infections and environmental factors are implicated in many

---

TABLE 13-1.

Severe asthma (forced expiratory volume in 1 minute [FEV$_1$] <1 L) presentation and treatment

Presentation
- Heart rate >120 beats/min
- Respiratory rate >40 breaths/min
- Pulsus paradoxus (>10 mm Hg difference)
- Accessory muscle use
- ABG Pao$_2$ <60 mm Hg
- ABG Paco$_2$ >42 mm Hg
- Peak expiratory flow rate <50% or inability to perform

Initial Treatment
- Oxygen
- Nebulized β-agonist
  - Levalbuterol, 1.25 mg every 30 min × 3 doses or continuous
  - Racemic albuterol, 2.5–5 mg every 20–30 min or continuous 10 mg in 70 mL normal saline
- Nebulized anticholinergic
  - Ipratropium, 0.5 mg every 20–30 min × 3 doses
- Corticosteroids
  - Prednisone, 60 mg orally
  - Methylprednisolone, 60–125 mg IV (or equivalent)
- Magnesium sulfate, 2–3 g IV over 20 min
- Heliox (60%–80% helium blend with 40%–20% oxygen)

TABLE 13-2.

Severe COPD (FEV$_1$ <30% predicted) presentation and treatment

Presentation
- Respiratory rate >35 breaths/min
- Dyspnea
- Accessory muscle use (abdominal muscles)
- Confusion, somnolence

Initial Treatment
- Controlled oxygen (goal oxygen saturation 90%)
- Nebulized β-agonist with anticholinergic
  - Racemic albuterol, 2.5 mg every 20–30 min or
  - Ipratropium, 0.5 mg every 20–30 min × 3 doses
- Methylprednisolone, 60–125 mg IV (or equivalent)
- Consider antibiotic therapy for chronic bronchitis or pneumonia
- Early application of NPPV

COPD exacerbations, but as many as one third cannot be linked to an inciting factor. COPD typically shows slow and progressive debilitation until cor pulmonale and significant functional limitation are present. Patients with COPD can be stratified on a continuum between chronic obstructive bronchitis and chronic emphysema. Cough, bronchial secretions, and polycythemia mark the progression to ventilation failure, chronic carbon dioxide retention, and cor pulmonale in patients with chronic obstructive bronchitis. Chronic emphysema presents as tachypneic, dyspneic, pursed-lip breathing with hyperinflation, flattened diaphragm, and relatively preserved oxygenation without carbon dioxide retention.

The mainstay of treatment for COPD exacerbation in the emergency department is support of impaired ventilation. Immediate airway support with endotracheal intubation and mechanical ventilation is necessary for the cyanotic, gasping, or unconscious patient in ventilatory failure. Fortunately, many patients arrive with progressive dyspnea, so there is opportunity for NPPV with continuous positive airway pressure (CPAP) or bilevel positive airway pressure (BiPAP) ventilation via full-face or nasal mask. Patient selection for NPPV over intubation remains somewhat subjective regarding who will benefit. An absolute contraindication to NPPV is the inability to be cooperative and to protect the airway. In various studies and systematic reviews, both CPAP and BiPAP have been shown to reduce mortality, the need for intubation, and the length of hospital stay.[20–26]

Pharmacologic treatment of COPD exacerbations centers on bronchodilators, corticosteroids, antibiotics, and NPPV. Most COPD exacerbations (78%) are caused by viral and bacterial infections; environmental changes can trigger them as well.[27] Inhaled and systemic steroids and β-agonists reduce inflammation, the severity of exacerbations, morbidity, and mortality.[28,29] The administration of antibiotics, guided by local resistance patterns and clinical strategies, is indicated in patients with purulent sputum.[10,30–32] In moderate to severe exacerbations with risk factors for poor outcome, the increasing drug resistance of

Streptococcus pneumoniae, Haemophilus influenzae, and *Moraxella catarrhalis* should be considered, suggesting that first-line antibiotics should include coverage against *Klebsiella pneumoniae, Escherichia coli, Proteus, Enterobacter,* and *Pseudomonas aeruginosa.* Best choices include β-lactam and fluoroquinolones with activity against *Pseudomonas* and second- and third-generation cephalosporins.[31,33,34]

Clinical Decision for Airway Support

The decision to intubate for severe asthma remains primarily a clinical decision, preferably made earlier rather than later in the clinical course in the emergency department. Aggressive intervention with intravenous steroids and inhaled continuous bronchodilators remains the mainstay of treatment. Adjunctive therapies for those without impending respiratory failure include heliox, intravenous magnesium sulfate, and leukotriene inhibitors. The utility of peak flow measurements in severe asthma is limited.

In the past decade, NPPV has become accepted as an early intervention for severe COPD exacerbations.[22,35–38] Early application of NPPV, which includes BiPAP and CPAP, by a prehospital or emergency department care provider experienced in its use has been shown to be efficacious, to prevent intubation, and to reduce morbidity. Controversy remains on patient selection for NPPV. The greatest benefit is seen in patients with moderate to severe ventilation failure; endotracheal intubation is preferred for respiratory arrest. Contraindications to the procedure are listed in Table 13-3.

KEY POINT

Early airway and ventilation support for severe asthma

- Early application of NPPV is effective in preventing intubation and reducing morbidity.
- The decision to intubate is a clinical decision, preferably made earlier rather than later.

A good response to NPPV will be evident by a decrease in work of breathing (resolution of abdominal and accessory muscle use, cessation of diaphoresis) and improvement of vital sign abnormalities such as tachycardia, hypertension, and tachypnea. Most modern machines provide measurement of exhaled tidal volume, calculate minute ventilation, and sound alarms for mask leaks. ABG measurement can assist but is not mandatory in assessing the response to NPPV. Improvement in clinical examination findings (ie, improved mental status and work of breathing) will become evident within 1 hour after initiation of treatment. Failure to see improvements in vital signs, mental status, and work of breathing within that time frame suggests the need for endotracheal intubation.

KEY POINT

Failure to see improvements in vital signs, mental status, and work of breathing within 1 hour after initiation of NPPV suggests the need for endotracheal intubation.

TABLE 13-3.

Contraindications to noninvasive positive-pressure ventilation

Absolute
- Severe agitation
- Severely altered mental status
- Copious secretions
- Vomiting
- Hemoptysis or hematemesis
- Cardiac or respiratory arrest
- Upper airway obstruction
- Apnea
- Patient intolerance

Relative
- Uncooperative but redirectable patient
- Hemodynamic instability
- Pregnancy
- Recent upper gastrointestinal surgical anastomosis

Intubation of Asthmatic and COPD Patients

Asthmatic patients with severe hypoxemia or acidemia should be intubated prior to respiratory failure (Table 13-4). Two percent of patients with asthma exacerbation require endotracheal intubation and mechanical ventilatory support. Rapid sequence induction (RSI) provides the safest method to secure the airway. For induction, ketamine (1.5 mg/kg IV), a phencyclidine derivative that provides bronchial smooth muscle relaxation and bronchodilation, is the agent of choice for severe asthma. Propofol (1.5 mg/kg IV in a euvolemic patient) is an alternative agent that also provides bronchodilation. Paralytic choices include depolarizing and nondepolarizing neuromuscular blockers. When using succinylcholine (1.5 mg/kg IV), vigilance is required for hyperkalemia, rhabdomyolysis, and arrhythmia side effects. A smooth, controlled elective airway experience provided to the anxious patient with severe asthma is important for prevention of further air trapping and bronchospasm.

PEARL
RSI in the unstable patient with asthma/COPD

- Ketamine, 1.5 mg/kg IV, or etomidate, 0.3 mg/kg IV
- Succinylcholine, 1.5 mg/kg IV, or rocuronium, 1 mg/kg IV

Many patients with severe COPD requiring intubation exhibit altered mental status from hypercarbic respiratory failure or agitation from increased work of breathing. RSI is the safest method to secure the airway, although some patients may be so obtunded from respiratory acidosis that sedation only or no drugs may be adequate. For cardiovascular reasons, etomidate (0.3 mg/kg IV) is the preferred drug for COPD patients, who frequently have coexisting cardiac disease and pulmonary hypertension.[39]

Confirmation of endotracheal tube placement with end-tidal carbon dioxide detectors is important. Breath sounds can be quite distant or absent in patients with severe bronchospasm and air trapping, making confirmation via auscultation difficult. Excessive or aggressive bag-valve-mask ventilation immediately following endotracheal tube placement can cause air trapping, sometimes significant enough to cause hemodynamic instability from increased intrathoracic pressure caused by severe intrinsic positive end-expiratory pressure (PEEP), resulting in bradycardia, hypotension, and asystole.

KEY POINT
Caution with ventilation after intubation

- Watch the frequency, rate, and force of bag-valve-mask ventilation following endotracheal tube placement, as air trapping can cause hemodynamic instability, seen as bradycardia, hypotension, hypoxia, and asystole.

Ventilatory Support of COPD Patients

Severe COPD exacerbations are characterized by primary ventilatory failure and subsequent hypoxemia and atelectasis. NPPV started in the emergency department has been shown to reduce the need for intubation, thereby reducing cost, complications, and mortality.[22,35,40–46] CPAP increases alveolar recruitment and improves ventilation-perfusion matching, while BiPAP uses two levels of CPAP to provide additional support for respiratory muscle work. Extrinsic PEEP, or expiratory positive airway pressure (EPAP), is set above intrinsic PEEP, or inspiratory positive airway pressure (IPAP), in order to provide the minute ventilation required to reverse the hypercarbic respiratory failure of COPD. IPAP can be set high (20–25 cm H_2O) and then decreased to optimal patient comfort and tidal volume, or it can be set lower (8–10 cm H_2O) and then gradually increased to relieve dyspnea and assist ventilation. Increasing the difference between IPAP and EPAP essentially increases

TABLE 13-4.
Clinical markers for elective intubation

Severe Asthma	Severe COPD
Impending respiratory failure • Decreasing level of consciousness • Confusion, agitation • Exhaustion	Unable to tolerate NPPV • Failure of improvement of respiratory acidosis with brief trial of NPPV
Work of breathing • Weak breathing efforts • "Silent chest"	Severe life-threatening hypoxemia
Hypercapnia and respiratory acidosis	Somnolence, impaired mental status with inability to protect airway
Hypoxemia and cyanosis (oxygen saturation <90%)	Respiratory arrest
Cardiovascular • Hypotension • Arrhythmia	Multisystem organ collapse • Cardiovascular hypotension/shock • Distributive/septic shock • Pulmonary complications (pneumonia, pleural effusion, empyema, pulmonary embolism, pneumothorax)

ventilation, and assessment of adequacy requires vigilance to tidal volume, mask fit, minute ventilation, ABG levels, and neurologic status.[47–49] Close observation by the physician and respiratory therapist for response to NPPV is needed during the first 1 to 2 hours, making NPPV slightly more labor intensive but certainly feasible for initiation and monitoring in the emergency department.[50]

Mechanical Ventilation in the Emergency Department

Mechanical ventilation of the patient with severe asthma requires careful attention to treatment of the primary problem—dynamic hyperinflation—and prevention of ventilator trauma. Severe asthma is primarily a resistance problem of medium to large airways, with obstruction caused by mucus plugging and bronchospasm. COPD is primarily a problem of inflammation, resulting in protease-mediated destruction of elastin connective tissue of lung parenchyma, leading to peripheral airway narrowing and air trapping.

Permissive hypercapnia, or controlled hypoventilation, is the primary modality for mechanically ventilating asthmatics.

Volume cycle ventilation with low respiratory rate (<10 breaths/min), low tidal volume (6 mL/kg), and normal to low PEEP produces respiratory acidosis that is well tolerated. Hypercarbia to values as high as a $Paco_2$ of 80 mm Hg and acidosis to a pH as low as 7.15 typically do not cause deleterious effects. Adequate time for exhalation is achieved with a low respiratory rate and setting the tidal volume for permissive hypercapnia; increased inspiratory flow times will also allow greater time for exhalation. Inspiratory flow is usually set at 60 L/min for normal minute ventilation of normal patients. Asthmatic patients usually require 80 to 100 L/min for inspiratory flow, as this will allow a longer time for exhalation.

Sedation of the intubated patient with severe asthma is vitally important to allow patient–ventilator synchrony and prevent breath stacking and further air trapping. Deep sedation provided by benzodiazepines and propofol via continuous infusion allows ease in mechanical ventilation and prevents further barotrauma. Ventilator peak pressure alarms require assessment of airway resistance problems versus airway compliance problems. Peak pressure alarms are the most common ventilator alarm encountered, requiring troubleshooting of causes, including moisture in ventilator tubing; mucus plugging; worsening bronchospasm; kinked tubing; an endotracheal tube that is too small, requiring higher inspiratory flow rates; or high set tidal volumes. Deepening sedation often helps, although some patients require paralytics to tolerate safe mechanical ventilation. However, avoiding neuromuscular blockade is ideal unless paralysis is absolutely necessary, as the combination of steroids and a paralytic significantly increases the incidence of critical illness polyneuropathy.

Complications of positive-pressure ventilation include hypotension and barotrauma. Most patients are relatively hypovolemic because of the gradually increasing intrathoracic trapped pressure combined with decreased enteral intake, reduction of work of breathing, and catecholamine drive after endotracheal intubation. Hypotension can be mitigated by administering fluid boluses ahead of the RSI. If hypotension persists despite intravenous fluids, phenylephrine can be administered (20 mg in 250 mL of normal saline mixed, drawn up in a 10-mL syringe; each 1–2 mL of 80–160 mcg can be given in a peripheral intravenous line). The most significant barotrauma complication is pneumothorax, which should be in the differential diagnosis during any desaturation, persistent unexplained agitation, or high peak pressure alarm.

Similar to ventilation of the asthmatic patient, prevention of barotrauma with low tidal volume, low respiratory rate, and long expiratory times constitutes the mainstay of ventilating patients with COPD. Unlike asthmatics, many patients with COPD can be mechanically ventilated with relatively low sedation on modes of ventilation that are spontaneous, such as pressure support, and newer modes (proportional-assist ventilation or neural-assist ventilation) designed to improve patient–ventilator synchrony.[51,52] Adequate attention to ventilator waveforms allows assessment of air trapping (auto-PEEP) or breath stacking—two common, preventable causes of barotrauma. Modern ventilators provide a variety of combinations of waveforms, of which flow-time and volume-time can be used to assess synchrony. Air trapping is best seen in the flow-time waveform, where the flow in exhalation does not return to baseline, resulting in auto-PEEP (Figure 13-1).

Breath stacking is seen in the volume-time or pressure-time waveforms, where another tidal volume breath is initiated before full exhalation has occurred. Breath stacking will eventually result in increased residual volume, worsening air trapping. Subsequently, the patient begins to have difficulty triggering the ventilator and an increased work of breathing, clinically seen as agitation and abdominal breathing.

In summary, severe air trapping and ventilatory failure characterize asthma and COPD. Early treatment with bronchodilation to improve air flow, administration of corticosteroids to reduce inflammation, and use of appropriate ventilatory support to unload respiratory muscle work are the primary goals of treatment. Patients with severe acute asthma will benefit from early control of the airway, deep sedation to tolerate mechanical ventilation, and prevention of ventilator-induced barotrauma and patient–ventilator dyssynchrony. Patients with severe COPD will benefit from early application of NPPV combined with systemic and inhaled steroids, bronchodilators, and antibiotics when warranted.

KEY POINTS

Prevention of ventilator injury in asthma and COPD

- Low tidal volume (6 mL/kg ideal body weight)
- Low respiratory rate
- Use permissive hypercapnia.
- Check for auto-PEEP with end-expiratory pause maneuver.
- Check peak and plateau pressures with end-inspiratory pause maneuver.
- Provide adequate sedation.
- Minimize oxygen free radical toxicity by using minimal F_{IO_2} (35%–40%).

Conclusion

Critically ill emergency department patients with acute exacerbations of asthma or COPD are some of the most challenging patients to treat. Mismanaged medical and ventilator (invasive and noninvasive) therapy can quickly lead to increased morbidity and mortality. For patients with acute exacerbations of

asthma, early bronchodilator and steroid therapy are indicated, with consideration of heliox, magnesium, and intubation with mechanical support for respiratory failure. For patients with acute exacerbations of COPD, early use of NPPV combined with steroids, bronchodilators, and possible antibiotics are the mainstays of emergency department therapy. For both asthma and COPD, it is crucial to prevent ventilator-induced lung injury through the use of permissive hypercapnia, attention to patient–ventilator synchrony, and prevention of barotrauma.

References

1. Environmental Protection Agency. Asthma Facts, 2010. Available at www.epa.gov/asthma/pdfs/asthma_fact_sheet_en.pdf. Accessed on June 3, 2010.
2. National Center for Environmental Health. Asthma at a Glance. Centers for Disease Control and Prevention, 1999. Available at www.cdc.gov/nchs/fastats/asthma.htm. Accessed on June 3, 2010.
3. Moorman JE, Rudd RA, Johnson CA, et al. National surveillance for asthma—United States, 1980–2004. *MMWR Surveill Summ.* 2007;56(SS08);154.
4. Kearney S, Graham D, Atherton S. Acute severe asthma treated by mechanical ventilation: a comparison of the changing characteristics over a 17 yr period. *Respir Med.* 1998;92(5):716-721.
5. Seneff MG, Wagner DP, Wagner RP, Zimmerman JE, Knaus WA. Hospital and 1-year survival of patients admitted to intensive care units with acute exacerbation of chronic obstructive pulmonary disease. *JAMA.* 1995;274(23):1852-1857.
6. McFadden ER. Acute severe asthma. *Am J Respir Crit Care Med.* 2003;168:740-759.
7. Wark PAB, Gibson PG. Asthma exacerbations. 3: pathogenesis. *Thorax.* 2006;61:909-915.
8. Elias J, Zhu Z, Chupp G, Homer R. Airway remodeling in asthma. *J Clin Invest.* 1999;104:1001-1006.
9. Fabbri LM, Caramori G, Beghé B, Papi A, Ciaccia A. Physiologic consequences of long-term inflammation. *Am J Respir Crit Care Med.* 1998;157(5 Pt 2):S195-198.
10. Global Initiative for Chronic Obstructive Lung Disease (GOLD). *Global Strategy for the Diagnosis, Management, and Prevention of Chronic Obstructive Pulmonary Disease,* 2009. Available at www.goldcopd.com. Accessed on June 4, 2010.
11. Barnes P. Mechanisms in COPD: differences from asthma. *Chest.* 2000;117(2 suppl):10S-14S.
12. Sciurba FC. Physiologic similarities and differences between COPD and asthma. *Chest.* 2004;126(2 suppl):117S-124S; discussion 159S-161S.
13. Hodder R, Lougheed MD, Fitzgerald JM, Rowe BH, Kaplan AG, McIvor RA. Management of acute asthma in adults in the emergency department: assisted ventilation. *CMAJ.* 2010;182:265-272.
14. Ameredes BT, Calhoun WJ. Levalbuterol versus albuterol. *Curr Allergy Asthma Rep.* 2009;9:401-409.
15. Dalonzo GE. Levalbuterol in the treatment of patients with asthma and chronic obstructive lung disease. *J Am Osteopath Assoc.* 2004;104:288-293.
16. Nowak R. Single-isomer levalbuterol: a review of the acute data. *Curr Allergy Asthma Rep.* 2003;3:172-178.
17. Nowak R, Emerman C, Hanrahan JP, et al. A comparison of levalbuterol with racemic albuterol in the treatment of acute severe asthma exacerbations in adults. *Am J Emerg Med.* 2006;24:259-267.
18. Truitt T, Witko J, Halpern M. Levalbuterol compared to racemic albuterol: efficacy and outcomes in patients hospitalized with COPD or asthma. *Chest.* 2003;123:128-135.
19. Molfino NA, Slutsky AS. Near-fatal asthma. *Eur Respir J.* 1994;7:981-990.
20. Confalonieri M, Parigi P, Scartabellati A, et al. Noninvasive mechanical ventilation improves the immediate and long-term outcome of COPD patients with acute respiratory failure. *Eur Respir J.* 1996;9:422-430.
21. Conti G, Antonelli M, Navalesi P, et al. Noninvasive vs. conventional mechanical ventilation in patients with chronic obstructive pulmonary disease after failure of medical treatment in the ward: a randomized trial. *Intensive Care Med.* 2002;28:1701-1707.
22. Keenan SP, Sinuff T, Cook DJ, Hill NS. Which patients with acute exacerbation of chronic obstructive pulmonary disease benefit from noninvasive positive-pressure ventilation? A systematic review of the literature. *Ann Intern Med.* 2003;138:861-870.
23. Peter JV, Moran JL, Phillips-Hughes J, Warn D. Noninvasive ventilation in acute respiratory failure—a meta-analysis update. *Crit Care Med.* 2002;30:555-562.
24. Ram FSF, Picot J, Lightowler J, Wedzicha JA. Non-invasive positive pressure ventilation for treatment of respiratory failure due to exacerbations of chronic obstructive pulmonary disease. *Cochrane Database Syst Rev.* 2004(3):CD004104.
25. Sinuff T, Cook DJ, Randall J, Allen CJ. Evaluation of a practice guideline for noninvasive positive-pressure ventilation for acute respiratory failure. *Chest.* 2003;123:2062-2073.
26. Sinuff T, Keenan SP; Department of Medicine, McMaster University. Clinical practice guideline for the use of noninvasive positive pressure ventilation in COPD patients with acute respiratory failure. *J Crit Care.* 2004;19:82-91.

FIGURE 13-1.

Flow-time waveform, showing that flow in exhalation does not return to baseline, resulting in auto-PEEP

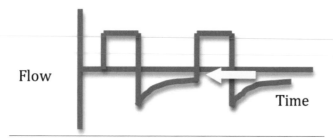

Flow

Time

27. Papi A, Bellettato CM, Braccioni F, et al. Infections and airway inflammation in chronic obstructive pulmonary disease severe exacerbations. *Am J Respir Crit Care Med.* 2006;173:1114-1121.

28. Macie C, Wooldrage K, Manfreda J, Anthonisen NR. Inhaled corticosteroids and mortality in COPD. *Chest.* 2006;130:640-646.

29. Sin DD, Wu L, Anderson JA, et al. Inhaled corticosteroids and mortality in chronic obstructive pulmonary disease. *Thorax.* 2005;60:992-997.

30. Allegra L, Blasi F, de Bernardi B, et al. Antibiotic treatment and baseline severity of disease in acute exacerbations of chronic bronchitis: a re-evaluation of previously published data of a placebo-controlled randomized study. *Pulm Pharmacol Ther.* 2001;14:149-155.

31. Celli BR, Macnee W, Force AET. Standards for the diagnosis and treatment of patients with COPD: a summary of the ATS/ERS position paper. *Eur Respir J.* 2004;23:932-946.

32. Nouira S, Marghli S, Belghith M, et al. Once daily oral ofloxacin in chronic obstructive pulmonary disease exacerbation requiring mechanical ventilation: a randomised placebo-controlled trial. *Lancet.* 2001;358(9298):2020-2025.

33. Sethi S, Evans N, Grant BJB, Murphy TF. New strains of bacteria and exacerbations of chronic obstructive pulmonary disease. *N Engl J Med.* 2002;347(7):465-471.

34. Woodhead M, Blasi F, Ewig S, et al. Guidelines for the management of adult lower respiratory tract infections. *Eur Respir J.* 2005;26:1138-1180.

35. Brochard L, Mancebo J, Wysocki M, et al. Noninvasive ventilation for acute exacerbations of chronic obstructive pulmonary disease. *N Engl J Med.* 1995;333(13):817-822.

36. British Thoracic Society Standards of Care Committee. Non-invasive ventilation in acute respiratory failure. *Thorax.* 2002;57:192-211.

37. Evans TW. International Consensus Conferences in Intensive Care Medicine: non-invasive positive pressure ventilation in acute respiratory failure. Organised jointly by the American Thoracic Society, the European Respiratory Society, the European Society of Intensive Care Medicine, and the Société de Réanimation de Langue Française, and approved by the ATS Board of Directors, December 2000. *Intensive Care Med.* 2001;27:166-178.

38. Mehta S, Hill NS. Noninvasive ventilation. *Am J Respir Crit Care Med.* 2001;163:540-577.

39. Walls RM, Murphy MF. *Manual of Emergency Airway Management.* 3rd ed. Philadelphia, PA: Lippincott Williams & Wilkins; 2008.

40. Bott J, Carroll MP, Conway JH, et al. Randomised controlled trial of nasal ventilation in acute ventilatory failure due to chronic obstructive airways disease. *Lancet.* 1993;341(8860):1555-1557.

41. Kramer N, Meyer TJ, Meharg J, et al. Randomized, prospective trial of noninvasive positive pressure ventilation in acute respiratory failure. *Am J Respir Crit Care Med.* 1995;151:1799-1806.

42. Meyer TJ, Hill NS. Noninvasive positive pressure ventilation to treat respiratory failure. *Ann Intern Med.* 1994;120:760-770.

43. International Consensus Conferences in Intensive Care Medicine. Noninvasive positive pressure ventilation in acute respiratory failure. *Am J Respir Crit Care Med.* 2001;163:283-291.

44. Plant PK, Owen JL, Elliott MW. Early use of non-invasive ventilation for acute exacerbations of chronic obstructive pulmonary disease on general respiratory wards: a multicentre randomised controlled trial. *Lancet.* 2000;355(9219):1931-1935.

45. Pollack C, Torres MT, Alexander L. Feasibility study of the use of bilevel positive airway pressure for respiratory support in the emergency department. *Ann Emerg Med.* 1996;27:189-192.

46. Yeow M-E, Santanilla JI. Noninvasive positive pressure ventilation in the emergency department. *Emerg Med Clin North Am.* 2008;26:835-847.

47. Díaz GG, Alcaraz AC, Talavera JCP, et al. Noninvasive positive-pressure ventilation to treat hypercapnic coma secondary to respiratory failure. *Chest.* 2005;127:952-960.

48. Scala R, Naldi M, Archinucci I, et al. Noninvasive positive pressure ventilation in patients with acute exacerbations of COPD and varying levels of consciousness. *Chest.* 2005;128:1657-1666.

49. Scala R, Nava S, Conti G, et al. Noninvasive versus conventional ventilation to treat hypercapnic encephalopathy in chronic obstructive pulmonary disease. *Intensive Care Med.* 2007;33:2101-2108.

50. Hill NS. Noninvasive ventilation for chronic obstructive pulmonary disease. *Respir Care.* 2004;49:72-89.

51. Gay PC, Hess DR, Hill NS. Noninvasive proportional assist ventilation for acute respiratory insufficiency. Comparison with pressure support ventilation. *Am J Respir Crit Care Med.* 2001;164:1606-1611.

52. Wysocki M, Richard J-C, Meshaka P. Noninvasive proportional assist ventilation compared with noninvasive pressure support ventilation in hypercapnic acute respiratory failure. *Crit Care Med.* 2002;30:323-329.

CHAPTER 14

The Critically Ill Poisoned Patient

Daniel M. Lugassy and Fermin Barrueto, Jr.

IN THIS CHAPTER

Approach to the critically ill poisoned patient

Gastrointestinal decontamination

ACLS/cardiorespiratory acute toxicology
Acute arrhythmias
Antihypertensive overdose

Neuromuscular toxicology
Toxin-induced seizures
Hyperthermic syndromes
Cholinergic crisis

Severe/increasing anion gap acidosis
Cyanide
Toxic alcohols

Introduction

Caring for the critically ill poisoned patient in the emergency department can be extremely challenging, gratifying, and frustrating all at once. The sickest patients arrive without the ability to communicate and have no family members or friends accompanying them to provide clues to recent events or medical history. We must use our skills of physical diagnosis, electrocardiographic analysis, and laboratory interpretation to piece together a unifying diagnosis. Although most poisoned patients do well with general supportive care, in some instances supportive care is inadequate or potentially harmful. This chapter reviews several clinical toxicologic scenarios that require immediate, specific, and appropriate intervention.

Assessment, Physical Examination, and Monitoring

The approach to all critically ill poisoned patients begins with aggressive care. Establishing intravenous access, providing supplemental oxygen, monitoring vital signs and pulse oximetry, stabilizing the ABCs, and obtaining a bedside glucose measurement and ECG are all critical actions. A thorough but brief physical examination should be performed and must include close examination of the skin (color, dry, diaphoretic), oral and respiratory secretions, reflexes, eyes (ocular clonus or nystagmus), muscle tone, bowel sounds, and bladder size. A constellation of symptoms can point to a toxidrome and lead to a diagnosis.

For routine low-risk exposures, a minimal laboratory assessment includes a basic metabolic panel and measurement of liver enzyme levels. In addition, the serum acetaminophen concentration should be checked in any patient who reports ingestion of that compound. Even among patients who report no ingestion of products containing acetaminophen, 1 in 500 will have a concentration warranting antidotal therapy.[1] Urine toxicology screens are often ordered, but their results are inconsistent, yielding many false positives and negatives, and their results rarely alter management.[2] No clinical scenario discussed in this chapter will benefit from a routine urine drug screen.

When assessing a critically ill poisoned patient, early consultation with a poison control center or local medical toxicologist can provide useful guidance regarding current management strategies.

Gastrointestinal Decontamination

Not long ago, patients with toxic ingestions routinely received syrup of ipecac to induce emesis as well as gastric lavage and activated charcoal. Syrup of ipecac is no longer indicated[3] and has been removed from almost all clinical settings. The instillation of a single dose of activated charcoal has yet to show significant improvement in morbidity or mortality rates, and its use can be complicated by aspiration, leading to life-threatening chemical pneumonitis.[4] Charcoal is contraindicated in caustic ingestions, as it will obscure the visualization of the esophagus and gastrointestinal (GI) tract during endoscopy. Data regarding the benefit of orogastric lavage in poisoned patients are limited and controversial.[5,6] There appears to be a benefit if the procedure is performed within 1 hour after ingestion for severe, or potentially severe, exposures.[5]

Despite limited clinical evidence, GI decontamination should be considered when the suspected toxicity carries a high risk of morbidity and mortality and in critically ill patients who are displaying severe and life-threatening symptoms. This chapter focuses on poisonings associated with the highest mortality—the patients who have the greatest potential to benefit from GI decontamination. Early consultation with a medical toxicologist will assist with decision making regarding the administration of charcoal and the use of gastric lavage or whole bowel irrigation (WBI).

KEY POINT

Despite limited clinical evidence, GI decontamination should be considered when the suspected toxicity carries a high risk of morbidity and mortality and in critically ill patients who are displaying severe and life-threatening symptoms.

Cardiopulmonary Support

Acute Arrhythmias

In the evaluation of a critically ill poisoned patient, the electrocardiogram (ECG) can provide vital clues and indicate the need for emergent antidotal treatment. Several key features of the ECG must be examined closely: QRS prolongation (wide complex tachycardia) caused by sodium channel blockade, torsade de pointes/QT interval prolongation, and arrhythmias induced by digoxin/cardioactive steroids.

QRS Prolongation/Wide Complex Tachycardia

Widened QRS complexes and a rightward axis on an ECG can represent cardiotoxicity from drugs that induce Vaughan Williams type IA antiarrhythmia or have a quinidine-like effect (amantadine, cocaine, diphenhydramine, quinine, tricyclic antidepressants).[7] Through blockade of fast-acting sodium channels of the His-Purkinje system and ventricular myocardium, a delay in depolarization (at phase 0 of the action potential) results in widening of the QRS complex. Clinically, patients with type IA poisoning have decreased inotropy and cardiac output, which manifests as severe hypotension or life-threatening arrhythmias.[8]

Wide complex tachycardias caused by toxins can be difficult to distinguish from true ventricular tachycardia (VT) and other mimics such as hyperkalemia, atrial fibrillation with bundle-branch block, and supraventricular tachycardia (SVT) with aberrancy.[9] Figure 14-1 demonstrates ECG findings suggestive of cardiotoxicity from type IA drugs as follows: tachycardia, a QRS complex greater than 100 msec, terminal 40-msec changes (R' in aVR, S in I and aVL), right bundle-branch block,

---

FIGURE 14-1.

Tricyclic antidepressant poisoning, QRS 148 msec. Note deep S wave in I and aVL and R' wave in aVR.

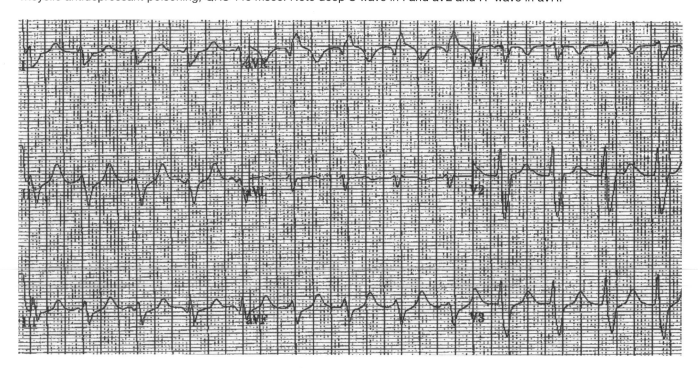

and right axis deviation. These cardiotoxic effects are often seen in patients with tricyclic antidepressant overdose.[10] A variety of other toxins produce similar sodium channel blocking effects, and each displays unique clinical symptoms. For example, acute cocaine intoxication and diphenhydramine overdose present with contrasting sympathomimetic and anticholinergic toxidromes, respectively, but they both carry type IA cardiotoxicity that causes wide complex tachycardia.

Emergent treatment is indicated for patients who manifest ECG signs of type IA toxicity along with hypotension or life-threatening arrhythmias (Table 14-1). Toxin-induced wide complex arrhythmias can be refractory to traditional therapies such as electrical cardioversion, adenosine, and amiodarone.[11] Sodium bicarbonate provides extracellular sodium that can overcome the sodium channel blockade. A bolus of sodium bicarbonate at a dose of 1 or 2 mEq/kg should be given.[9] The ECG must be monitored continuously while sodium bicarbonate is administered to observe for narrowing of the QRS complex (which can narrow and then lengthen within moments after initiation of treatment). The end point of treatment should be QRS narrowing, with improvement in blood pressure and cessation of arrhythmia. Patients who respond to a bolus of sodium bicarbonate may be placed on a continuous infusion. Severely poisoned patients receiving a continuous infusion of sodium bicarbonate can require additional boluses if the QRS widening persists. The serum pH must be monitored to maintain a safe level of less than 7.55.[8,9]

KEY POINT

The end point of treatment should be QRS narrowing, with improvement in blood pressure and cessation of arrhythmia. Patients who respond to a bolus of sodium bicarbonate may be placed on a continuous infusion.

PEARL

Toxin-induced wide complex arrhythmias can be refractory to traditional therapies such as electrical cardioversion, adenosine, and amiodarone.[11]

TABLE 14-1.

Treatment of type IA poisoning manifesting as QRS prolongation, hypotension, or arrhythmias

---

Fluid resuscitation with normal saline or lactated Ringer solution

---

Sodium bicarbonate: 1–2 mEq/kg as a bolus over 1–2 min
- Monitor response with continuous ECG to observe for narrowing of the QRS complex
- If response: initiate sodium bicarbonate infusion
- Repeat bolus as needed

Vasopressors: norepinephrine is the preferred agent, but others may be used (ie, epinephrine, vasopressin)

For refractory arrhythmias
Lidocaine, 1–1.5 mg/kg IV bolus over 2–3 minutes, followed by 1–4 mg/min IV infusion

Sodium bicarbonate ampules are commonly packaged in 50-mL vials, at a concentration of either 8.4% or 7.5% (50 or 44 mEq of sodium bicarbonate, respectively). Therefore, when treating a 100-kg patient, four ampules (200 mL of the 8.4% solution) would be needed to achieve a bolus dose of 2 mEq/kg. A continuous sodium bicarbonate infusion can be made by placing three ampules (150 mL of either 8.4% or 7.5% solution) of sodium bicarbonate into a 1-liter bag of D_5W run at two or three times the maintenance rate.[9] Water should be used for the dilution, not a sodium-containing solution (eg, 0.9% or 0.45% normal saline), which would create a dangerously hypertonic and hypernatremic solution. Other complications of sodium bicarbonate therapy include excessive alkalemia, hypervolemia, hypokalemia, and hypernatremia. Frequent monitoring of electrolytes and serum pH (avoiding values >7.55) is warranted.

If the QRS interval does not narrow with a bolus of sodium bicarbonate, ensure that an appropriate weight-based bolus was administered. If a repeat bolus fails to correct the arrhythmia, lidocaine may be used.[11] Although the administration of this drug might seem counterintuitive given its sodium channel properties, as a type IB agent, it can actually antagonize a type IA agent. Type IA and type IC antiarrhythmics are always contraindicated in the treatment of wide complex arrhythmias. Human and animal data have demonstrated the safety and benefit of lidocaine in treating cocaine-induced wide complex tachycardia, but its use in countering other type IA toxins is still unclear. β-Blockers and calcium channel blockers should be avoided, as they can further blunt cardiac conduction. Amiodarone, which blocks β-receptors as well as sodium, potassium, and calcium channels, has no defined role in toxin-induced wide complex tachycardias. It presents more potential for harm and should be avoided until the causative agent is clearly identified.[8]

PEARL

When treating a suspected poisoned patient who has QRS prolongation (>100 msec) and signs of cardiovascular toxicity, consider administration of sodium bicarbonate if traditional interventions such as cardioversion and defibrillation have been ineffective.

PEARL

Amiodarone, which blocks β-receptors as well as sodium, potassium, and calcium channels, has no defined role in toxin-induced wide complex tachycardias.

Prolonged QT Interval/Torsade de Pointes

The QT interval represents the period of ventricular depolarization and repolarization. Measured from the onset of the QRS complex to the end of the T wave, the length of the QT interval shortens in the presence of tachycardia and lengthens with bradycardia. Although controversial, the Bazett formula, which takes heart rate into account, is commonly accepted as an accurate measure of the QT interval, known as the "corrected QT" or "QTc."[12,13] It is calculated by measuring the longest QT interval and dividing it by the square root of the preceding RR interval. Computer analysis of QTc measurements is reliable if the rhythm is regular and T waves are clear; if those conditions are not present, the interval should be calculated manually.

The normal range of the QTc interval varies with age, sex, and race. Values below 440 msec are considered normal.[14] Accepted upper limits are 440 to 460 msec in men and 440 to 470 msec in women.[13,14]

When considering the approval of a new drug, the US Food and Drug Administration (FDA) meticulously assesses its effect on the QT interval.[15] Prolongation of this interval represents an increased risk of polymorphic VT, which can degenerate to torsade de pointes (TdP). Literally a "twisting of the points," TdP describes the characteristic undulating pattern that the QRS complexes undergo in a sinusoidal type pattern. The ECG of a patient on methadone who presented for treatment of syncope is shown in Figure 14-2. It illustrates an extremely prolonged QTc with runs of polymorphic VT and a characteristic slow-fast-slow pattern seen with QTc prolongation. Electrocardiographic analysis for TdP and assessment of QTc should be performed in patients presenting with cardiovascular complaints such as lightheadedness, dizziness, syncope, palpitations, or even cardiac arrest. Intermittent episodes of apparent VT should prompt close investigation of the QTc.

Fortunately, the number of patients in whom TdP develops after drug-induced prolongation of the QT interval is small. TdP is a nonperfusing rhythm that can degenerate into ventricular fibrillation and therefore must be identified and managed rapidly. Specific therapy is necessary because the traditional means of managing VT may be unsuccessful.

It is unclear how the risk of TdP increases as QTc values rise. There is clinical evidence that a QTc interval of more than 500 msec increases the risk for TdP significantly.[12-14] Nevertheless, TdP never develops in many patients with QTc values well above normal (500–600 msec), and it has been observed in some with only minimal elevation (<500 msec).

Hundreds of commonly used drugs can cause QT prolongation in single dose, overdose, and therapeutic use. Some of the most common are listed in Table 14-2.[13,14] Up to 3% of non-cardiac drugs can prolong the QT interval.[12] The Arizona Center for Education and Research on Therapeutics maintains a Web site (www.azcert.org) that lists drugs that have been confirmed to cause QTc prolongation or that probably or conditionally induce it.

Risk Factors for Drug-Induced Torsade de Pointes

Patients with a congenital long QT interval are at higher risk for TdP when exposed to drugs that cause QT prolongation.[14] Electrolyte abnormalities such as hypokalemia, hypomagnesemia, and hypocalcemia can independently prolong the QT interval.[13] The concurrent use of multiple QT-prolonging drugs and drug–drug interactions that alter the metabolism of such drugs also increase the risk of TdP.[14] Alterations in liver or kidney function can affect the metabolism of certain drugs, leading to abnormally elevated serum concentrations. Other recognized risk factors include bradycardia, female sex, and atrioventricular blockade.[12-14]

Treatment of Torsade de Pointes/QTc Prolongation

If a patient presents with TdP, be prepared to perform immediate electrical cardioversion because this rhythm can degenerate into ventricular fibrillation and unstable VT. An immediate bolus of intravenous magnesium, 1 to 2 g over 1 to 2 minutes, is the first-line agent.[14] Magnesium acts as a calcium channel blocker, preventing spontaneous depolarization during the ventricular repolarization that is responsible for causing TdP. An infusion of magnesium should be initiated after the

---

FIGURE 14-2.

Severe QTc prolongation with polymorphic VT caused by methadone

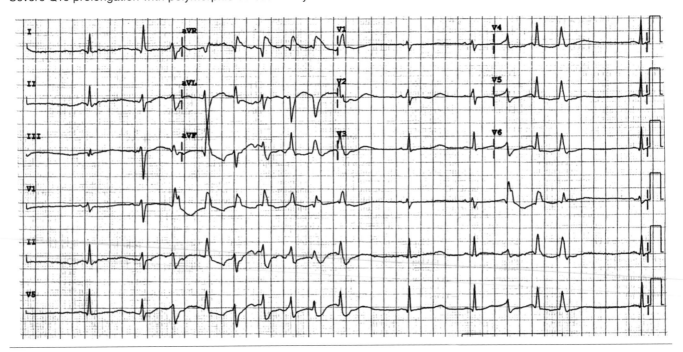

bolus to continue suppression of TdP until the QTc interval shortens. Aggressive repletion of potassium, magnesium, and calcium may shorten the QT interval. The magnesium bolus may be repeated. If the patient remains in refractory TdP, the heart rate may be stimulated to beat faster by one of two interventions—overdrive pacing (cutaneous or transvenous) or administration of isoproterenol. After electrical and mechanical capture is obtained, the target heart rate is 90 to 110 beats/min. This increased rate decreases the QTc interval. Isoproterenol, a β_1-agonist, also increases the heart rate. The infusion should be titrated to achieve a heart rate of more than 90 beats/min. Once the patient is stabilized, the next step is to identify the offending agent and consider GI decontamination or another form of removal. Hemodialysis can be used for medications that are cleared via the kidneys (eg, sotalol).[13,14]

KEY POINT

For a patient presenting with TdP, an immediate bolus of intravenous magnesium, 1 to 2 g over 1 to 2 minutes, is the first-line agent.[15]

Antihypertensive Overdose

Hypertension is one of the most prevalent diseases worldwide. Nearly 30% of Americans above the age of 18 have this condition, and about 68% of them are taking an antihypertensive medication.[16] Many different types of antihypertensive medications are available, and patients commonly take more than one class. Although most antihypertension medications can cause hypotension in overdose, calcium channel blockers and β-blockers are associated with significant morbidity and mortality because they induce severe hypotension that is refractory to traditional therapies. Their toxicity and the approach to management of overdoses are discussed here.

Calcium channel blockers, which block calcium channels on the surface of cells, are used to treat hypertension, arrhythmias, angina, and migraine headaches. They are further broken down into two subsets: the non-dihydropyridines (which act on the peripheral vasculature and the myocardium) and the dihydropyridines (which are selective for the peripheral vasculature). In the periphery, calcium channel blockers cause smooth-mus-

cle relaxation and vasodilation; in the myocardium, channel blockade decreases contractility and conduction. At therapeutic dosing, these actions result in the desired effects of decreasing blood pressure and serving as an antiarrhythmic. β-Blockers block β-adrenergic surface receptors throughout the body (in the heart, eye, peripheral vascular smooth muscle, and liver). They vary in their selectivity of β_1-, β_2-, and β_3-receptor activities, and some have α-receptor-blocking properties as well (eg, labetalol and carvedilol).

Only a few medications cause hypotension and bradycardia. A calcium channel blocker, a β-blocker, digoxin, and clonidine should be considered in the differential diagnosis of a poisoned patient with those clinical signs. The non-dihydropyridines will induce hypotension with paradoxic bradycardia, given their effect on the heart. It is expected that the dihydropyridines will manifest hypotension with reflex tachycardia, although in a large overdose they may lose selectivity and act like a non-dihydropyridine.[17] Individuals with β-blocker overdose are also likely to present with hypotension and bradycardia.[18]

The difference between the clinical manifestations of overdoses of calcium channel blockers and β-blockers is subtle. We address the management of them concurrently because, in acute overdose, it can be impossible to distinguish them, the treatments overlap, and the clinical history may be unknown.

After aggressive intravenous fluid resuscitation, atropine, glucagon, and calcium may be administered to patients experiencing persistent hypotension and bradycardia. Specific dosing regimens for these interventions are listed in Table 14-3. Atropine can be used to treat bradycardia and thereby improve cardiac output and blood pressure, but it is often ineffective.

Glucagon

Glucagon is a specific antidote for β-blocker poisoning, but it can also provide some benefit in the treatment of hypotension induced by a calcium channel blocker. It bypasses β-blockade and leads to activation of adenyl cyclase, the very action of a β-agonist. If the glucagon bolus elicits a favorable response, then a continuous infusion must follow at a rate based on that initial response. For example, if a response is observed at 5 mg, then the infusion should begin at 5 mg/hr. Most patients who receive large doses of glucagon will have emesis. This reaction can preclude its use in a severely ill patient with depressed mental status and an unprotected airway. Glucagon is a tachyphylactic drug, meaning that its clinical effect diminishes over a short time.

Calcium

Intravenous boluses of calcium should be given for refractory hypotension in patients with confirmed or suspected overdose of a calcium channel blocker or β-blocker. Increasing the extracellular calcium concentration elevates the gradient across the cell membranes, allowing more calcium to enter the cell. This appears to improve mean arterial pressure more than the negative chronotropy. Recommendations for the management of patients suspected of calcium channel blocker poisoning call for the administration of 13 to 25 mEq of calcium (Table 14-3) in the form of either calcium gluconate or calcium chloride salts. As with glucagon, patients should receive a continuous

TABLE 14-2.

Drugs that can cause QTc prolongation and torsade de pointes

Amiodarone	Ibutilide
Clarithromycin	Methadone
Disopyramide	Procainamide
Erythromycin	Quinidine
Fluconazole	Sotalol
Fluoxetine	Terfenadine
Haloperidol	Terodiline

infusion of calcium after the bolus. Aggressive administration is warranted in cases of severe refractory hypotension, but there are no clear guidelines on how high to push the limit of total measured serum calcium. In case reports of severe calcium channel blocker overdose, total calcium concentrations have risen as high as 15 to 20 mg/dL. This permissive hypercalcemia is not without risk, as it can cause nausea, vomiting, flushing, and constipation. Rigorous monitoring of the serum calcium and phosphorus levels for calculation of the calcium-phosphate product will give the clinician a sense of the likelihood of crystallization. Medical toxicology consultation is suggested to help guide continued management.

KEY POINT

Recommendations for the management of patients suspected of calcium channel blocker poisoning call for the administration of 13 to 25 mEq of calcium (Table 14-3) in the form of either calcium gluconate or calcium chloride salts.

Vasopressors

After interventions with intravenous fluids, atropine, glucagon, and calcium, the management of refractory hypotension may require infusion of catecholamines. No specific evidence-based recommendations have been formulated, but, theoretically, norepinephrine offers an advantage over other vasopressors in that it provides myocardial stimulation at β_1-receptors of the heart. In addition, it has potent α_1-adrenergic effects on the peripheral vasculature. Vasopressin, phenylephrine, dopamine, and dobutamine have all been used to treat overdoses of calcium channel blockers and β-blockers with varying success. Invasive monitoring and echocardiography will provide insight into which vasopressors might provide optimal hemodynamic function.

Alternative Therapies for Refractory Hypotension in β-Blocker/Calcium Channel Blocker Toxicity

Hyperinsulinemia Euglycemia Therapy

Despite maximal therapy with intravenous fluids, atropine, glucagon, and vasopressors, patients with severe calcium channel blocker/β-blocker overdose could still be profoundly hypotensive. For years, insulin has been known to have beneficial inotropic and chronotropic effects. Hyperinsulinemia euglycemia therapy (HIET) uses the effects of high-dose insulin infusions, while maintaining serum glucose within normal limits. The dosing protocol is presented in Table 14-4.

The exact mechanism of action for this therapy is unclear. One theory suggests that the poisoned myocardium is in a stressed state that prefers glucose as a substrate instead of the free fatty acids that it normally uses.[19,20] There is convincing animal evidence and anecdotal human case reports that HIET improves hemodynamic function.[18,20–23] Given the grave nature of these poisonings, HIET should be considered concurrently with the initiation of vasopressors or even earlier in patients who do not respond to fluids, glucagon, and calcium.

TABLE 14-3.

Dosing of atropine, glucagon, and calcium in calcium channel blocker and β-blocker toxicity

Atropine
   Adults: 0.5–1 mg IV
   Children: 0.02 mg/kg (minimum 0.1 mg) IV
   May be repeated every 2 or 3 minutes, up to a total dose of 3 mg

Glucagon
   Adults: 2–5 mg slow IV push, repeated every 5–10 minutes, up to a total dose of 10 mg, followed by an infusion at the hourly rate of response (ie, if 5 mg provided a response, then start a continuous infusion at 5 mg/hr)
   Children: 50–150 mcg/kg slow IV push, then 50 mcg/kg/hr up to the maximum adult dosing

Calcium: bolus with 13–25 mEq of calcium
   1 g of calcium gluconate (4.3 mEq of calcium)[a,b]
   1 g of calcium chloride (13.4 mEq of calcium)[a,b]
   Adults: Slow IV push over 5–10 minutes of 30–60 mL of 10% of calcium gluconate or 10–20 mL of 10% calcium chloride
   Children: 0.1 mL/kg of 10% calcium gluconate
   Continuous infusions of 0.5 mEq/kg/hr of calcium may be initiated after 3 or 4 doses of bolus dosing (described above) but should be preceded by checking calcium and phosphorus concentrations

[a]One ampule usually contains 10 mL of a 10% solution of either calcium chloride or calcium gluconate; confirm before administering.

[b]Calcium chloride has about three times the molar amount of calcium as calcium gluconate but is associated with a significant risk of sclerosis.

TABLE 14-4.

Hyperinsulinemia euglycemia therapy (HIET) dosing

Begin HIET with the following:
- Intravenous bolus of regular insulin at a dose of 1 unit/kg
- If serum glucose >250 mg/dL, concurrently administer a bolus of dextrose, 25–50 g (or 0.5–1 g/kg) IV

After bolus, start regular insulin at a rate of 0.5–1 unit/kg/hr, along with continuous infusion of dextrose at 0.5 g/kg/hr and titrate to maintain glucose levels of 110–150 mg/dL. Monitor serum glucose every 30 minutes for the first 1 or 2 hours until euglycemia is maintained. Potassium should also be monitored closely and repleted to maintain within normal limits.

Insulin bolus and infusion can take 20–30 minutes to induce a clinical inotropic/chronotropic effect. Increase insulin infusion by 0.5–1 unit/kg/hr every 60 minutes (similar to administration of a pressor to maintain desired hemodynamic effect).

Optimal insulin dosing is unknown, but patients have been maintained on insulin infusion rates as high as 2–5 units/kg/hr.

PEARL

High-dose boluses and infusions of insulin can be very safe in the treatment of refractory calcium channel blocker/β-blocker overdose. This therapeutic approach is associated with a low incidence of clinically significant hypoglycemia and hypokalemia.

The safety of this therapy is often questioned, but clinical experience demonstrates that it can be quite safe, not inducing significant episodes of hypoglycemia. In a 100-kg person, a bolus of 100 units of insulin followed by 50 to 100 units/hr would be an initial starting regimen.[21] Other physicians, nurses, and staff members may balk at these doses, given that they represent a 10-fold increase in the insulin regimens used for diabetic ketoacidosis. However, there appears to be a dose-response effect. Low-dose insulin does not provide an inotropic or chronotropic benefit.[22]

Many patients can be maintained on HIET alone without vasopressors, thus avoiding the severe complications associated with vasopressor therapy such as tachyarrhythmias or ischemic injury to the bowel, limbs, or vital organs. If the patient responds to HIET, hemodynamic monitoring will show an increase in ejection fraction and cardiac function.[18] HIET may not increase the heart rate. In cases of severe peripheral vasodilation, vasopressors may still be needed to augment decreased systemic vascular resistance.

Despite adequate boluses and infusion of dextrose, recurrent episodes of hypoglycemia can signal resolution of calcium channel blocker poisoning. Calcium channels facilitate exocytosis in β-islet cells and are thus responsible for baseline-mediated insulin release.[21] This is the reason patients without underlying diabetes can display hyperglycemia in calcium channel blocker overdose, which may be an initial clue to this exposure. Improved hemodynamics and decreased vasopressor requirement are other indications that the insulin infusion may be titrated down.

Intralipid Infusion

The use of 20% intravenous lipid emulsion therapy in calcium channel blocker/β-blocker overdose is still in an experimental phase, but animal evidence and limited anecdotal human experience suggest that intralipid infusion improves hemodynamic function in this clinical scenario.[24,25] This therapy was first discovered as an antidote to cardiac arrest after unintentional bupivacaine intravenous injection.[26] Two theories about its action have been postulated. One is that it acts as a "lipid sink," soaking up lipophilic drugs such as bupivacaine. The other theory contrasts intralipid infusion and HIET, suggesting that since the heart normally prefers free fatty acids as an energy source, intralipid can provide this substrate at a high concentration.[24,25] Intralipid preparations and recommended dosing regimens are presented in Table 14-5.

Intralipid can be found on many anesthesia carts because of its obvious benefit in cases of acute bupivacaine toxicity. At this time, the use of intralipid is reserved for the most severe cases of calcium channel blocker/β-blocker overdose that are refractory to all other therapies and involve impending or current cardiac arrest. There is only limited human experience with intralipid; the rate and extent of complications are unknown. Lipid emboli have been observed in animal trials. Intralipid therapy is under active investigation, so new indications or dosing regimens may be elucidated in the near future. Poison control centers and medical toxicologists are good sources of information about the use of this compound.

Other Therapies to Consider in Severe β-Blocker/Calcium Channel Blocker Poisoning

A few animal studies and case reports have reported the use of additional therapies. Phosphodiesterase inhibitors such as milrinone and amrinone have been used to improve myocardial inotropy, but they can cause hypotension.[27] Extracorporeal membrane oxygenation has been used successfully in some pediatric poisonings.[28] Cardiopulmonary bypass, transvenous pacemakers, and intraaortic balloon pumps have also been used. Despite limited evidence of the efficacy of these adjuncts,

---

TABLE 14-5.

Intralipid therapy for calcium channel blocker/β-blocker overdose[a]

Obtain a prepared infusion, if available, or request an infusion made from intravenous lipid preparations used in total parenteral nutrition from the pharmacy.

For patients with severe refractory cardiovascular collapse or impending or current cardiac arrest:

- Bolus: 1–1.5 mL/kg over 1 minute, using a 20% intravenous lipid emulsion solution
- Repeat every 3 to 5 minutes to a maximum dose of 3 mL/kg
- Some clinicians begin an infusion after the initial bolus at a rate of 0.25 mL/kg/min until hemodynamic recovery is achieved.

[a]Discuss the latest indications with your local poison control center or medical toxicologist.

TABLE 14-6.

Seizure-inducing toxins

Amphetamines	Isoniazid
Antihistamines	Lidocaine
Antipsychotics	Lindane
Bupropion	MDMA (ecstasy)
Caffeine	Organophosphate
Camphor	Phencyclidine (PCP)
Carbon monoxide	Theophylline
Cocaine	Tramadol
Hydrazines	Tricyclic antidepressants

they may be life-saving measures to bridge patients through acute toxicity. Early discussion with consultants may expedite such heroic measures.

Neuromuscular Excitation

Toxin-Induced Seizures/Status Epilepticus

The main inhibitory neurotransmitter is γ-aminobutyric acid (GABA), which binds to the GABA receptor, which is linked to a chloride channel. The opening of this channel by GABA binding allows an influx of chloride into the cell, resulting in inhibitory hyperpolarization. Other drugs that affect chloride influx or attenuate the GABA receptor are ethanol, benzodiazepines, barbiturates, and propofol.

The primary excitatory neurotransmitter is glutamate, which binds to kainite, AMPA, and NMDA receptors. Additional neurotransmitters and channels (eg, adenosine and sodium channels) are also involved in the pathology of toxin-induced seizures. A wide range of drugs and toxins can cause acute seizures (Table 14-6) or lower the seizure threshold, uncovering underlying epileptic disease.

The emergency department management of seizures is the same regardless of their cause. The patient should be stabilized, intravenous access should be established, and the airway should be protected. Alterations in glucose, electrolytes, oxygen, blood pressure, and temperature should be addressed, and eclampsia should be considered until a woman's pregnancy status is known. Severe hyponatremia—toxin-induced or primary metabolic—must be considered in patients experiencing seizures and can be caused by a variety of toxins (eg, MDMA and other amphetamines). Withdrawal syndromes associated with the abrupt cessation of ethanol or benzodiazepine use in adults can present as seizures. Opioid withdrawal does not usually cause seizures in adults, but it might in neonates.

TABLE 14-7.

Treatment of toxin-induced seizures

First line: benzodiazepines
- Diazepam may offer slight benefit and synergy with pyridoxine in seizures induced by isoniazid; otherwise, no specific agent is preferred.

Second line: pyridoxine (vitamin B$_6$)
- Empiric treatment in adults is 5 g slow IV push; if seizure terminates before completion of bolus, allow the rest of the dose to be infused over the next 30 minutes.
- In children, 70 mg/kg (maximum 5 g)
- In isoniazid overdose, pyridoxine can be given in an amount equal to the dose of isoniazid ingested.

Third line: barbiturates and propofol
- Both will likely require intubation.

Special consideration: tricyclic antidepressants in overdose can cause acute seizures that may be responsive to benzodiazepines, but special consideration must be given to administering sodium bicarbonate (discussed in the section on toxin-induced wide complex tachycardia).

Management of Seizures

Patients who are actively seizing should receive rapidly escalating doses of benzodiazepines to terminate the convulsions. When seizures do not respond to benzodiazepines, or if they are recurrent and meet clinical criteria for status epilepticus, pyridoxine (vitamin B$_6$) should be given emergently as an intravenous push. There are very few causes of true toxin-induced convulsive status epilepticus, and fewer that are benzodiazepine resistant. Isoniazid, *Gyromitra* mushroom species, and rocket fuel are hydrazines that produce benzodiazepine-resistant seizures and, without pyridoxine therapy, status epilepticus.[29]

TABLE 14-8.

Clinical features of several toxin-induced hyperthermic syndromes[a]

Serotonin syndrome: caused by excess serotonin stimulation
- Develops within minutes to hours after a combination, initiation, or increase of pro-serotonergic drugs (eg, selective serotonin reuptake inhibitors, monoamine oxidase inhibitors, dextromethorphan, meperidine, lithium, linezolid)
- Tremor, spontaneous or inducible clonus of extremities or eyes, hyperreflexia (which may be greater in lower extremities than upper)

Neuroleptic malignant syndrome: caused by excess blockade of dopamine or withdrawal from dopaminergic agents
- Insidious onset, developing over days to weeks of chronic or high-dose neuroleptics (eg, haloperidol, phenothiazines, or withdrawal from dopaminergic medications for parkinsonism)
- Early symptoms can be mistaken for psychiatric illness, as facial muscles may portray a flat affect and patients might move more slowly than usual
- Tremor, trismus, drooling, "lead pipe" muscle rigidity, hyperreflexia caused by severe muscle rigidity, elevated creatine kinase

Malignant hyperthermia: inherited disorder affecting intracellular calcium release from the sarcoplasmic reticulum
- Typically develops in the operating room within minutes to hours after exposure to succinylcholine and inhalation anesthetics (halothane)
- An early finding in an intubated patient may be increased end tidal CO_2 and difficulty ventilating because of chest wall rigidity
- Severe muscle rigidity and masseter spasm during intubation are associated with the development of malignant hyperthermia

Sympathomimetic excess: severe agitation caused by drug-induced excess catecholamine release
- Cocaine, amphetamines, MDMA (ecstasy)
- Severe agitation, diaphoresis, mydriasis

[a]All of these disorders can present with autonomic instability, usually manifested by hypertension, tachycardia, arrhythmias, agitation, and delirium.

KEY POINT

Patients who are actively seizing should receive rapidly escalating doses of benzodiazepines to terminate the convulsions.

PEARL

Isoniazid, *Gyromitra* mushroom species, and rocket fuel are hydrazines that produce benzodiazepine-resistant seizures and, without pyridoxine therapy, status epilepticus.[29]

Hydrazines inhibit the metabolic pathway responsible for the normal production of GABA metabolized from glutamate. This leads to excess glutamate and decreased GABA, causing increased excitation and decreased inhibition; this imbalance leads to severe acute convulsions. Although pyridoxine therapy is specific to this group of toxins, it is prudent to empirically administer at least one dose of pyridoxine to patients presenting to the emergency department with status epilepticus when any of the following conditions applies: a toxin-induced seizure is suspected, the patient has a history of tuberculosis (TB) or resides in an area of endemic TB, or the cause of the seizures cannot be explained. The dose of pyridoxine for seizures is extremely high compared with routine replacement (Table 14-7), but its adverse-effect profile is low and complications are expected only with chronic continuous elevated dosing regimens. Most drug-induced hyponatremia can be approached in the typical manner for patients with the syndrome of inappropriate antidiuretic hormone secretion because this is the primary mechanism of action for the hyponatremia. In patients with toxin-induced seizures, phenytoin will be unsuccessful at terminating convulsions and can be detrimental if the toxin is cocaine, tricyclic antidepressants, or theophylline.[29]

Hyperthermic Syndromes

Several syndromes and exposures can lead to toxicologically induced hyperthermia. Emergency physicians should be familiar with the clinical presentations of serotonin syndrome, neuroleptic malignant syndrome, malignant hyperthermia, and sympathomimetic overdose (Table 14-8). Although each entity has a different mechanism of action, they share the ability to cause excess neuromuscular activity. This leads to an increase in heat production, which can cause a patient's core temperature to rise rapidly.

Toxin-induced hyperthermia can be indistinguishable from temperature elevation caused by an infection.[30] One of the key differences between them is that infection produces an inflammatory response, causing the endogenous release of cytokines and interleukins, which will reset the thermoregulation center of the hypothalamus, raising the body's temperature (a "fever"). Hyperthermia resulting from exposure to a toxin is universally caused by extreme muscular rigidity or activity. Until an infectious process is definitively ruled out, it is most appropriate to treat the patient empirically for a potential exposure to a toxin along with standard measures for infectious causes of an elevated temperature.

It is imperative to obtain a rectal temperature or core body temperature immediately on any patient suspected of hyperthermia. Oral and axillary temperatures are unreliable. A common pitfall is to assume that a normal core body temperature rules out these toxin-induced hyperthermic syndromes.

All of these syndromes except malignant hyperthermia can present with a wide spectrum of clinical severity. Early recognition of neuroleptic malignant syndrome and cessation of neuroleptic therapy are likely to decrease morbidity and mortality.[31]

TABLE 14-9.

Critical actions in the management of toxin-induced hyperthermia: STOP, CALM, and COOL!

1) STOP all drugs and refrain from administering any drugs that could exacerbate current hyperthermic syndrome (eg, haloperidol to sedate the patient with possible neuroleptic malignant syndrome).

2) CALM with benzodiazepines; endpoint should be control of agitation and muscular rigidity; intubate and paralyze if needed.

3) COOL; if the interventions listed above do not decrease core temperature, immediately initiate cooling, best performed by packing the patient in ice from head to toe, anteriorly and posteriorly.

Antidotes
- Serotonin syndrome: cyproheptadine, serotonin antagonist
- Neuroleptic malignant syndrome: bromocriptine, dopamine agonist
- Malignant hyperthermia: dantrolene, a direct skeletal muscle relaxant, decreases calcium release from the sarcoplasmic reticulum.

Of all these antidotes, only dantrolene for malignant hyperthermia is warranted for emergent use that may be life saving. Cyproheptadine and bromocriptine are available only in oral preparations, have not been shown to improve outcomes, and do not replace the principles of aggressive sedation and cooling.

TABLE 14-10.

Features of cholinergic toxicity

Muscarinic
- SLUDGE: salivation, lacrimation, urination, diarrhea, GI cramps, emesis
- Killer B's: bronchorrhea, bronchospasm, bradycardia
- Some patients have miosis

Nicotinic: autonomic ganglia
- Diaphoresis, tachycardia, hypertension, mydriasis

Nicotinic: neuromuscular junction
- Muscle fasciculation, weakness, and paralysis

Depending on the stage of toxicity and the location and chemical binding features of each specific agent, the patient could exhibit tachycardia or bradycardia, so no one symptom should rule in or rule out clinical suspicion of organophosphate or carbamate toxicity.

The complications associated with toxin-induced hyperthermia include rhabdomyolysis, seizures, disseminated intravascular coagulopathy, arrhythmias, multisystem organ failure, and death.[30] The length of time a patient spends in a hyperthermic state correlates with the likelihood of complications; only 30 minutes at temperatures above 39°C (102.2°F) increases morbidity and mortality.[32]

The approach to critically ill hyperthermic patients is detailed in Table 14-9. The most critical action when patients are significantly hyperthermic is to aggressively sedate and cool them. Muscular rigidity and agitation can be halted with appropriate benzodiazepine administration. If this does not lower the patient's core temperature, the patient must be intubated, paralyzed, and rapidly cooled. Active cooling must be initiated immediately to decrease core temperature below 39°C within 15 to 20 minutes. In patients with heat stroke, ice water bath immersion is clearly the superior method of cooling. The most practical method is to pack the patient in ice from head to toe, posteriorly and anteriorly. New technologies such as endovascular coils used to control hypothermia after cardiac arrest have not been studied in the treatment of heat stroke or toxin-induced hyperthermia, but they may have benefit.

KEY POINT

The most critical action when patients are significantly hyperthermic is to aggressively sedate and cool them.

Other toxins such as cyanide, carbon monoxide, and even salicylate can cause hyperthermia by poisoning mitochondria and uncoupling oxidative phosphorylation, leading to hyperthermia due to resulting inefficiency in the normal processes responsible for ATP production. This effect is usually a very late or pre-terminal finding.[33]

Cholinergic Crisis

Organophosphates and carbamates are toxins that can cause acute and life-threatening cholinergic toxicity. Most commonly used as insecticides and pesticides, they have also been used to assist in suicide, as agents of terrorism, and in chemical warfare.[34] Organophosphates and carbamates bind to cholinesterases, preventing the metabolism of acetylcholine, resulting in significant cholinergic excess. The features of classic cholinergic excess can be broken down by the effect of excess acetylcholine at three different receptors (Table 14-10). Unlike organophosphates, carbamates do not "age," meaning they can reversibly bind and spontaneously release cholinesterases. In addition, carbamates are less toxic to the central nervous system.

Exposure to organophosphates and carbamates can occur via inhalation, ingestion, or dermal, ocular, or parenteral routes. Health care providers receiving patients who have been exposed to these compounds must ensure their own safety. Appropriate decontamination of patients and the use of personal protective gear are critical.

Atropine is the mainstay of treatment, inducing competitive antagonism of acetylcholine at muscarinic sites. Aggressive treatment of bronchorrhea by achieving adequate atropinization is the defined clinical end point. The recommended dosing regimen is presented in Table 14-11. Pralidoxime should be administered to all patients with suspected or confirmed organophosphate exposure who present with severe signs of toxicity, who have neuromuscular weakness, or who have required a significant amount of atropine. Although evidence suggests that pralidoxime may not be beneficial in all types of organo-

TABLE 14-11.

Initial atropine and pralidoxime dosing for cholinergic toxicity

Atropine
- Administer atropine IVP: 0.5–2 mg in adults, and 0.02 mg/kg in children, depending on severity
  - Minimum doses (0.5 mg in adults and 0.1 mg in children) should be given to avoid paradoxic bradycardia
- Aggressively repeat dose every 3–5 minutes, doubling each subsequent dose in severe cases
- Titrate to drying of bronchial secretions
- Tachycardia is *not* a contraindication and should not suppress aggressive therapy

Pralidoxime (2-PAM)
- Give 1–2 g in 100 mL of normal saline over 15–30 minutes to adults and 20–40 mg/kg (maximum 2 g) to children.
- These doses may be repeated in 1 hour if muscle weakness and fasciculation are not relieved.
- Initial dose may be repeated every 3–6 hours as needed for severe poisoning.

or

- Continuous infusion may be initiated for severe cases:
  - Adults and children: 10–20 mg/kg/hr, up to a maximum of 500 mg/hr
  - Expert medical consultation should be sought to direct appropriate dosing.

TABLE 14-12.

Increased anion gap differential diagnosis using the CAT MUDPILES mnemonic

C = Carbon monoxide, Cyanide

A = Aspirin (salicylate), Alcoholic ketoacidosis

T = Toluene

M = Methanol, Metformin

U = Uremia

D = Diabetic ketoacidosis

P = Propylene glycol

I = Iron, Isoniazid

L = Lactic acidosis

E = Ethylene glycol

S = Starvation ketoacidosis

phosphate poisoning, such as that caused by carbamates, the associated morbidity/mortality of such exposures warrants its continued use.[35]

PEARL

Seizures after organophosphate exposure should be treated with benzodiazepines emergently, as they may not be halted by atropine and pralidoxime.

Severe Metabolic Acidosis

In all critically ill poisoned patients, the anion gap must be measured quickly. The gap is calculated using the following formula:

$$[Na^+] - [Cl^- + HCO_3^-]$$

Depending on laboratory technique, the normal range for the anion gap is 6 to 14 mEq/L. An increase in the gap beyond the accepted normal range, accompanied by metabolic acidosis, represents an increase in unmeasured endogenous (ie, lactate) or exogenous (ie, salicylates) anions.[36] Several toxins produce an elevated anion gap. The mnemonic CAT MUDPILES is not complete, but it can be used to consider toxicologic causes of an increased anion gap (Table 14-12).

A thorough history, along with careful analysis of laboratory data, may provide all the necessary information to confirm the suspected diagnosis; however, in some cases, routine laboratory data can be insufficient. Clues to the diagnosis can be ascertained from additional laboratory assessments, as follows: measurement of arterial and/or venous blood gases; serum/urine ketone concentrations; blood urea nitrogen; and creati-

nine, lactate, and salicylate levels. Normal renal function and an undetectable salicylate concentration quickly rule out uremia and salicylate toxicity, respectively. The absence of ketones does not rule out diabetic/starvation/alcoholic ketoacidosis but makes it less likely. Lactic acidosis is responsible for elevated anion gaps in carbon monoxide, cyanide, metformin, propylene glycol, iron, and isoniazid (seizures) toxicity. Toluene is a rare toxin that causes anion gap elevation by hippuric acid formation. The management of exposures to methanol and ethylene glycol is discussed below.

Three important and relatively common causes of elevated anion gap metabolic acidosis are cyanide toxicity, toxic alcohol ingestion, and severe salicylate toxicity. Even with adequate airway support, oxygenation, and fluid resuscitation, patients with these types of poisonings may not survive without toxin-specific management.

Cyanide

Cyanide is a mitochondrial toxin that inhibits the function of cytochrome oxidase at the α_3 portion. This disrupts the electron transport chain at a critical step in the utilization of oxygen. Despite adequate oxygenation, oxygen cannot be used, resulting in cellular hypoxia. A shift toward anaerobic metabolism produces metabolic acidosis with an increase in the serum lactic acid concentration.[37]

Cyanide is known for inducing extremely rapid neurologic and cardiovascular collapse. Neurologic symptoms can progress rapidly from headache to agitation, seizures, and coma. Cyanide poisoning can initially produce the cardiovascular effects of hypertension and bradycardia, but most patients present with hypotension and tachycardia. Bradycardia may represent a preterminal event. Diagnostically, cyanide concentrations usually are not available quickly enough to aid in management. Increased anion gap metabolic acidosis and an elevated lactate (>8 mmol/L) should raise suspicion of cyanide poisoning.[37] Given the patient's inability to use oxygen, "arterialization" of venous blood can be indicated by elevated venous (>90%) oxygenation.

Patients can be exposed to cyanide by inhalation, ingestion, or dermal or parenteral routes. The rate of onset of symptoms is related to the route of exposure, with inhalation of gaseous

TABLE 14-13.

Cyanide antidote kit and hydroxocobalamin dosing

Cyanide antidote kit

1) Amyl nitrite pearls[a]
- Crack open and place under patient's nose; may use while intravenous line is being established

2) Sodium nitrite[a]
- Adult: 10 mL (300 mg)
- Children: 0.33 mL/kg (maximum dose 10 mL)
- Infuse over 3–5 minutes

3) Sodium thiosulfate[b]
- Adult: 50 mL (12.5 g)
- Children: 1.65 mL/kg (maximum 50 mL)
- Infuse over 3–5 minutes

Hydroxocobalamin[b]

- Adult: 5 g (2 vials lyophilized)
- Children: 70 mg/kg (maximum 5 g)
- Infuse over 15 minutes

[a]Do *not* give the amyl nitrite or sodium nitrite portions of the cyanide antidote kit to fire victims.
[b]Sodium thiosulfate and hydroxocobalamin may be given together for possible synergistic effect, but they should never run concurrently through the same intravenous line.

TABLE 14-14.

Osmolar gap calculation and clinical utility for toxic alcohol ingestion

Osmolar Gap = Measured Osmolarity – Calculated Osmolarity

Measured osmolarity is obtained from clinical laboratory analysis.

Calculated osmolar gap =
(2 x [Na⁺]) + glucose/18 + BUN/2.8 + ethanol/4.6

Units: Na (mEq/L), Glucose (mg/dL), BUN (mg/dL), Ethanol (mg/dL)

Osmolar gap >50 is highly specific for toxic alcohol ingestion.

A "normal" osmolar gap never rules out a toxic alcohol ingestion.[45]

hydrogen cyanide resulting in nearly immediate collapse, while ingestion of a cyanide salt such as sodium cyanide can induce clinical effects in 20 minutes. Cyanide salts are commonly found in chemical laboratories, photographic chemical processing, and jewelers' supplies. A history of such occupations or exposure should raise clinical suspicion for cyanide toxicity. Fire victims can be exposed to hydrogen cyanide gas liberated from the burning of the wool, plastics, nylon, and polyurethane found in automobiles, carpets, home furniture, and appliances. A lactate concentration higher than 10 mmol/L on arrival in the emergency department in fire victims without significant cutaneous burns is a sensitive marker for an elevated blood cyanide concentration.[37] These patients tend to have concurrent carbon monoxide poisoning, asphyxia, trauma, and thermal injury—all of which can be indistinguishable from cyanide poisoning.

PEARL

A lactate concentration higher than 10 mmol/L on arrival in the emergency department in fire victims without significant cutaneous burns is a sensitive marker for an elevated blood cyanide concentration.[37]

The "original" cyanide antidote kit contains amyl nitrite, sodium nitrite, and sodium thiosulfate (Table 14-13). The amyl and sodium nitrites cause the production of a small amount of methemoglobin, which removes cyanide from the mitochondria. Sodium thiosulfate provides cofactors for rhodanese, an enzyme that assists in metabolizing cyanide to thiocyanate, a relatively nontoxic metabolite that is eliminated via the kidneys. Fire victims who may have elevated carboxyhemoglobin concentrations should not receive the amyl and sodium nitrite portions of the kit. The production of a small amount of methemoglobinemia in these patients is potentially devastating, as neither carboxyhemoglobin nor methemoglobin can deliver oxygen to the tissues.

In 2006, hydroxocobalamin was approved by the FDA for the treatment of cyanide poisoning. A precursor to cyanocobalamin (vitamin B_{12}), it contains an OH group in place of a CN group. Hydroxocobalamin binds cyanide, displacing the OH, to form the vitamin, which is rapidly eliminated in the urine.[38] Hydroxocobalamin is marketed as Cyanokit (King Pharmaceuticals, Bristol, TN) and is packaged as a lyophilized powder that requires reconstitution with normal saline (Table 14-13). In fire victims, hydroxocobalamin appears to be safer than the traditional cyanide antidote kit.[39] Hydroxocobalamin may be used in conjunction with sodium thiosulfate, but they should not be administered concurrently through the same intravenous line.[40]

TABLE 14-15.

Dosing regimen for fomepizole

Loading dose of 15 mg/kg IV, followed by 10 mg/kg every 12 hours for 4 doses

Each dose is infused over 30 minutes.

If the patient requires dialysis, increase the dosing frequency to every 4 hours.

Toxic Alcohol Ingestion

Methanol and ethylene glycol are "toxic" alcohols because their degradation leads to extremely toxic metabolites that produce significant metabolic acidosis and specific end-organ damage. Methanol is used as a denaturant for ethanol, windshield washer fluid, a solvent, and fuel (ie, buffet can heaters). Ethylene glycol is found in antifreeze, solvents, deicers, and air conditioning units. Both methanol and ethylene glycol produce inebriation similar to and often mistaken for ethanol intoxication, but the absence of central nervous system depression does not exclude a potentially life-threatening exposure. Methanol is metabolized to formic acid, an ocular toxin that produces a spectrum of visual changes from blurred vision to blindness, and the pathognomonic "snowfield vision." Ethylene glycol's toxic metabolites include oxalic acid, which causes renal failure, hypocalcemia, and calcium oxalate crystalluria.[41]

Toxic alcohol ingestion should be suspected in patients who present after known ingestion of products containing toxic alcohols, those with unexplained metabolic acidosis or a significantly elevated osmolar gap (>50) (Table 14-14) and those who do not respond to treatment for another presumed cause of an elevated anion gap acidosis (eg, thiamine and dextrose for alcoholic ketoacidosis).[42] The serum lactate concentration can be falsely elevated in patients with ethylene glycol poisoning, given that one of its metabolites, glycolic acid, can be misinterpreted as lactate.[43]

PEARL

The serum lactate concentration can be falsely elevated in patients with ethylene glycol poisoning, given that one of its metabolites, glycolic acid, can be misinterpreted as lactate.[43]

The parent compounds of ethylene glycol and methanol are osmotically active, but their metabolites, oxalic acid and formic acid, are not.[44] Therefore, as time passes and metabolism occurs, the osmolar gap will fall and the metabolites will cause the anion gap to rise.

Theoretically, patients who present very early after exposure will have an elevated osmolar gap and may have no elevation in their anion gap. Conversely, late presenters who have metabolized the alcohol will display an elevated anion gap and a very low to normal osmolar gap.[45] This progression will be halted in the presence of ethanol because alcohol dehydrogenase preferentially metabolizes ethanol over ethylene glycol or methanol. This "protective" effect is the reason ethanol can be used to treat toxic alcohol ingestions. Today, ethanol should be used only when fomepizole is not readily available.[46]

PEARL

Without treatment and with no concurrent ethanol intoxication, the natural progression of toxic alcohol ingestions, despite resuscitation, is a declining osmolar gap mirrored by an increasing anion gap.

Fomepizole (4-methyl-pyrazole, Antizol [Paladin Labs, Quebec, Canada]) is an alcohol dehydrogenase inhibitor that prevents the metabolism of ethylene glycol and methanol to their toxic metabolites. It should be administered as soon as possible in all confirmed cases of ethylene glycol or methanol poisoning and when one of these conditions is suspected (Table 14-15). Fomepizole will stop the creation of the toxic metabolites of ethylene glycol and methanol and may be the only therapy needed for patients with mild to moderate exposures. Critically ill patients warrant immediate nephrology consultation because emergent hemodialysis is indicated in patients with severe metabolic acidosis, end-organ toxicity, renal failure, and methanol or ethylene glycol concentrations greater than 25 mg/dL; unfortunately, this intervention is not readily available in most hospitals.[41]

Conclusion

We have discussed some of the more common and complex medications and chemicals that can cause severe toxicity. Any drug can cause a patient to become critically ill. Consultation with a medical toxicologist or poison control center can assist with management. Treatment of the critically poisoned patient requires immediate identification of the toxicant, anticipation of the toxicity, and administration of antidotal therapy when appropriate.

References

1. Ashbourne JF, Olson KR, Khayam-Bashi H. Value of rapid screening for acetaminophen in all patients with intentional drug overdose. *Ann Emerg Med.* 1989;18:1035-1038.
2. Tenenbein M. Do you really need that emergency drug screen? *Clin Toxicol.* 2009;47:286-291.
3. Seger D, Muelenbelt J. Position paper: ipecac syrup. *J Toxicol Clin Toxicol.* 2004;42:133-143.
4. Chyka PA, Seger D, Krenzelok EP, et al. Position paper: single-dose activated charcoal. *Clin Toxicol.* 2005;43:61-87.
5. Kulig K, Bar-Or D, Cantrill SV, et al. Management of acutely poisoned patients without gastric emptying. *Ann Emerg Med.* 1985;14:562-567.
6. Vale JA, Kulig K. Position paper: gastric lavage. *J Toxicol Clin Toxicol.* 2004;42:933-943.
7. Sharma A, Hexdall A, Chang E, et al. Diphenhydramine-induced wide complex dysrhythmia responds to treatment with sodium bicarbonate. *Am J Emerg Med.* 2003;21:212-215.
8. Kalimullah E, Bryant S. Case files of the medical toxicology fellowship at the toxikon consortium in Chicago: cocaine-associated wide-complex dysrhythmias and cardiac arrest—treatment nuances and controversies. *J Med Toxicol.* 2008;4:277-283.
9. Hollowell H, Mattu A, Perron A, et al. Wide-complex tachycardia: beyond the traditional differential diagnosis of ventricular tachycardia vs supraventricular tachycardia with aberrant conduction. *Am J Emerg Med.* 2005;23:876-889.
10. Thanacoody HKR, Thomas SHL. Tricyclic antidepressant poisoning: cardiovascular toxicity. *Toxicol Rev.* 2005;24:205-214.
11. Wood D, Dargan P, Hoffman R. Management of cocaine-induced cardiac arrhythmias due to cardiac ion channel dysfunction. *Clin Toxicol.* 2009;47:14-23.
12. Roden D. Clinical practice. Long-QT syndrome. *N Engl J Med.* 2008;358:169-176.
13. Yap Y, Camm AJ. Drug induced QT prolongation and torsades de pointes. *Heart.* 2003;89:1363-1372.
14. Gupta A, Lawrence A, Krishnan K, et al. Current concepts in the mechanisms and management of drug-induced QT prolongation and torsade de pointes. *Am Heart J.* 2007;153:891-899.
15. Yap YG, Camm J. Risk of torsades de pointes with non-cardiac drugs. Doctors need to be aware that many drugs can cause QT prolongation. *BMJ Br Med J (Clin Res).* 2000;320:1158-1159.
16. Ostchega Y, Dillon C, Hughes J, et al. Trends in hypertension prevalence, awareness, treatment, and control in older U.S. adults: data from the National Health and Nutrition Examination Survey 1988 to 2004. *J Am Geriatr Soc.* 2007;55:1056-1065.
17. Smith S, Ferguson K, Hoffman R, et al. Prolonged severe hypotension following combined amlodipine and valsartan ingestion. *Clin Toxicol.* 2008;46:470-474.
18. Mgarbane B, Karyo S, Baud F. The role of insulin and glucose (hyperinsulinaemia/euglycaemia) therapy in acute calcium channel antagonist and beta-blocker poisoning. *Toxicol Rev.* 2004;23:215-222.
19. Kline JA, Leonova E, Raymond RM. Beneficial myocardial metabolic effects of insulin during verapamil toxicity in the anesthetized canine. *Crit Care Med.* 1995;23:1251-1263.
20. Kline JA, Tomaszewski CA, Schroeder JD, et al. Insulin is a superior antidote for cardiovascular toxicity induced by verapamil in the anesthetized canine. *J Pharmacol Exp Ther.* 1993;267:744-750.
21. Greene S, Gawarammana I, Wood D, et al. Relative safety of hyperinsulinaemia/euglycaemia therapy in the management of calcium channel blocker overdose: a prospective observational study. *Intensive Care Med.* 2007;33:2019-2024.
22. Nickson C, Little M. Early use of high-dose insulin euglycaemic therapy for verapamil toxicity. *Med J Aust.* 2009;191:350-352.
23. Yuan TH, Kerns WP, Tomaszewski CA, et al. Insulin-glucose as adjunctive therapy for severe calcium channel antagonist poisoning. *J Toxicol Clin Toxicol.* 1999;37:463-474.
24. Cave G, Harvey M. Intravenous lipid emulsion as antidote beyond local anesthetic toxicity: a systematic review. *Acad Emerg Med.* 2009;16:815-824.
25. Jamaty C, Bailey B, Larocque A, et al. Lipid emulsions in the treatment of acute poisoning: a systematic review of human and animal studies. *Clin Toxicol.* 2010;48:1-27.
26. Weinberg G. Lipid infusion therapy: translation to clinical practice. *Anesth Analg.* 2008;106:1340-1342.
27. Love JN, Leasure JA, Mundt DJ, et al. A comparison of amrinone and glucagon therapy for cardiovascular depression associated with propranolol toxicity in a canine model. *J Toxicol Clin Toxicol.* 1992;30:399-412.
28. Hendren WG, Schieber RS, Garrettson LK. Extracorporeal bypass for the treatment of verapamil poisoning. *Ann Emerg Med.* 1989;18:984-987.
29. Wills B, Erickson T. Drug- and toxin-associated seizures. *Med Clin North Am.* 2005;89:1297-1321.
30. Boyer E, Shannon M. The serotonin syndrome. *N Engl J Med.* 2005;352:1112-1120.
31. Strawn J, Keck P, Caroff S. Neuroleptic malignant syndrome. *Am J Psychiatr.* 2007;164:870-876.
32. Dematte JE, O'Mara K, Buescher J, et al. Near-fatal heat stroke during the 1995 heat wave in Chicago. *Ann Intern Med.* 1998;129:173-181.
33. Temple AR. Pathophysiology of aspirin overdosage toxicity, with implications for management. *Pediatrics.* 1978;62:873-876.
34. Roberts D, Aaron C. Management of acute organophosphorus pesticide poisoning. *BMJ Br Med J (Clin Res).* 2007;334:629-634.
35. Nelson LS, Perrone J, DeRoos F, et al. Aldicarb poisoning by an illicit rodenticide imported into the United States: Tres Pasitos. *J Toxicol Clin Toxicol.* 2001;39:447-452.
36. Chabali R. Diagnostic use of anion and osmolal gaps in pediatric emergency medicine. *Pediatr Emerg Care.* 1997;13:204-210.
37. Baud FJ, Barriot P, Toffis V, et al. Elevated blood cyanide concentrations in victims of smoke inhalation. *N Engl J Med.* 1991;325:1761-1766.
38. Forsyth JC, Mueller PD, Becker CE, et al. Hydroxocobalamin as a cyanide antidote: safety, efficacy and pharmacokinetics in heavily smoking normal volunteers. *J Toxicol Clin Toxicol.* 1993;31:277-294.
39. Borron SW, Baud FJ, Barriot P, et al. Prospective study of hydroxocobalamin for acute cyanide poisoning in smoke inhalation. *Ann Emerg Med.* 2007;49:794-801.
40. Shepherd G, Velez LI. Role of hydroxocobalamin in acute cyanide poisoning. *Ann Pharmacother.* 2008;42:661-669.
41. Brent J. Fomepizole for ethylene glycol and methanol poisoning. *N Engl J Med.* 2009;360:2216-2223.
42. Hoffman RS, Smilkstein MJ, Howland MA, et al. Osmol gaps revisited: normal values and limitations. *J Toxicol Clin Toxicol.* 1993;31:81-93.
43. Morgan TJ, Clark C, Clague A. Artifactual elevation of measured plasma L-lactate concentration in the presence of glycolate. *Crit Care Med.* 1999;27:2177-2179.
44. Glaser DS. Utility of the serum osmol gap in the diagnosis of methanol or ethylene glycol ingestion. *Ann Emerg Med.* 1996;27:343-346.
45. Soghoian S, Sinert R, Wiener S, et al. Ethylene glycol toxicity presenting with non-anion gap metabolic acidosis. *Basic Clin Pharmacol Toxicol.* 2009;104:22-26.
46. Mgarbane B, Borron S, Baud F. Current recommendations for treatment of severe toxic alcohol poisonings. *Intensive Care Med.* 2005;31:189-195.
47. Galbois A, Ait-Oufella H, Baudel J-L, et al. An adult can still die of salicylate poisoning in France in 2008. *Intensive Care Med.* 2009;35:1999.
48. Stolbach A, Hoffman R, Nelson L. Mechanical ventilation was associated with acidemia in a case series of salicylate-poisoned patients. *Acad Emerg Med.* 2008;15:866-869.
49. Dart R, Borron S, Caravati EM, et al. Expert consensus guidelines for stocking of antidotes in hospitals that provide emergency care. *Ann Emerg Med.* 2009;54:386-394.

CHAPTER 15

The Crashing Trauma Patient

Michael A. Gibbs and Robert J. Winchell

Introduction

It may seem ambitious to attempt a summary of the evaluation and management of a disease as complex and heterogeneous as trauma in the few pages that follow, and presenting a comprehensive description of trauma care in a single chapter is indeed a challenge. To cover this broad topic succinctly, we propose that a series of concise, goal-directed recommendations can help the clinician manage the "crashing trauma patient":

1) Develop a rapid and effective method of identifying and prioritizing critical injuries.
2) Employ rational resuscitative strategies that address critical physiologic derangement.

These actions are driven by the answers to two very basic questions: 1) What do I need to know? and 2) What do I need to do?

Emergency management of the critically injured patient is fast moving, complex, and diverse. The clinician is often confronted with multiple, simultaneous, life-threatening conditions with divergent diagnostic and therapeutic pathways. To maximize a patient's functional outcome, it is essential to correctly prioritize studies and interventions and to avoid delay. To further complicate matters, these decisions must be made rapidly, in the high-stress environment of the trauma resuscitation room. With a lot at stake for the patient and the team, it is essential to follow a simple algorithm that adheres to basic principles, while at the same time providing the flexibility to adapt to changes in clinical status.

Few disease states are more demanding of a collaborative, team approach. Each member of the team must understand his or her specific role, the constantly changing resuscitative priorities, and the overall management plan in the context of multiple, coincident injuries. Effective care also requires a clearly identified leader to oversee and guide the team. As the "conductor of the orchestra," the team leader remains constantly vigilant; receiving input from the team and from consultants, reassessing the patient's clinical status, and making minute-to-minute decisions about the most important "next test," "next intervention," or "next stop" along the care continuum.

Injury Identification—What Do I Need to Know?

The Basic Approach

The series of decisions involved in the initial resuscitation of the critically injured patient can be reduced to a straightforward strategy, as follows: problems must be identified and treated first in the order of their immediate threat to life, followed by the immediacy of their threat to functional outcome. This process can be distilled to the steps listed in Figure 15-1, which are independent of the specific injuries involved. Throughout the process, both the team leader and the resuscitation team must be focused on adhering strictly to these priorities and must not be distracted by potential "efficiencies" such as undertaking noncritical diagnostic studies or noncritical therapeutic interventions.

Step 1: Identify the need to immediately control the airway.

Control of the airway is the first and most critical component of resuscitation. The decision to intubate is complex and is influenced by several factors (Table 15-1). Because the clinical picture often evolves rapidly in the setting of acute injury, the general dictum to "intubate early" applies much more often than not. This is particularly true for patients with injuries likely to cause abrupt anatomic distortion of the airway and for those whose overall physiologic reserve is threatened. The one mitigating factor that must be considered is the patient's volume status. Rapid sequence intubation (RSI) and institution of positive-pressure ventilation could cause severe and refractory hypotension in the hypovolemic patient. This risk must be weighed against the potential benefits of temporizing to allow for fluid resuscitation or to prepare for surgical intervention.

Consider the patient with a small stab wound to the neck, stable vital signs, and no overt clinical evidence of airway compromise. Although this seemingly innocuous initial presentation could reassure the clinician at the bedside, airway obstruction can develop rapidly and with little warning. As a second example, consider the patient with a severe, displaced pelvic ring fracture, who is being prepared for transfer. As hemorrhage continues unabated, the patient is likely to decompensate abruptly in the back of the ambulance. Lastly, consider the elderly patient with blunt chest trauma and multiple rib fractures. Increased work of breathing, hypercarbia, and progressive respiratory failure are almost unavoidable. In each of these examples, early airway management is both prudent and protective. This philosophy allows the treating clinician to approach the intervention when the patient's physiology is at its best, not at its worst. The cognitive and technical aspects of trauma airway management are discussed in more detail later in this chapter.

KEY POINTS
Airway management in the crashing trauma patient

- **Preparation**
  - Perform a focused airway assessment to predict difficulty.
  - Identify surgical airway landmarks ahead of time.
  - Be sure appropriate airway rescue equipment is nearby.
  - Perform a brief neurologic examination *before* intubation.
  - Maximize preload in hypotensive patients and those with traumatic brain injury.

- **Drug selection**
  - Choose neuroprotective agents for patients with brain injury.
  - Be cautious with agent selection and dosage to avoid hypotension.
  - Ensure appropriate postintubation sedation with or without neuromuscular blockade.

- **Rescue**
  - Choose the approach/device most likely to be successful in your hands.
  - Know when to call for help.

Step 2: Identify and control immediate threats to maintaining central perfusion.

The clinical picture of impending cardiovascular collapse is not generally subtle. The patient is typically profoundly hypotensive, with clear clinical signs of inadequate perfusion. If the patient fails to respond to initial volume resuscitation and control of external hemorrhage, a very rapid assessment must be done to find the most likely cause of bleeding and to intervene immediately, often surgically. Physical examination may be sufficient, as is the case with penetrating injuries, or it may be augmented by rapid and basic diagnostic tests, including a focused assessment with sonography for trauma (FAST) and plain films of the chest and pelvis (Table 15-2). Control of hemorrhage and stabilization of perfusion outweigh all other concerns.

FIGURE 15-1.
Injury identification: the basic approach

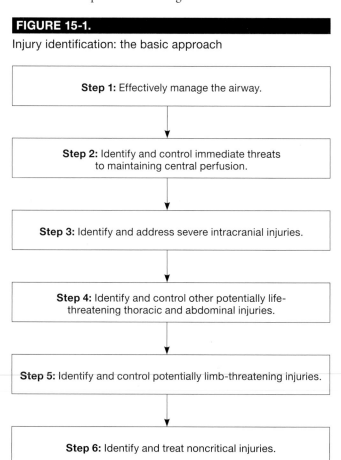

Step 1: Effectively manage the airway.

Step 2: Identify and control immediate threats to maintaining central perfusion.

Step 3: Identify and address severe intracranial injuries.

Step 4: Identify and control other potentially life-threatening thoracic and abdominal injuries.

Step 5: Identify and control potentially limb-threatening injuries.

Step 6: Identify and treat noncritical injuries.

The diagnostic approach will vary somewhat based on the mechanism of injury. In the crashing patient with blunt multisystem trauma, it is safest to assume that shock could come from any source or a combination of sources (Table 15-3). The assessment of a patient with penetrating trauma is somewhat different, based on an understanding of trajectory (Table 15-4). In a patient with stab wounds, the location of injury can generally be predicted with accuracy. The trajectory of bullets or other missiles is much less predictable, so it is wise to cast a very wide diagnostic net.

Step 3: Identify and address severe intracranial injuries.

If the patient has adequate perfusion with ongoing resuscitation, the next critical step is assessment of the likelihood of an intracranial lesion requiring neurosurgical intervention (Table 15-5). Physical examination and assessment of the Glasgow Coma Scale (GCS) score are the primary tools in initial triage. Patients with a GCS score of less than 8, especially in the presence of lateralizing signs, must be presumed to have a surgical lesion, and computed tomography (CT) of the head must be prioritized, even above interventions targeted at ongoing but manageable hemorrhage, a presumed intraabdominal injury, or compromise of an extremity. Patients with a GCS score of more than 13 have a very slight probability of requiring neurosurgical intervention, so CT of the head should be delayed. Patients with GCS scores between 8 and 13 should be triaged based on individual circumstances.

Step 4: Identify and control potentially life-threatening intrathoracic and intraabdominal injuries.

After establishment of sustainable perfusion and determination of intracranial pathology, attention should be directed toward diagnosis and management of other life-threatening issues (Table 15-6). This is the primary phase for more sophisticated diagnostic imaging techniques. Potential problems are listed below:

- Ongoing hemorrhage in the chest, abdomen, or pelvis
- Hollow viscus injuries
- Contained aortic injuries
- Other contained major vascular injuries

Step 5: Identify and control potentially limb-threatening injuries.

Once potentially life-threatening injuries have been addressed, injuries threatening limb function may be addressed (Table 15-7). This is another area in which specific diagnostic

---

TABLE 15-1.

Identify the need to immediately control the airway[a]

Indications for Intubation of the Trauma Patient
- Loss of airway or inability to protect the airway due to facial and/or neck injuries
- Severe head injury with a GCS score ≤8 (higher if head injury is obvious and the patient is combative)
- Significant chest injury with inadequate oxygenation/ventilation
- Insufficient ventilatory effort
- Low preexisting physiologic reserve
- Significant inhalation injury

[a]The patient's *anticipated course* should contribute to the decision to intubate early. Examples:
- The patient's injuries predict that airway obstruction is likely.
- The patient's injuries predict that cardiopulmonary deterioration is likely.
- The patient will be in a less secure environment soon (eg, radiology, interfacility transfer).
- The patient is bound for immediate surgery.

Pitfalls
- Failure to predict the patient's anticipated course
- Failure to protect the airway before interfacility transfer
- Intubation of the severely hypotensive patient with adequate airway and ventilation prior to volume resuscitation

---

TABLE 15-2.

Identify and control immediate threats to maintaining central perfusion

Differential Diagnosis
- Hemorrhagic causes
  - External bleeding
  - Intrathoracic bleeding
  - Intraperitoneal bleeding
  - Pelvic fracture
- Nonhemorrhagic causes
  - Pericardial tamponade
  - Tension pneumothorax
  - Myocardial contusion
  - Coincident medical condition (eg, acute myocardial infarction)

Physical Examination
- Identify sites of external hemorrhage
- Identify all penetrating wounds
- Identify major external evidence of injury

Diagnostic Strategy
- Bedside testing options
  - Chest film
  - Pelvic film
  - FAST
  - Diagnostic peritoneal lavage
- Definitive testing option—surgical exploration

Pitfalls
- Failure to recognize the need for immediate surgical exploration
- Delays caused by diagnostic testing (eg, computed tomography imaging)
- Inadequate resuscitation
- Failure to initiate early transfusion
- Failure to consider nonhemorrhagic causes of traumatic shock
- Failure to consider more than one cause of shock in the patient with multisystem injury
- Failure to consider coincident medical causes of shock in the injured patient

testing will be necessary. Injuries in this category include the following:

- Injuries associated with neurovascular compromise
- Open fractures
- Massive soft-tissue injuries
- Compartment syndrome

Step 6: Identify and treat noncritical injuries.

Injuries of a noncritical nature should be addressed only as time allows, after all issues identified in Steps 1 through 5 have been addressed (Table 15-8). Examples include the injuries listed below:

- Simple long-bone fractures
- Facial fractures
- Lacerations

The Diagnostic Toolbox

With advances in technology, the number of diagnostic options for the evaluation of trauma patients is growing. When an injured patient is crashing and time is of the essence, emergency physicians must be able to select the right tool to get the right information. Each approach and each modality have strengths and weaknesses, which are reviewed below.

Physical Examination

For decades, the foundation of the advanced trauma life support (ATLS) assessment has been the physical examination. It is important to recognize that physical assessment of the trauma patient, although valuable, has limitations. For example, large studies describe a 5% to 10% rate of "occult" abdominal injuries when patients are evaluated with physical examination alone.[1-3] Missed abdominal injuries are especially common in patients with neurologic impairment resulting from brain injury or alcohol, patients with multiple coincident injuries or severe "distracting" injuries, and patients at the extremes of age. It is logical that the same pitfalls apply to other organ systems.

We strongly support the performance of a careful, targeted examination in the crashing trauma patient. The missed-injury data presented above should not tempt the clinician to bypass

this important step on the way to the CT scanner. The challenge is to understand when the physical examination is enough, and when additional diagnostic information is needed.

Laboratory Testing

Laboratory tests are easy to obtain and relatively inexpensive. Unfortunately, the information they provide seldom provokes a change in the acute management plan. In a prospective review of 200 injured patients at a Level I trauma center, where the treating clinician was asked to generate a management plan prior to and after the availability of point-of-care test results, the plan was almost never altered. Serum electrolytes and blood

---

TABLE 15-4.

Rapid evaluation of the crashing patient with penetrating trauma

---

Step 1: Find all the holes and mark them prior to radiography

Step 2: Understand the trajectory

- Neck wound
  - Is there a major vascular injury?
  - Is the airway compromised?
  - Has the chest cavity been penetrated (see below)?

Testing: Chest film, surgical exploration; strong consideration for CT or plain film angiography in injuries involving Zone I or Zone III

- Chest wound
  - Is there a major vascular injury?
  - Does the patient have pericardial tamponade?
  - Does the patient have a tension pneumothorax?
  - Has the abdominal cavity or neck been penetrated (see below)?

Testing: Chest film, FAST, surgical exploration

Approach: If the patient is unresponsive to resuscitation, immediate surgical exploration is warranted. In patients with adequate perfusion, tube thoracostomy is the initial step.

- Abdominal/flank wound
  - Is there a major vascular injury?
  - Has the chest cavity been penetrated (see above)?

Testing: FAST (limited sensitivity for abdominal injury), DPL, chest film, surgical exploration

Approach: If the patient is unresponsive to resuscitation, immediate surgical exploration is warranted. In patients with adequate perfusion, further evaluation is warranted for stab wounds or tangential gunshot wounds. Most patients with abdominal gunshot wounds should undergo surgical exploration based on the high probability of injury.

- Extremity wound
  - Is there a major vascular injury?
  - Has the chest or abdominal cavity been penetrated (see above)?

Testing: Ankle-brachial index, surgical exploration

Approach: Hard signs of injury (eg, expanding hematoma, distal compromise, active arterial bleeding) warrant immediate surgical intervention, with imaging in the operating room as needed. Soft signs (hematoma, proximity) warrant further investigation.

TABLE 15-3.

Causes of shock in the critically injured trauma patient

Hemorrhagic Shock

- Intraabdominal
- Intrathoracic
- Retroperitoneal
- Long-bone fractures
- External
- Scalp (infants and small children)

Nonhemorrhagic Shock

- Tension pneumothorax
- Pericardial tamponade
- Myocardial contusion
- Spinal cord transection
- Coexistent medical condition (eg, acute myocardial infarction, gastrointestinal bleed, medications)

urea nitrogen were never influential. Changes were made based on hemoglobin in 3.5% of cases, a blood gas parameter in 3% of cases, and glucose in 0.5% of cases.[4]

Laboratory data are more useful to establish trends rather than pinpoint a diagnosis or sway a course of action. In the crashing trauma patient, it is reasonable to obtain "standard" laboratory studies, acknowledging that they will be most useful for downstream providers. The serum lactate level is a useful marker of global perfusion. In the critically ill patient, serial measurements every 2 to 4 hours can be used to assess the adequacy of resuscitation.[5,6]

Plain Film Imaging

Many practitioners remember the "c-spine, chest, pelvis" imaging triad of years past. As the experience with CT imaging grows, many centers have questioned the need for plain film imaging. For example, some authors have challenged the need for routine chest radiography, favoring CT imaging instead.[7] Others have argued to retain the chest film because of its speed and simplicity and the value of the information provided.[8] Others point to the overall low yield of chest CT, favoring clinically based selection of the right test.[9]

As the debate rages on with reasonable arguments to support all positions, it is useful to return to the critical question: in the crashing trauma patient, how will the information obtained affect patient management? If the chest film shows a massive hemothorax, this is useful information that can be acted on immediately. If a pelvic radiograph shows an "open-book" injury with 5 cm of pubic diastasis, this is useful information that can be acted on immediately. So, the question becomes, will plain films provide information the clinician must know *before* leaving the trauma room?

Plain films of the spine or the extremity are generally of very little value in the crashing trauma patient. Obtaining these images wastes precious time, especially if transfer to a tertiary center is imminent. Instead, maintain spinal immobilization at all times and reduce and splint obvious extremity fractures.

Bedside Ultrasonography

In experienced hands, bedside ultrasonography can be a very useful adjunct in the management of the injured patient.[10] Applied correctly, it serves as an extension of the physical examination.[11] Thus, it is important for clinicians to understand the following caveats to maximize effectiveness and avoid false-negative studies:

1) The FAST detects free fluid as a surrogate for injury, not the injury itself. The detection of fluid may be only the first step, with the second step being better definitive characterization of specific injuries (ie, using CT, angiography, or laparotomy).

TABLE 15-5.

Identify and address severe intracranial injuries

Differential Diagnosis
- Extra-axial collections (epidural hematoma, subdural hematoma)
- Intracerebral hemorrhage
- Subarachnoid hemorrhage
- Diffuse axonal injury
- Cerebrovascular injury

Physical Examination
- Signs of external head trauma
- GCS score <8
- GCS motor component <5
- Pupillary or motor asymmetry

Diagnostic Strategy
- Bedside testing options — none
- Definitive testing options
  - Noncontrast head CT
  - Head CT/CT-angiogram

Pitfalls
- Failure to consider reversible causes such as hypoglycemia, hypoxia, shock
- Failure to manage overall patient with respect to perfusion and oxygenation
- Attribution of neurologic dysfunction to intoxication
- Delays in transfer to obtain a head CT in the patient with severe neurologic dysfunction
- Failure to consider cerebrovascular disease in the at-risk patient

TABLE 15-6.

Identify and control potentially life-threatening thoracic and abdominal injuries

Differential Diagnosis
- Ongoing hemorrhage in the chest, abdomen, or pelvis
- Contained aortic injury
- Hollow viscus injuries, including bladder
- Other contained major vascular injuries

Physical Examination
- External signs of injury, chest asymmetry, crepitus, seat-belt sign
- Penetrating injuries
- Signs of decreased ventilation
- Peritoneal signs
- Pelvic instability or deformity

Diagnostic Strategy
- Bedside testing options
  - Chest film
  - Pelvic film
  - FAST
- Definitive testing options
  - CT
  - CT or plain film angiography

Pitfalls
- Failure to diagnose aortic injury in a timely fashion
- Failure to diagnose hollow viscus injury
- Failure to appreciate potential for pelvic bleeding
- Failure to appreciate potential for chest or abdominal bleeding
- Inadequate drainage of hemothorax or pneumothorax
- Inadequate resuscitation

2) Ultrasonography provides the highest yield in patients who are in shock. A grossly positive (or a grossly negative) FAST in the hypotensive blunt trauma patient gives you valuable information regarding the best next step. In this population, sensitivities and specificities exceed 95%.[10–13]

3) Ultrasonography is highly sensitive for detecting the presence or absence of hemopericardium and should be used early in the evaluation of patients with penetrating torso trauma.[14,15] Exceptions include patients with large pericardial lacerations that can evacuate into the left chest. Hemopericardium should be considered in patients with penetrating chest trauma, a "negative" FAST, and fluid in the left hemithorax. Serial FAST examinations can increase diagnostic accuracy.[16]

4) In patients with bladder rupture, the detection of free intraabdominal fluid could reflect the presence of urine,

not blood.[16] This is especially likely in patients with anterior pelvic ring fractures.[17] Diagnostic peritoneal lavage (DPL) or CT imaging can help in these cases.

5) Recent data suggest that thoracic ultrasonography provides higher sensitivity for detecting pneumothorax than a single anteroposterior (AP) chest film. As is the case for the abdominal and cardiac examinations, sonographic evaluation of the chest relies on surrogate measures of the disease (ie, the presence or absence of lung sliding and comet tails) (see Chapter 3, "The Crashing Ventilated Patient").[18,19]

Computed Tomography Imaging

The use of CT imaging in trauma has flourished. Third- and fourth-generation multidetector technology offers superior image quality, rapid acquisition time, and impressive reformatting capabilities. Injuries for which CT imaging was previously thought to be insensitive (eg, pancreas, bowel, diaphragm) can now be interrogated with a high degree of precision. In many large trauma centers, the use of routine "pan CT scanning" involving the head, neck, chest, abdomen, and pelvis has been promoted.[20,21] However, this approach has not been well studied in critically ill trauma patients. In this population, the question is less "Will I get enough information?" and more "Is the patient stable enough to travel to radiology?"

Diagnostic Peritoneal Lavage

DPL was first described by Root et al in 1965 as a rapid method of detecting intraperitoneal hemorrhage.[22] Since then, numerous authors have demonstrated the utility of DPL, especially in a hemodynamically unstable patient.[23,24] Although bedside ultrasonography has largely supplanted DPL, DPL remains a valuable tool in the evaluation of unstable patients.[25] In the crashing patient with suspected abdominal injury, DPL should be considered when 1) ultrasonography is not available, 2) FAST results are equivocal, or 3) a positive FAST result has a likelihood of being a false positive (eg, pelvic trauma with possible bladder rupture and uroperitoneum).[16,17]

TABLE 15-7.

Identify and control potentially limb-threatening injuries

Differential Diagnosis
- Arterial injury
- Compartment syndrome
- Severe fracture and/or dislocation

Physical Examination
- Limb deformity
- Evidence of inadequate perfusion
- Hard signs of vascular injury
  – Expanding hematoma
  – Loss of distal pulses
  – Active arterial bleeding
- Soft signs of vascular injury
  – Proximity of penetrating wounds or high-risk fractures
  – Nonexpanding hematoma
  – Evidence of associated peripheral nerve injury
- Open wounds, especially in proximity to fractures
- Tight compartments, especially lower leg

Diagnostic Strategy
- Bedside testing options
  – Ankle-brachial index
  – Bedside assessment of compartment pressure
  – Plain films
- Definitive testing options
  – CT
  – CT or plain film angiography
  – Surgical exploration

Pitfalls
- Failure to proceed directly to surgery with hard signs of vascular injury
- Failure to control ongoing bleeding from extremity wounds
- Failure to perform an ankle-brachial index with soft signs of vascular injury or knee dislocation
- Failure to consider and evaluate for compartment syndrome, especially in unconscious patients
- Failure to reduce and splint long-bone fractures
- Failure to reduce dislocations

TABLE 15-8.

Identify and treat noncritical injuries

Physical Examination
Once life-threatening injuries have been identified and stabilized, a thorough head-to-toe secondary survey should be performed.

Diagnostic Strategy
- Definitive imaging of facial fractures
- Plain film imaging of extremity fractures

Pitfalls
- Failure to perform a thorough secondary survey once the critically ill patient has been stabilized
- Delayed diagnosis of closed fractures
- Failure to address lacerations and open wounds
- Failure to fully examine wounds for potential complications, including injury to underlying structures or retained foreign bodies

Clinical Decision Rules

Well-studied clinical decision rules have been developed to guide imaging of the spine,[26,27] brain,[28] and pelvis[29,30] in *stable* patients. These processes have been incorporated into the most recent ATLS guidelines. Preliminary studies have explored the use of clinical decision rules to guide management of chest and abdominal injury, again, in the stable patient.

There are currently no clinical decision rules to support imaging decisions in the crashing trauma patient. It is logical that the sicker the patient, the less room there is for error. Therefore, liberal use of imaging in this patient population should be considered.

Resuscitation Essentials—What Do I Need To Do?

Managing the Trauma Airway

In critically injured patients, early effective management of the airway is fundamental. Systematic reviews reveal that delayed or ineffective airway management is associated with significant increases in mortality. Failure to manage the airway has been repeatedly cited as one of the most common causes of preventable death in trauma.[31–33]

Once the decision to intubate has been made (Step 1 of the basic approach, discussed above), a successful strategy combines sophisticated assessment skills, the ability to predict physiologic derangement, and technical proficiency with a rapidly growing number of airway management devices. In the heat of the moment, the clinician must be a quick planner and rapidly answer two related questions:

- Will the procedure be difficult?
- What is the best airway management strategy?

Predicting the Difficult Airway

A number of systems have been developed to predict the difficult airway. The "LEMON" mnemonic represents a practical, systematic assessment that can be performed rapidly at the bedside. Based on anatomic features, this approach was developed as a tool to predict difficult laryngoscopy and intubation.[34] The mnemonic refers to assessing five predictors of difficulty: looking at the external features; evaluating the geometry of the airway; the Mallampati score; obstruction; and neck mobility. Recent studies have validated the predictive utility of this mnemonic,[35] which is endorsed in the most recent edition of the ATLS guidelines.[36] (See Chapter 2, "The Difficult Airway in the Critically Ill Patient.")

Choosing an Airway Management Strategy

An effective airway management strategy combines two independent predictive steps: 1) *anticipation* of the technically difficult airway and selection of the most appropriate technique to overcome it and 2) *anticipation* of the physiologic response to intubation and the drugs used to facilitate the procedure.

Once the airway has been assessed for potential technical difficulty, questions about physiology can be guided by the "Trauma ABCs," a mnemonic developed by one of the authors of this chapter (M.A.G.).[37]

A – Airway Injury?

Injury to the airway mandates that the clinician recognize the inherent risk of neuromuscular blockade. In this situation, a number of alternatives may be considered, including sedative-assisted "awake" orotracheal intubation, fiberoptic or videolaryngoscopic intubation with topical anesthesia and sedation, surgical cricothyroidotomy, or a "double setup" technique (RSI with surgical airway equipment at the ready).

B – Brain Injury?

The overriding priorities during intubation of the patient with severe head injury are 1) to avoid hypotension and/or hypoxia and resultant secondary injury and 2) to employ a neuroprotective pharmacologic regimen. RSI is the standard in this population, unless it is contraindicated by airway injury or anatomic difficulty.

A number of premedication strategies (using lidocaine, fentanyl, and defasciculation) have been proposed to decrease the sympathetic response to laryngoscopy, but studies demonstrating any outcome benefit are lacking. Therefore, a simple strategy using a neuroprotective induction agent and a short-acting neuromuscular blocking agent seems logical, practical, and safe.

C – Cervical Injury?

All blunt trauma patients have cervical injury until proven otherwise. Because a single cross-table lateral cervical spine radiograph has limited sensitivity for fracture, interrupting the resuscitation to obtain this image offers no value and should be avoided. The spine should be held in line at all times during airway management, and this should be documented in the medical record.

C – Chest Injury?

Acute chest injury markedly limits respiratory reserve and virtually ensures rapid desaturation on paralysis. Decompensation should be anticipated in patients with significant blunt or penetrating chest trauma, and deliberate steps should be taken to maximally preoxygenate the patient, execute RSI rapidly, and have an airway rescue plan at the ready.

Risks persist after successful laryngoscopy, when positive-pressure ventilation rapidly converts a simple pneumothorax into a tension pneumothorax. Should this injury be known or suspected, the team should be prepared to perform an immediate needle chest decompression or chest tube thoracostomy.

S – Shock?

In the hemodynamically compromised patient, multiple factors can worsen shock during airway management. Induction agents decrease vascular tone and cardiac output. Loss of muscle tone following paralysis and positive-pressure ventilation both decrease venous return and cardiac output.

When patients are in overt or subclinical shock, several steps can be taken to avoid decompensation. When time permits, fluids should be administered rapidly to augment preload. Induction drugs with the most favorable hemodynamic profile (eg, etomidate, ketamine) should be selected over those more likely to decrease vascular tone and cardiac output (eg, thiopental, propofol, midazolam). When a patient is in frank shock, no matter which agent is selected, dosing should be reduced by 50%.

The use of etomidate for trauma intubations has been questioned recently.[38–40] Described as the "etomidate paradox," the favorable hemodynamic profile of the drug in compromised patients is offset by the risk of subsequent adrenal suppression.[41] Until well-designed, randomized, controlled trials demonstrate a clear detrimental effect, it is difficult to ignore the superiority of this drug in the acute setting.[42]

Ketamine is an attractive alternative to etomidate in the injured patient.[40] Because ketamine augments sympathetic outflow and therefore increases heart rate and blood pressure, it is considered by many to be the induction agent of choice in hypotensive trauma patients without brain injury. The traditional concern about using ketamine in brain-injured patients stems from the observation that the drug increases cerebral blood flow and cerebral metabolic rate and therefore has the potential to increase intracranial pressure (ICP). More recent data challenge this assertion, citing demonstrated reductions in ICP in children with brain trauma.[43]

Optimizing Resuscitation

General Principles

Failure to recognize and adequately treat shock is an important problem during the early phases of trauma management. It represents one of the top causes of preventable and potentially preventable mortality.[44]

Clinicians must develop a unique resuscitative strategy for each acutely injured patient based on known or suspected injuries, the evolving clinical status, and the patient's preinjury condition. This strategy must be fluid, changing from minute to minute in tandem with careful assessment and reassessment of the patient.

Recent data suggest that the physical examination is insensitive for detection of ongoing hemorrhage and subclinical shock. This is especially true in elderly trauma patients with decreased physiologic reserve.[45,46] The addition of serum markers (eg, lactate, base deficit) significantly improves the ability to assess tissue perfusion and hypoxia across all age groups.[6,47] Serial measurements of these markers will help guide the resuscitation. Bedside sonographic assessment of the diameter of the inferior vena cava can also be useful to assess preload and response to fluid therapy.[48]

Fluid and Transfusion Therapy

Normal saline and lactated Ringer solution remain the fluids of choice for initial trauma resuscitation. There is no compelling evidence from randomized trials that colloid therapy offers any outcome benefit.[49] The decision to transfuse is complex and should be based on the patient's clinical status, the response to crystalloid, and the anticipated ongoing blood loss.

There is increasing study of massive transfusion, defined as the administration of 10 or more units of packed red blood cells (PRBCs) within 24 hours. Because massive transfusion is required in only 1% to 3% of civilian trauma patients, institutional protocols should be developed to facilitate effective execution of this low-frequency intervention. Under ideal circumstances, massive transfusion begins in the emergency department and continues in the operating room, angiography

suite, or intensive care unit (ICU).

When massive transfusion is anticipated, all efforts should be made to achieve a 1:1:1 ratio of PRBCs to platelets to fresh frozen plasma. This aggressive approach lowers overall transfusion requirements, forestalls coagulopathy, and decreases mortality.[50–53] (See Chapter 16, "Emergency Transfusions," for additional discussion.)

Hypovolemic Resuscitation

Resuscitation of the crashing patient with penetrating torso wounds should follow a different resuscitative paradigm. Overzealous fluid administration in this setting, with the aim of achieving a "normal" blood pressure, increases intracavitary bleeding and mortality. The practice of hypovolemic resuscitation is based on the Houston experience, where immediate transport to the operating room with minimal fluid therapy was associated with increased survival and fewer complications.[54] A target systolic blood pressure of 80 to 90 mm Hg is reasonable, provided rapid surgical control of bleeding can be achieved. This strategy should not be applied to patients with coincident brain injury or to those who have sustained multisystem blunt trauma.

Neuroresuscitation

Early resuscitation of the patient with severe traumatic brain injury (TBI) can have a profoundly beneficial effect on survival. In the landmark study of 717 patients with severe TBI, Chesnut and colleagues observed that a single episode of hypotension was associated with a 150% increase in mortality.[55] During the early management of these patients, the main objective should be to maintain adequate central nervous system (CNS) perfusion at all times to minimize secondary brain injury.[56]

In the emergency department, this translates into a diligent search for hemorrhagic and nonhemorrhagic causes of shock, adequate fluid and transfusion therapy, careful drug selection to avoid iatrogenic hypotension (eg, during RSI), and planning for the definitive control of bleeding. These decisions must be made in close collaboration with neurosurgical colleagues to effectively stage hemorrhage-controlling surgery with definitive head-injury management.

Effective Early Management of Severe Traumatic Brain Injury

Severe TBI is the primary cause of death and serious disability after trauma. Each year, 50,000 patients die from head injury and another 80,000 are left with permanent neurologic disability.[56,57] It is critical for acute care physicians to have a sophisticated understanding of the imperatives of early TBI care. Adherence to published evidence-based guidelines decreases variability and improves outcomes.[58,59]

Initial management should focus on the following:
1) Effective management of the airway
2) Careful maintenance of adequate tissue perfusion
3) Medical treatment of clinically evident intracranial hypertension
4) Timely consultation with and transfer to a trauma center

At the center of an effective TBI management strategy is the prevention of secondary injury brought on by hypotension and/

or hypoxemia. Even transient drops in blood pressure or oxygen saturations are associated with markedly worsened outcomes.[55] At the bedside, this translates into aggressive airway management and fluid resuscitation, caution with all vasoactive medications, and prompt hemorrhage control.

Once the airway is secure and resuscitation is ongoing, attention can be turned to assessing whether or not the patient has intracranial hypertension, and if so, what should be done to manage it. In the hemodynamically stable patient with clear signs of impending herniation (rapid neurologic decline, pupillary asymmetry, motor posturing), medical therapy to reduce elevated ICP is indicated. In this setting, the Brain Trauma Foundation's TBI guidelines (www.braintrauma.org) recommend early mannitol therapy as the initial approach, with a target dose of 1 to 1.5 g/kg. Consistent with the goal of avoiding secondary injury, mannitol should be given with caution or should be withheld entirely from patients who are hypotensive and those with significant ongoing hemorrhage.[56]

The role of hyperventilation in the management of severe TBI has evolved considerably. Once a mainstay of early therapy, hyperventilation is now known to cause considerable morbidity. Hyperventilation reduces ICP at the expense of cerebral blood flow. In an acutely injured patient, in whom CNS perfusion is already threatened, hyperventilation causes additional impairment in regional blood flow and significant issue ischemia.[60,61] Thus, marked hyperventilation should generally be avoided in patients with severe TBI. Mild hyperventilation, with target $Paco_2$ of 35 to 40 mm Hg, should be used, but more aggressive hyperventilation should be reserved for patients with unequivocal signs of impending herniation who fail to respond to mannitol and for those with significant hypotension, when mannitol is contraindicated. Aggressive hyperventilation should be as brief as clinically possible, typically with a target of no lower than 30 mm Hg.[56]

The anticoagulated patient with TBI deserves special mention. When controlled for injury severity, studies have demonstrated markedly worse outcomes for patients taking warfarin.[62,63] Whenever possible, reversal of anticoagulation should be initiated as early as possible, preferably *before* transfer.

Timely transfer of severely brain-injured patients to centers capable of providing operative and intensive care is essential. When severe TBI is clinically evident, time should not be wasted obtaining a head CT scan, only to find critical lesions that cannot be managed. Sound clinical judgment, early communication, and regional referral protocols will bring efficiency to the process.

KEY POINTS
Effective management of traumatic brain injury

- **Airway Management**
  - Even transient hypoxemia dramatically worsens outcomes; therefore, *intubate early.*
  - Rapid-sequence intubation is the preferred technique.
  - Use a neuroprotective sedative (eg, etomidate).
  - Pretreatment (lidocaine, fentanyl, defasciculation) is controversial, with no proven benefit.

- **Resuscitation**
  - Even transient hypotension dramatically worsens outcome; therefore, *resuscitate aggressively.*
  - Rapid identification of coincident hemorrhage is crucial.
  - Resuscitative goal is to maintain CNS perfusion.
  - Be cautious with medications that can precipitate hypotension.

- **Diagnostic Testing**
  - Do not delay patient transfer to get a head CT if severe TBI is clinically evident.
  - The goal of early testing is to identify injuries that require immediate surgical management.

- **Management of Intracranial Hypertension**
  Mannitol
  - Effectively reduces elevated ICP
  - Recommended dose, 1–1.5 g/kg
  - Can precipitate hypotension:
  - Withhold if blood pressure is 90 mm Hg or lower.
  - Use with caution if blood pressure is above 90 mm Hg and tenuous and/or if there is ongoing hemorrhage.
  - Administer small sequential boluses (0.25–0.5 g/kg) if hypotension is a risk.

  Hyperventilation
  - Effectively reduces elevated ICP
  - Potential for local CNS hypoperfusion
  - Mild hyperventilation ($Paco_2$ of 35–40 mm Hg) for all patients with TBI
  - Aggressive hyperventilation:

    Only as a temporizing measure if clear clinical signs of herniation are present (blown pupil, motor posturing, rapid neurologic decline + coma) or signs of herniation are visible on CT.

    Use in conjunction with other measures (eg, mannitol, sedation) whenever possible.

    Use for the shortest duration possible.

    Maintain end-tidal Pco_2 above 30 mm Hg.

Preparing the Patient for Definitive Management

The first minutes after patient arrival are focused on initial resuscitation and rapid diagnostic evaluation. In the very critical patient, this evaluation could lead directly to definitive care in the operating room or the ICU, and the patient may never return to the resuscitation bay. Often, however, patients remain in the resuscitation space for a time while therapeutic decisions are made and resources marshaled. In this circumstance, there is a natural tendency for the level of engagement to wane and a risk for the intensity of care to decrease as providers shift their perception of the situation and their role in patient care. There is also a possible transition between teams with primary responsibility for the patient. It is imperative that the resuscitative team maintain vigilance and active management of the injured patient until definitive hand-off to another team. In many emergency departments, this means essentially providing an ICU level of care within the resuscitation space, with appropriate attention to details of neurologic care, medications, active warming, correction of coagulopathy and metabolic derangements, ongoing resuscitation, and preparations for surgical intervention.

Preparing the Patient for Transfer

For a significant majority of injured patients, care begins outside a regional trauma center. Clinicians working in community hospitals, therefore, play a pivotal role in trauma care. Trauma systems that connect community hospitals with regional trauma centers have superior patient outcomes, especially for the critically injured.[64-66]

The decision to transfer, which is based primarily on local resources, is complex and unique to each institution. The challenge is to give just the right amount of stabilizing care, without delaying transfer and definitive therapy unnecessarily. Although the solution to this dilemma is not always self-evident or easy to achieve, a minimalistic approach is logical; once the decision to transfer has been made, do only what must be done and request tests only if the results will be acted upon. In a study that illustrates the second point, Onzuka and colleagues reviewed the care of 249 consecutive adult trauma patients who were transferred to a regional Canadian trauma center over a 2-year period. Roughly one third of these patients had CT imaging performed prior to transfer. In no case was the CT result used to determine the need for transfer, and in no case did it lead to a decision to perform surgery before transfer.[67] Interventions that should and should not be done prior to transfer are listed in the key points.

Another essential element of the transfer process hinges on effective communication. This is grounded on basic principles as follows: 1) establish transfer policies and procedures ahead of time, 2) communicate early, 3) ensure that all relevant documents and test results are available for downstream care providers, and 4) participate in the ongoing regional quality assurance process.

KEY POINTS

Preparing the patient for transfer

- **Interventions: should be done before transfer**
  - Manage the airway.
  - Secure adequate intravenous access and begin resuscitation.
  - Control external bleeding.
  - Begin PRBC transfusion if the patient is persistently hypotensive after 2 liters of crystalloid, with potential for ongoing hemorrhage.
  - Begin anticoagulation reversal for intracranial, major intracavitary, or external hemorrhage.
  - Perform tube thoracostomy for symptomatic pneumothorax/hemothorax.
  - Stabilize grossly displaced pelvic ring fractures and provide external compression.
  - Reduce dislocations with clear vascular compromise.
  - Splint extremity fractures.
  - Protect the patient from hypothermia.

- **Interventions: should not delay transfer and definitive management**
  - In general, once the decision to transfer has been made, further diagnostic imaging is unlikely to be of benefit and is likely to be repeated at the receiving institution, unless there is strong interfacility sharing of image data.
  - May consider only if they will cause absolutely no delay in transfer:
    Cranial CT
    Body CT
    Plain films of the extremities for obvious fractures
    Cervical imaging when the spine is properly immobilized
    Specific laboratory testing

- **Communication and the transfer process**
  - When clinical instability or the nature of the injuries mandates transfer, communicate early. Do not wait for test results.
  - Ensure the transfer of all notes, images, test results, and summary of interventions.

Conclusion

Emergency department management of the critically ill trauma patient is complex, challenging, and, quite simply, stressful. To minimize morbidity and decrease mortality, a systematic approach to evaluation and management is essential. Injury identification begins with determining the need to immediately control the airway, followed by identification of central perfusion deficits, severe intracranial injuries, intrathoracic and intraabdominal injuries, and limb-threatening injuries. Successful resuscitation strategies must include management of the airway, appropriate fluid and transfusion therapy, and management of traumatic brain injury. Many critically ill trauma patients require transfer to a regional trauma center. For these patients, a number of critical interventions should be performed prior to transfer.

References

1. Schurink GW, Bode PJ, van Luijt PA, et al. The value of physical examination in the diagnosis of patients with blunt abdominal trauma: a retrospective study. *Injury.* 1997;29:261-265.

2. American College of Emergency Physicians. Clinical policy: critical issues in the evaluation of adult patients presenting to the emergency department with acute blunt abdominal trauma. *Ann Emerg Med.* 2004;43:278-290.

3. Holmes J, Nguyen H, Jacoby RC, et al. Do all patients with left costal margin injuries require radiographic evaluation for abdominal injury? *Ann Emerg Med.* 2005;46:232-236.

4. Asimos A, Gibbs MA, Marx JA, et al. Value of point-of-care blood testing in emergent trauma management. *J Trauma.* 2000;48:1101-1108.

5. Paladino L, Sinert R, Wallace D, et al. The utility of base deficit and arterial lactate in differentiating major from minor injury in trauma patients with normal vital signs. *Resuscitation.* 2008;77:363-368.

6. Callaway DW, Shapiro NI, Donnino MW, et al. Serum lactate and base deficit as predictors of mortality in normotensive elderly blunt trauma patients. *J Trauma.* 2009;66:1040-1044.

7. Wisbach GG, Sise MJ, Sack DI, et al. What is the role of chest X-ray in the initial assessment of stable trauma patients? *J Trauma.* 2007;62:74-79.

8. Cyer HM. Chest radiography in blunt trauma patients: is it necessary? *Ann Emerg Med.* 2006;47:422-423.

9. Plurad D, Green D, Demetriades D, et al. The increased use of chest computed tomography for trauma: is it being over utilized? *J Trauma.* 2007;62:631-635.

10. Shackford SR, Rogers FB, Osler TM, et al. Focused abdominal sonography for trauma: the learning curve of nonradiologist clinicians in detecting hemoperitoneum. *J Trauma.* 1999;46:553-556.

11. Rozycki GS, Root D. The diagnosis of intraabdominal injury. *J Trauma.* 2010;68:1019-1023.

12. Lee BC, Ormasby EL, McGahan JP, et al. The utility of sonography for the triage of blunt abdominal trauma patients to exploratory laparotomy. *Am J Roentgenol.* 2007;188:415-421.

13. Rozycki GS, Ballard R, Feliciano DV, et al. Surgeon-performed ultrasound for assessment of truncal injuries: lessons learned from 1,540 patients. *Ann Surg.* 1998;228:16-28.

14. Rozycki GS, Feliciano DV, Ochsner MG, et al. The role of ultrasound with possible penetrating cardiac wounds: a prospective multicenter study. *J Trauma.* 1999;46:543-552.

15. Rozycki GS, Feliciano DV, Schmidt JA, et al. The role of surgeon-performed ultrasound in patients with possible cardiac wounds. *Ann Surg.* 1996;223:737-746.

16. Jones AE, Mason P, Tayal VT, et al. Uroperitoneum presenting as a positive FAST in a patient with bladder rupture. *Am J Emerg Med.* 2003;25:373-377.

17. Tayal VS, Nielsen A, Jones AE, et al. Accuracy of trauma ultrasound in major pelvic injury. *J Trauma.* 2006;61:1453-1457.

18. Knudtson JL, Dort JM, Helmer SD, et al. Surgeon-performed ultrasound for pneumothorax in the trauma suite. *J Trauma.* 2004;56:527-530.

19. Wilkerson RG, Stone MB. Sensitivity of bedside ultrasound and supine anteroposterior chest radiography for the identification of pneumothorax after blunt trauma. *Acad Emerg Med.* 2010;17:11-17.

20. Salim A, Sangthong B, Martin M, et al. Whole body imaging in blunt multisystem trauma patients without signs of injury: results of a prospective study. *Arch Surg.* 2006;141:468-473.

21. Deunk J, Brink M, Dekker HM, et al. Routine versus selective multidetector-row computed tomography (MDCT) in blunt trauma patients: level of agreement on the influence of additional findings on management. *J Trauma.* 2009;67:1080-1086.

22. Root HD, Hauser CW, McKinley CR, et al. Diagnostic peritoneal lavage. *Surgery.* 1965;57:633-637.

23. Henneman PL, Marx JA, Moore EE, et al. Diagnostic peritoneal lavage: accuracy in predicting necessary laparotomy following blunt and penetrating trauma. *J Trauma.* 1990;30:1345-1355.

24. Blow O, Bassam D, Butler K, et al. Speed and efficiency in the resuscitation of blunt abdominal trauma patients with multiple injuries: the advantage of diagnostic peritoneal lavage over abdominal computerized tomography. *J Trauma.* 1998;44:287-290.

25. Cha JY, Kashuk JL, Sarin EL, et al. Diagnostic peritoneal lavage remains a valuable adjunct to modern imaging techniques. *J Trauma.* 2009;67:330-336.

26. Hoffmann JR, Mower WR, Wolfson AB, et al. Validity of a set of clinical criteria to rule out injury to the cervical spine in patients with blunt trauma. *N Engl J Med.* 2000;343:94-99.

27. Stiell IG, Clement CM, McKnight RD, et al. The Canadian C-spine rule versus the NEXUS low-risk criteria in patients with trauma. *N Engl J Med.* 2003;349:2510-2518.

28. Stiell IG, Wells GA, Vandemheen K, et al. The Canadian CT Rule for patients with minor head injury. *Lancet.* 2001;357:1391-1396.

29. Duane TM, Tan BB, Golay D, et al. Blunt trauma and the role of routine pelvic radiographs: a prospective analysis. *J Trauma.* 2002;53:463-468.

30. Gonzalez RP, Fried PQ, Bukhalo M. The utility of clinical examination in screening for pelvic fractures in blunt trauma. *J Am Coll Surg.* 2002;194:121-125.

31. Dunham MC, Barraco RD, Clark DE, et al. Guidelines for emergency tracheal intubation immediately after traumatic injury. *J Trauma.* 2003;55:162-179.

32. Esposito TJ, Sanddal ND, Hansen JD, et al. Analysis of preventable trauma deaths and inappropriate trauma care in a rural state. *J Trauma.* 1995;39:955-962.

33. Esposito TJ, Sanddal TL, Reynolds SA, et al. Effect of a voluntary trauma system on preventable death and inappropriate care in a rural state. *J Trauma.* 2003;54:662-670.

34. Murphy MF, Walls RM. Identification of the difficult and failed airway. In: Walls RM, Murphy MF, eds. *Manual of Emergency Airway Management.* 3rd ed. Philadelphia, PA: Lippincott Williams & Wilkins; 2008:81-93.

35. Reed MJ. Can an airway assessment score predict difficulty at intubation in the emergency department? *Emerg Med J.* 2005;22:99-110.

36. Kortbeek JB, Al Turki SA, Jameel A, et al. Advanced Trauma Life Support, 8th ed, the evidence for change. *J Trauma.* 2008;64:1638-1650.

37. Gibbs MA. Trauma. In: Walls RM, ed. *Manual of Emergency Airway Management.* 2nd ed. Philadelphia, PA: Lippincott Williams & Wilkins; 2004:251-261.

38. Hildreth AN, Mejia VA, Maxwell RA, et al. Adrenal suppression following a single dose of etomidate for rapid sequence intubation: a prospective randomized trial. *J Trauma.* 2008;65:573-579.

39. Warner KJ, Cuschieri J, Jurkovich GJ, et al. Single-dose etomidate for rapid sequence intubation may impact outcome after severe injury. *J Trauma.* 2009;67:45-50.

40. Fields AM, Rosbolt MB, Cohn SM. Induction agents for intubation of the trauma patient. *J Trauma.* 2009;67:867-869.

41. Andrade FM. Postintubation hypotension: the "etomidate paradox." *J Trauma.* 2009;67:417.

42. Oglesby AJ. Should etomidate be the induction agent of choice for rapid sequence intubation in the emergency department? *Emerg Med J.* 2004;21:655-659.

43. Bar-Joseph G, Guilburd Y, Tamir A, et al. Effectiveness of ketamine in decreasing intracranial pressure in children with intracranial hypertension. *J Neurosurg Pediatr.* 2009;4:40-46.

44. Teixeira PFR, Inaba K, Hadjizacharia P, et al. Preventable or potentially preventable mortality at a mature trauma center. *J Trauma.* 2007;63:1338-1347.

45. Jacobs DG, Plaisier BR, Barie PS, et al. EAST Practice Management Guidelines Work Group. Practice management guidelines for geriatric trauma: the EAST Practice Management Guidelines Work Group. *J Trauma.* 2003;54:391-416.

46. Callaway DW, Wolfe R. Geriatric trauma. *Emerg Med Clin North Am.* 2007;25:837-860.

47. Paladino L, Sinert R, Wallace D, et al. The utility of base deficit and arterial lactate in differentiating major from minor injury in trauma patients with normal vital signs. *Resuscitation.* 2008;77:363-368.

48. Yanagawa Y, Sakamoto T, Odaka Y. Hypovolemic shock evaluated by sonographic measurement of the inferior vena cava during resuscitation in trauma patients. *J Trauma.* 2007;63:1245-1248.

49. Perel P, Roberts I. Colloids versus crystalloids for fluid resuscitation in critically ill patients. *Cochrane Database Syst Rev.* 2007;(4):CD000567.

50. Gonzalez EA, Moore FA, Holcomb JB, et al. Fresh frozen plasma should be given early to patients requiring massive transfusion. *J Trauma.* 2007;62:112-119.

51. Teixeira PGR, Inaba K, Shulman I, et al. Impact of plasma transfusion in massively transfused trauma patients. *J Trauma.* 2009;66:693-697.

52. Dente CJ, Shaz BH, Nicholas JM, et al. Improvements in early mortality and coagulopathy are sustained better in patients with blunt trauma after institution of a massive transfusion protocol in a civilian Level I trauma center. *J Trauma.* 2009;66:1616-1624.

53. Perkins JG. An evaluation of the impact of apheresis platelets used in the setting of massively transfused trauma patients. *J Trauma.* 2009;26:S77.

54. Bickell WH, Wall MJ, Pepe PE, et al. Immediate versus delayed fluid resuscitation for hypotensive patients with penetrating torso injuries. *N Engl J Med.* 1994;331:1105-1109.

55. Chesnut RM, Marshall LF, Klauber MR, et al. The role of secondary brain injury in determining outcome from severe head injury. *J Trauma.* 1993;34:216-221.

56. Brain Trauma Foundation. Guidelines for the management of severe traumatic brain injury, 3rd edition. *J Neurotrauma.* 2007;24(suppl 1).

57. Langlois JA, Rutland-Brown W, Wald MM, et al. The epidemiology and impact of traumatic brain injury: a brief overview. *J Head Trauma Rehabil.* 2006;21:375-378.

58. Hesdorffer DC, Ghajar J. Marked improvement in adherence to traumatic brain injury guidelines in United States trauma centers. *J Trauma.* 2007;63:841-848.

59. Fakhry SM, Trask AL, Waller MA, et al, for the IRTC Neurotrauma Task Force. Management of brain-injured patients by an evidence-based medicine protocol improves outcomes and decreases hospital charges. *J Trauma.* 2004;54:492-500.

60. Coles JP, Minhas PS, Fryer TD, et al. Effect of hyperventilation on cerebral blood flow in traumatic head injury: clinical relevance and monitoring correlates. *Crit Care Med.* 2002;30:1950-1959.

61. Marion DW, Puccio A, Wisiniewski SR, et al. Effect of hyperventilation on extracellular concentrations of glutamate, lactate, pyruvate, and local cerebral blood flow in patients with severe traumatic brain injury. *Crit Care Med.* 2002;30:2619-2625.

62. Franko J, Kish KJ, O'Connell BG, et al. Advanced age and preinjury warfarin anticoagulation increase the risk of mortality after head trauma. *J Trauma.* 2006;61:107-110.

63. Pieracci FM, Eachempate SR, Shou J, et al. Degree of anticoagulation, but not warfarin use itself, predicts adverse outcomes after traumatic brain injury in elderly trauma patients. *J Trauma.* 2007;63:525-530.

64. Cudnik MT, Newgard CD, Sayre M, et al. Level I versus level II trauma centers: an outcomes-based assessment. *J Trauma.* 2009;66:1321-1326.

65. Hedges JR, Newgard CD, Veum-Stone J, et al. Early neurosurgical procedures enhance survival in blunt head injury: propensity score analysis. *J Emerg Med.* 2009;37:115-123.

66. Newgard CD, McConnell KJ, Hedges JR, et al. The benefit of higher level of care transfer of injured patients from nontertiary hospital emergency departments. *J Trauma.* 2007;63:965-971.

67. Onzuka J, Worster A, McCreadie B. Is computerized tomography of trauma patients associated with a transfer delay to a regional trauma centre? *Can J Emerg Med.* 2008;10:205-208.

CHAPTER 16

Emergency Transfusions

Joseph R. Shiber

IN THIS CHAPTER

Red blood cell transfusions

Massive transfusion protocols

Platelet transfusions

Plasma transfusions

Adverse effects of blood product transfusions

Introduction

Each year, 1.4 million units of red blood cell (RBC) concentrates, also known as packed RBCs, and 1.6 million units of platelets are transfused in the United States.[1] The total number of transfusions increased by 6% during the past decade, but the number of transfusions in ICUs declined slightly as physicians adopted more conservative transfusion policies.[2-4] In this chapter, the indications for blood product administration—whole blood, packed RBCs, platelets, fresh frozen plasma (FFP), cryoprecipitate, and albumin—are reviewed. Procedures for safe and expedient transfusion are described, along with the potential adverse effects associated with blood product administration and the recommended treatment of these complications.

The goals of transfusion are to prevent and treat shock, hypovolemia, and coagulopathy; to maintain oxygen-carrying capacity; and to maintain vascular oncotic pressure without causing adverse effects.[5-8] In the early stages of transfusion medicine, whole blood was commonly given, with a preference for "fresh" whole blood, which by definition is stored for less than 24 hours at 22°C.[6] A unit of whole blood (450 mL at collection, with 60 mL of anticoagulant added, for a total volume of 510 mL) has a shelf life of 35 days, but the platelet function and coagulant factor quickly degrade. Modern blood-banking practices, including the separation of whole blood into distinct components, lengthen the viability of blood products. For example, packed RBCs have a shelf life of 42 days, and frozen RBC concentrates, typically reserved for autologous donation or rare antibody cross-matched blood, can be kept for 10 years and must be used within 24 hours of thawing.[7] Currently, whole blood transfusion is rarely given outside combat hospital situations.[7,9]

A single unit of packed RBCs will raise the hemoglobin (Hgb) level by 1 g/dL and the hematocrit (Hct) by 3% in a 70-kg patient without ongoing blood loss.[3,7] The average half-life of a transfused RBC is 57.7 days. Patients with pure RBC aplasia require a two-unit transfusion approximately every 2 weeks.[7]

The North American population has the following blood types: O, 44%; A, 43%; B, 9%; and AB, 4%. Eighty-four percent of the population is Rh positive and the other 16% is Rh negative. For a critically ill or injured patient, "emergency release" blood is typically type O, the universal RBC donor; O Rh-negative blood is a precious resource and is reserved for girls and women with childbearing potential in order to prevent Rh(D) antibody complications.[1] Type-specific blood, which should be given, if necessary, for ongoing hemorrhage or uncorrected shock after the emergency release blood, is usually available 15 minutes after the specimen is received in the blood bank. Cross-matching will take 45 to 60 minutes if no antibodies are detected.[1,3] Platelets, plasma, and cryoprecipitate must be ABO compatible but do not require cross-matching. AB plasma is the universal plasma donor since it does not contain anti-A or anti-B antibodies. Platelets are usually available in 5 to 15 minutes, and plasma and cryoprecipitate in 5 to 30 minutes.[1,9]

Red Blood Cell Transfusion

Indications for RBC transfusion are listed in Table 16-1. RBC transfusion can increase oxygen delivery, expand blood volume, alleviate symptoms of acute blood loss anemia, and relieve cardiac ischemia.[10,11] A clear distinction needs to be made between chronic anemia, which can be well tolerated by otherwise healthy individuals, and acute hemorrhage, which represents loss of red cell mass and intravascular volume. The initial Hgb and Hct in acute blood loss do not reflect the actual extent of hemorrhage since the recruitment of interstitial and intracellular fluid into the intravascular space is not immediate. Unless crystalloid or colloid is given to replace the blood volume lost, the Hgb and Hct will underestimate the hemorrhage.[7,12] Clinical evaluation is required to judge the degree of acute blood loss by vital signs and physical examination findings such as tachycardia, orthostasis, decreased pulse pressure, pallor, cool extremities, and delayed capillary refill. Frank arterial hypotension is a late finding in acute blood loss.[3] In hypovolemic shock, the systolic pressure is decreased as a result of falling cardiac output caused by lowered filling pressures, and the diastolic pressure is increased in response to increased systemic vascular resistance. This compensation effect is only temporary and goes away with frank cardiovascular collapse.

PEARL

The initial Hgb and Hct in acute blood loss do not reflect the actual extent of hemorrhage since the recruitment of interstitial and intracellular fluid into the intravascular space is not immediate. Unless crystalloid or colloid is given to replace the blood volume lost, the Hgb and Hct will underestimate the hemorrhage.[7,12]

TABLE 16-1.

Indications for red blood cell transfusion

Evidence of hemorrhagic shock

Acute blood loss of >15%–20% estimated blood volume

Symptomatic anemia in a euvolemic patient

Hgb <7 g/dL in a critically ill patient

Hgb <8 g/dL in a patient with an acute coronary syndrome

Hgb <9 g/dL preoperatively with expected blood loss of >500 mL

Hgb <10 g/dL in a possibly euvolemic patient with evidence of tissue hypoxemia

Sickle cell acute chest syndrome if Hgb <10 g/dL or Hgb-SS >30%

In a healthy person at rest, oxygen delivery is four times greater than tissue utilization. Even with an isolated decrease in Hgb to 10 g/dL, oxygen delivery will still be twice that needed for resting consumption.[13] Signs and symptoms of anemia are unlikely to be evident at Hgb values above 7 or 8 g/dL in healthy patients. Even critically ill patients with chronic anemia can tolerate a Hgb of 7 g/dL, except those with preexisting coronary, pulmonary, or cerebrovascular disease.[5,7,11] The anemic patient has a diminished arterial oxygen content but is able to increase oxygen delivery by increasing cardiac output and increasing coronary blood flow through vasodilation. Myocardial oxygen extraction increases from 25% at baseline; at approximately 50%, the anaerobic threshold is reached and myocardial lactate levels increase.[7] Therefore, the current recommendations for packed RBC transfusions are more liberal in patients with coronary artery disease, particularly those with acute myocardial ischemia.[1,6,13,14] The likelihood of benefit from the transfusion of packed RBCs to nonbleeding patients is summarized in Table 16-2. Clinical judgment and data such as lactate levels and/or central venous oxygen saturation should be used to assess each case individually for the benefits and risks of transfusion versus the risks of ongoing anemia.[1,12,14]

PEARL

In a healthy person at rest, oxygen delivery is four times greater than tissue utilization. Even with an isolated decrease in Hgb to 10 g/dL, the oxygen delivered will still be twice that needed for resting consumption.[13]

In a previously healthy patient with blood loss of less than 20% to 25% of blood volume without ongoing blood loss, only volume restoration with crystalloid or colloid is needed.[3,6] If the total blood volume loss exceeds 20% to 25% (with a normal blood volume of 70 mL/kg), regardless of the presenting blood indices, RBC transfusion may be indicated. Transfusion can be indicated at even lower percentages of blood volume loss if there is a high risk of ongoing hemorrhage such as in a trauma patient, a woman with postpartum hemorrhage, or a patient with gastrointestinal bleeding, particularly one with cirrhosis. In such situations, group O packed RBCs are given because this is the most expedient blood product available. Type ABO specific blood may be given next if more blood is required, but eventually cross-matched blood should be administered. Patients with sickle cell anemia can require RBC transfusion to begin in the emergency department. In those who are critically ill, particularly with acute chest syndrome, a Hct of 30% and a Hgb-sickle of less than 30% should be the goal.[8]

TABLE 16-2.

Likelihood of benefit from transfusion of packed RBCs[7,10,13]

Hgb	Is transfusion beneficial?
>10 g/dL	Unlikely
7–10 g/dL	Potentially beneficial if other deficits in oxygen transport are present
<7 g/dL	Likely

Massive Transfusion

The term *massive transfusion* describes the administration of more than 10 units of blood, or an amount equal to the patient's circulating blood volume, within 24 hours.[3] Massive transfusion is needed by 1% to 3% of civilian trauma patients and has been used in patients with gastrointestinal bleeding, ruptured abdominal aortic aneurysm, ruptured ectopic pregnancy, and obstetric or postpartum hemorrhage.[9,15] Risk factors that predict the need for massive transfusion include any of the following: abnormal vital signs on presentation (tachycardia and hypotension), pH below 7.25, Hct less than 32%, a penetrating mechanism of trauma, and evidence of hemoperitoneum on bedside ultrasonography (FAST).[15] Critically ill or injured patients who have sustained significant blood loss are likely to present with coagulopathy resulting from platelet and clotting factor consumption as well as tissue hypoperfusion, acidosis, and hypothermia, all causing dysfunction of the remaining coagulation factors and platelets.[3,9,15] Resuscitation with crystalloid, colloid, or packed RBCs can cause further dilutional coagulopathy. The term *hemostatic resuscitation* (Table 16-3) describes the use of all blood components in order to give the equivalent of whole blood in an effort to prevent or treat the coagulopathy associated with massive transfusions.[15] Using an equal ratio of packed RBC units, FFP, and platelet units (1:1:1 resuscitation) is the nearest substitute for whole blood and has been associated with decreased mortality in trauma patients receiving massive transfusion.[3,9,15] A transfusion made up of this 1:1:1 solution actually has a Hct of 30%, a platelet count of 80×10^9/L, and approximately 60% of coagulation factors, which is clearly not equal to whole blood.[9] For this reason, crystalloid and colloid infusion should be limited in patients requiring massive transfusion to prevent further dilutional coagulopathy and thrombocytopenia, while allowing permissive hypotension until definitive control of hemorrhage has been achieved. The strategy of hemostatic resuscitation includes giving plasma and platelets early to prevent hemorrhagic exacerbation requiring more blood products.[9,15]

Platelet Transfusion

Platelet units are obtained by separating them from single donor units of whole blood or, more commonly, apheresis. An apheresis platelet unit, which contains 4.2×10^{11} platelets, is equivalent to four to six individual platelet units, each containing 8×10^{10} platelets.[2,12] Each unit also contains approximately 50 mL of plasma.[7] Platelets are stored at room temperature (22°C) for up to 5 days. Each platelet unit can be expected to increase the platelet count of a 75-kg patient by 5,000 to 10,000/μL, and an apheresis unit will raise the count by 20,000 to 40,000/μL.[8,16] Approximately one third of all circulating platelets, whether transfused or released from the marrow, are pooled in the spleen; this number is larger in patients with splenomegaly. The in vivo lifespan of a platelet is 9 to 10 days.[16]

The indications for platelet transfusion in the nonbleeding critically ill patient are different from the intent of transfusions to control bleeding. To maintain the integrity of the vascular endothelium by filling the gaps in the junctions between endothelial cells requires 7,000 platelets per microliter. When the number of circulating platelets falls below 7,000, mucosal surfaces start to bleed and measured blood in the stool increases.[7,16] The platelet count should be kept higher than 50,000/μL in a patient who is actively bleeding and even higher (>100,000/μL) if the patient has microvascular bleeding, particularly if it involves the central nervous system or retina.[6,7] To decrease the chance of hemorrhage in a patient without recognized risk factors for bleeding, platelets should be transfused when the count is below 10,000/μL. Platelet transfusion thresholds for other clinical scenarios are listed in Table 16-4.

TABLE 16-3.

Hemostatic resuscitation guidelines

Expedite control of hemorrhage to reduce the need for blood products and prevent consumptive coagulopathy and thrombocytopenia

Limit crystalloid infusion to prevent dilutional coagulopathy

Goal systolic blood pressure of 80–100 mm Hg until definitive hemorrhage control is achieved

Transfuse at 1:1:1 ratio of packed RBCs/FFP/platelets (1 apheresis unit = 5 platelet units)

Frequently monitor potassium, ionized calcium, lactate, and blood gas values

---

TABLE 16-4.

Guidelines for platelet transfusions in various clinical scenarios

Stable patient without increased bleeding risk: <10,000/μL

Patient with increased bleeding risk: <20,000/μL

For bedside procedure: <20,000–30,000/μL

For most surgery: <40,000–50,000/μL (except neurologic/ophthalmologic surgery: <100,000/μL)

For bleeding: <50,000/μL except central nervous system or retinal bleeding: <100,000/μL

Platelet transfusion is contraindicated in certain groups of patients with thrombocytopenia. Giving platelets to patients with thrombotic thrombocytopenic purpura, hemolytic uremic syndrome, or heparin-induced thrombocytopenia will "add fuel to the fire" and worsen the microvascular thrombosis. Platelet transfusion may not be deleterious but is unlikely to be effective in patients with thrombocytopenia caused by immune-mediated platelet destruction.[6,8,16]

Plasma Transfusion

One unit of plasma contains between 200 and 280 mL of fluid volume. After separation from whole blood, it can be frozen for up to 1 year but must be used within 24 hours after thawing (hence the name *fresh frozen plasma*).[7] Each milliliter of FFP contains approximately 1 unit of each coagulation factor and 2 mg of fibrinogen. One unit of FFP contains about 500 mg of fibrinogen, which is twice as much as is in a unit of cryoprecipitate but in a much larger volume. Plasma needs to be ABO compatible but does not require cross-matching. A critically ill hemorrhaging patient should receive AB plasma, which is usually immediately available.[7,8]

There is a difference between the use of plasma transfusion to prevent bleeding and to treat bleeding. Bleeding does not usually occur until the prothrombin time (PT), partial thromboplastin time (PTT), or international normalized ratio (INR) is more than 1.5 times higher than normal; therefore, there is little benefit to be gained from prophylactic plasma transfusion in a nonbleeding patient with coagulation function tests below these levels. The exception is patients in need of neurosurgical or ophthalmologic procedures, who may be at increased risk for devastating results of hemorrhage; in these situations, a value of 1.3 times higher than normal is the threshold for plasma transfusion.[8] The dose that will commonly achieve hemostasis is 10 to 20 mL/kg, but 30 mL/kg should be given if the patient is critically ill and bleeding.[7,8] This dose may be repeated in 4 to 6 hours to maintain adequate factor levels, or a constant infusion may be given until hemostasis is achieved.

The common clinical indications for plasma transfusion are listed in Table 16-5. It can take 12 to 18 hours for vitamin K to correct the factor deficiency (II, VII, IX, X) induced by warfarin, so in a symptomatic or high-risk patient, plasma transfusion is indicated for more rapid reversal. If a single factor deficiency is known to be present, it is preferable to use specific replacement factors that are purified, that are standardized in activity, and that carry an extremely low risk of infectious disease transmission (or no risk if they are made by a recombinant process).[7,8] Plasma transfusion is also indicated for treatment of thrombotic thrombocytopenic purpura, hemolytic uremic syndrome, and the syndrome of hemolysis, elevated liver enzymes, and low platelets. Plasmapheresis can also be required, but there can be a delay in obtaining vascular access and the staffing necessary for the plasmapheresis, so early administration of plasma in the emergency department can be lifesaving.[7,8] Acute angioedema, particularly if caused by C1 esterase inhibitor deficiency, is also an indication for plasma administration. Plasma transfusion may be necessary for disseminated intravascular coagulation if bleeding is the clinical feature causing the most concern.

Cryoprecipitate Transfusion

Cryoprecipitate is obtained when a unit of frozen plasma is thawed at 4°C. The 10 to 15 mL of plasma that precipitates out of this thawing contains fibrinogen, factor VIII, von Willebrand factor, and factor XIII. Each unit of cryoprecipitate contains 80 to 100 units of factor VIII activity and 150 to 200 mg of fibrinogen.[6,8,14] This is a smaller amount of fibrinogen than is contained in plasma but it is more concentrated, so cryoprecipitate can be a better choice when volume overload is a concern. As with FFP, cryoprecipitate requires ABO compatibility but not cross-matching.

A dose of 2 to 4 units/kg can be expected to raise the fibrinogen level by 60 to 100 mg/dL.[7] A fibrinogen level above 100 mg/dL is the goal of cryoprecipitate transfusion for any bleeding patient; below this level, PT and PTT values will be elevated despite sufficient clotting factors. Cryoprecipitate transfusion is indicated for any deficient fibrinogen state such as massive transfusion, disseminated intravascular coagulation, congenital hypofibrinogenemia, or reversal of thrombolytic therapy; it is

TABLE 16-5.

Indications for plasma transfusion

Massive transfusion protocol
Hemorrhage in liver disease
Disseminated intravascular coagulation
Multiple coagulation factor deficiency
Thrombotic thrombocytopenic purpura
Rapid reversal of warfarin effect
Prevention of bleeding if PT/PTT/INR >1.5 × normal (except for central nervous system or retinal bleeding, then >1.3 × normal)
Acute angioedema caused by C1 esterase inhibitor deficiency

TABLE 16-6.

Indications for albumin transfusion[8]

Nephrotic syndrome resistant to diuretics
Volume replacement with plasmapheresis
Fluid resuscitation for sepsis or burns associated with interstitial edema
Prevention of vascular collapse after large-volume paracentesis

also indicated for factor XIII deficiency.[7,8] Transfusion of cryo-precipitate is an option for factor VIII deficiency and von Willebrand disease if the respective factor concentrates are unavailable. It has also been given for bleeding abnormalities associated with uremia, but desmopressin is the preferred treatment for this disorder.[7,8]

Albumin Transfusion

Albumin provides 80% of intravascular oncotic pressure. Patients with disease states associated with low albumin levels such as cirrhosis and nephrotic syndrome can require albumin transfusion to aid in maintaining intravascular volume. Albumin is derived from human sources but is heat treated so that it is unable to transmit viruses. It is available as a 5% solution, which is oncotically equivalent to normal plasma, and a 25% solution, which is hyperoncotic and able to pull three to four times the volume administered into the vascular space.[8] The typical dose is 50 to 100 mL, but if the patient does not have adequate extravascular hydration, then additional isotonic fluids should also be given. After 4 hours, 50% of infused albumin is lost to the extravascular space. Indications for albumin transfusion are listed in Table 16-6.

PEARL

After 4 hours, 50% of infused albumin is lost to the extravascular space.

Adverse Effects of Transfusions

Complications from blood component therapy include acute immunologic transfusion reactions, allergic reactions, volume overload, viral or bacterial transmission, acute lung injury, and immunomodulating effects associated with an increased risk of nosocomial infection and multiorgan failure (Table 16-7).[11,14,16–18] The risk of a transfusion-related adverse event is 10%, and the risk of it being a serious event is 0.5%.[1] ABO incompatibility reactions, previously the leading cause of trans-fusion-related morbidity and mortality, have decreased with improved clerical and nursing documentation and verification policies. Unfortunately, they have been replaced by transfusion-related acute lung injury (TRALI).[19] The third most common cause of serious transfusion-related complications, including death, is bacterial contamination of blood products.[1]

Hemolytic transfusion reactions occur when preformed IgM against ABO antigens causes complement activation and intravascular hemolysis. Patients experience fever, chills, dyspnea, hypotension, tachycardia, and diffuse myalgias along with hemoglobinemia and hemoglobinuria. The haptoglobin level will be low and bilirubin will be elevated. The main causes of hemolytic transfusion reactions are patient misidentification and clerical errors.

Nonhemolytic transfusion reactions are caused by an amnestic response against non-ABO erythrocyte antigens that were not identified by the cross-match testing. Complement is not activated but RBCs are cleared by the reticuloendothelial system 2 to 10 days later. The clinical picture is less severe than with hemolytic transfusion reactions, and there is modest elevation of bilirubin without hemoglobinemia and hemoglobinuria.[1,8] Allergic reactions are common, occurring in about 1% of all transfusions. Most are mild, consisting of pruritus and hives; frank anaphylaxis is rare.

The risk of disease transmission per unit of blood transfused is 1:2 million for HIV, 1:500,000 for hepatitis B, and 1:2 million for hepatitis C.[8,16] The risk for bacterial infection transmission (which is highest for platelets, since they are stored at room temperature to keep their activity) is 1:2,000 to 3,000 platelet units. Fortunately, only 1 in 5,000 contaminated units causes sepsis.[16,20] Bacteria can be transferred if the skin preparation at the phlebotomy site was unsterile, if the donor had transient bacteremia, if a blood-banking procedure was not sterile, or if the integrity of the bag or tubing was breeched. Gram-negative rods (*Serratia, Pseudomonas, Yersinia, Enterobacter,* and *Salmonella*) and gram-positive cocci (*Staphylococcus* and *Streptococcus*) are the most common organisms.[7]

TRALI occurs after 1 in 1,000 to 5,000 units of blood products are transfused, the highest risk being associated with plasma-containing transfusions.[7,21,22] It is caused by the transfusion recipient's having neutrophils that are already "primed" by a prior stimulus (eg, trauma, infection, malignancy) and adherent to the pulmonary endothelium, which are then stimulated by donor antileukocyte antibodies in the blood product.[23] The activated neutrophils cause diffuse pulmonary capillary leak, leading to noncardiogenic pulmonary edema. Dyspnea, decreased oxygen saturation, and bilateral fluffy pulmonary infiltrates, with a normal left ventricular end-diastolic pressure, occur within 6 hours after transfusion. TRALI typically resolves within 72 hours but has a mortality rate of up to 20%.[24,25]

Prevention of adverse effects is crucial and begins with scrupulous adherence to blood-bank policies to prevent incompatibility reactions. Irradiation of blood products, which prevents donor leukocytes from replicating, should be ordered for patients at risk for graft-versus-host disease as follows: those with severe cellular immunodeficiency (but not AIDS), those on potent chemotherapeutic regimens, and those receiving transfu-

TABLE 16-7.

Clinical presentation of the transfusion reaction types

Acute hemolytic	Fever, chills, dyspnea, tachycardia, hypotension, back/flank pain
Febrile	Fever, chills (patient not ill appearing)
Mild allergic	Urticaria, pruritus
Anaphylactic	Bronchospasm, dyspnea, angioedema, tachycardia, hypotension
TRALI	Dyspnea, decreased arterial oxygen saturation, fever, hypotension, normal/low central venous pressure
Hypervolemic	Dyspnea, headache, tachycardia, hypertension, elevated central venous pressure
Septic	Fever, chills, hypotension, tachycardia, vomiting

sions from biologic relatives. Graft-versus-host disease has no effective treatment and a 90% mortality rate.[6-8] All blood products should be given with an isotonic non–calcium-containing solution such as normal saline to prevent hemolysis and clotting.[8] Unless the patient is in hemorrhagic shock, the transfusion should be started at a slow rate for the first 15 minutes while the patient is monitored closely for signs of a transfusion reaction since the main determinant of the severity of such a reaction is the volume of blood transfused.[7]

If any signs or symptoms suggesting a transfusion reaction emerge (Table 16-8), the blood product should be halted immediately, while the patient is assessed and the blood bank is notified. If the allergic reaction is mild, the patient should be treated with acetaminophen and diphenhydramine, and the transfusion can be continued safely. An anaphylactic reaction should be treated appropriately, and the patient should not be re-challenged by continuing the transfusion. Treatment for hemolytic transfusion reactions includes intravenous volume expansion and diuretics to maintain urine output at more than 100 mL/hr and bicarbonate to raise the urinary pH above 7.0. The treatment of TRALI is supportive: oxygen and positive-pressure ventilation are effective, but there is no role for diuretics or steroids.[24,25]

KEY POINT

During transfusion, if signs or symptoms of a transfusion reaction emerge, the blood product should be halted immediately, while the patient is assessed and the blood bank is notified. If the allergic reaction is mild, the patient should be treated with acetaminophen and diphenhydramine, and the transfusion may be continued. An anaphylactic reaction should be treated appropriately; the patient should not be re-challenged by continuing the transfusion.

Each blood product should be given over a maximum of 4 hours to decrease bacterial contamination.[7,8] If the patient's volume status is labile or if there is concern about congestive heart failure, each unit can be split by the blood bank so it can be given even more slowly. Diuretics may be administered.[24] Rapid transfusion, as in a massive transfusion protocol, can be associated with hypothermia if more than 100 mL/min of volume is given for more than 30 minutes without using a blood-warming device. Other complications of rapid transfusion include hypocalcemia due to citrate toxicity, alkalosis due to citrate conversion, and hyperkalemia due to potassium release from stored erythrocytes.[6-8] Each 1 mL of blood contains 1 mg of iron, so there are about 250 mg in a unit of packed RBCs.[7] This iron load can be helpful in a patient with iron deficiency, but it could be deleterious to a patient who requires frequent transfusions.

Transfusions activate an inflammatory cascade and have immunomodulating effects that are associated with immunosuppression, increased risk of nosocomial infections, acute lung injury, and increased mortality. Intensive care patients who received fewer units of blood products had less serious infections, shorter lengths of stay, and a lower mortality rate than did similar patients who received more transfusions.[2,14,17] An example of the importance of considering the risk versus the benefit of the

transfusion is demonstrated by one study that found that patients hospitalized for acute coronary syndrome had improved outcome if they received an RBC transfusion for a Hgb of less than 8 g/dL, particularly if they were elderly, but they had a worse outcome if they were transfused for a Hgb above 8 g/dL.[13]

TABLE 16-8.

Treatment of transfusion reactions

Reaction	Treatment
General Fever (1°C increase in temperature) Chills Rigors Urticaria Dyspnea Tachycardia Hyper/hypotension Chest/abdominal/back pain Unwell feeling	Stop transfusion immediately. Rapidly assess patient. Verify compatibility of blood product with patient. Notify blood bank of possible problem. Maintain crystalloid infusion. Support respiratory function.
Mild allergic reaction (most common)	Diphenhydramine IV Acetaminophen Consider slowly restarting transfusion after patient is asymptomatic.
Anaphylaxis	Epinephrine IM/IV Albuterol nebulizer Isotonic fluids Diphenhydramine
ABO incompatibility	Isotonic fluids Diuretics to maintain urine output above 100 mL/hr Bicarbonate infusion to keep urine pH above 7 Treat clinically evident disseminated intravascular coagulation.
TRALI	Oxygen and mechanical ventilation strategies as in acute respiratory distress syndrome
Fluid overload	Diuretics IV Oxygen Continuous positive airway pressure Slower rate for further transfusion
Bacterial infection	Culture all remaining blood products. Administer broad-spectrum antibiotics. Provide supportive care.

Adjunctive Therapies

Several nonblood products may be considered to augment or replace a transfusion strategy. Recombinant activated factor VII (rFVIIA) initiates the extrinsic coagulation pathway when complexed with tissue factor at sites of injury. Currently, rFVIIA is approved by the US Food and Drug Administration (FDA) only for the treatment of hemophilia and factor VII deficiency; however, it has been used with some success in coagulopathic trauma patients, decreasing the need for massive transfusion, the amount of total blood products transfused, and the incidence of organ failure. An increase in vascular thromboembolic events in treated patients has been documented.[9,15] Desmopressin increases endothelial cell release of von Willebrand factor molecules. Desmopressin is FDA approved for the treatment of hemophilia A and von Willebrand disease type 1, but it is also used clinically for uremic bleeding. Aminocaproic acid inhibits plasmin and is approved by the FDA for the enhancement of hemostasis in any hyperfibrinolytic state such as certain acute leukemias or after fibrinolytic therapy.[9,15]

Conclusion

The transfusion of blood products is common practice in the management of critically ill patients. As many critically ill patients remain in the emergency department for exceedingly long periods awaiting an ICU bed, it is imperative that emergency physicians know the indications for transfusion of blood products. Equally important is the ability to recognize and manage complications of blood product transfusion, namely allergic reactions, hemolytic reactions, anaphylaxis, and TRALI.

References

1. Despotis GJ, Zhang L, Lublin DM. Transfusion risks and transfusion-related pro-inflammatory responses. *Hematol Oncol Clin North Am.* 2007;21:147-161.
2. Brandt MM, Rubinfeld I, Jordan J, et al. Transfusion insurgency: practice change through education and evidence-based recommendations. *Am J Surg.* 2009;197:279-283.
3. Peterson SR, Weinberg JA. Transfusions, autotransfusions, and blood substitutes. In: Feliciano DV, Mattox KL, Moore EE, eds. *Trauma.* 6th ed. New York, NY: McGraw-Hill; 2008:235-242.
4. American Association of Blood Banks. National Blood Bank Data Resource Center. Available at: www.aabb.org. Accessed on July 6, 2010.
5. Hebert PC, Tinmouth A. Anemia and red blood cell transfusion in critically ill patients. In: Fink MP, ed. *Textbook of Critical Care.* 5th ed. Philadelphia, PA: Elsevier Saunders; 2005:1421-1426.
6. Isbister JP. Blood component therapy. In: Fink MP, ed. *Textbook of Critical Care.* 5th ed. Philadelphia, PA: Elsevier Saunders; 2005:1427-1435.
7. Cushing MM, Ness PM. Blood cell components. In: Hoffman R, ed. *Hematology: Basic Principles and Practice.* 5th ed. Philadelphia, PA: Churchill Livingstone; 2008:146-154.
8. McPherson M, Pincus P. Transfusion administration. In: Henry S, ed. *Clinical Diagnosis and Management by Laboratory Methods.* 21st ed. Philadelphia, PA: W.B. Saunders; 2006:486-499.
9. Perkins JG, Cap AP, Weiss BM, et al. Massive transfusion and nonsurgical hemostatic agents. *Crit Care Med.* 2008;36:S325-S339.
10. Napolitano LM, Corwin HL. Efficacy of red blood cell transfusion in the critically ill. *Crit Care Clin.* 2004;20:255-268.
11. Napolitano LM, Kurek S, Luchette FA, et al. Clinical practice guideline: red blood cell transfusion in adult trauma and critical care. *Crit Care Med.* 2009;37:3124-3139.
12. Isbister JP. Decision making in perioperative transfusion. *Transfus Apheresis Sci.* 2002;27:19-28.
13. Aronson D, Dann EJ, Bonstein L, et al. Impact of red blood cell transfusion on clinical outcomes in patients with acute myocardial infarction. *Am J Cardiol.* 2008;102:115-119.
14. Marik PE, Corwin HL. Efficacy of red blood cell transfusion in the critically ill: a systematic review of the literature. *Crit Care Med.* 2008;36:1654-1667.
15. Sihler KC, Napolitano LM. Massive transfusion: new insights. *Chest.* 2009;136:1654-1667.
16. Slichter SJ. Platelet transfusion therapy. *Hematol Oncol Clin North Am.* 2007;21:697-729.
17. Wahl WL, Hemmila MR, Maggio PM, Arbabi S. Restrictive red blood cell transfusion: not just for the stable intensive care unit patient. *Am J Surg.* 2008;195:803-806.
18. Beale E, Zhu J, Chan L, et al. Blood transfusion in critically injured patients: a prospective study. *Injury.* 2006;37:455-465.
19. Chaiwat O, Lang JD, Vavilala M, et al. Early packed red blood cell transfusion and acute respiratory distress syndrome after trauma. *Anesthesiology.* 2009;110:351-360.
20. MacLennan S, Williamson LM. Risks of fresh frozen plasma and platelets. *J Trauma.* 2006;60:S46-S50.
21. Marik PE, Corwin HC. Acute lung injury following blood transfusion: expanding the definition. *Crit Care Med.* 2008;36:3080-3084.
22. Benson AB, Moss M. Trauma and acute respiratory distress syndrome: weighing the risks and benefits of blood transfusions. *Anesthesiology.* 2009;110(2):216-217.
23. Silliman CC. The two-event model of transfusion-related acute lung injury. *Crit Care Med.* 2006;34:S124-S131.
24. Skeate RC, Eastlund T. Distinguishing between transfusion related acute lung injury and transfusion associated circulatory overload. *Curr Opin Hematol.* 2007;14:682-687.
25. Triulzi DJ. Transfusion-related acute lung injury: current concepts for the clinician. *Anesth Analg.* 2009;108:770-776.

CHAPTER 17

Intracerebral Hemorrhage

Dale S. Birenbaum

IN THIS CHAPTER

Hematoma enlargement and its effect on mortality

Airway management and mechanical ventilation

Blood pressure control

Hemostatic therapy

Management of increased intracranial pressure

Surgical therapy

Introduction

Spontaneous intracerebral hemorrhage (ICH) is a devastating disease that occurs predominantly as a result of chronic hypertension and degenerative changes in cerebral arterioles.[1] Medical references to this condition date back to Hippocrates (400 BC), who alluded to sanguineous apoplexy.[2] Most ICHs occur during activity and manifest with the sudden onset of a neurologic deficit. ICHs account for approximately 10% of all cerebral vascular accidents (CVAs) and have a 30-day mortality rate of 35% to 50%.[1,2] Half of all deaths occur within the first 48 hours.[1-5]

Ultimately, patient outcome depends on several factors, including age; initial Glasgow Coma Scale (GCS) score; and the cause, location, and size of the ICH. The presence of intraventricular hemorrhage (IVH), hematoma expansion, and hydrocephalus substantially increases patient morbidity and mortality. In fact, the patient with an ICH volume of more than 85 mL has an almost uniformly fatal condition, while the patient with an initial hematoma volume of less than 30 mL has a 30-day mortality rate of just 19%.[1-5] All of these factors are intimately related to the pathophysiology of this lethal disease.

Pathophysiology

The initial hemorrhage causes a direct elevation of the local hydrostatic pressure and direct trauma to the brain tissue. When critical areas of the brain are affected, even a small amount of bleeding can have a dramatic effect. Trauma to the brainstem and reticular activating system can lead to apnea and sudden cardiovascular collapse. As the hematoma retracts, serum leaks out of the capillaries and causes perihematomal edema. Blood that is released from the capillaries activates the coagulation cascade, and thrombin is released. The lysis of red blood cells releases hemoglobin and other inflammatory mediators, resulting in irritation and chemical meningitis.

Larger hemorrhages cause an external mass effect by placing pressure on the third or fourth ventricle, causing them to become obstructed and leading to dilation of the lateral ventricles and frontal horns (Figure 17-1). Hydrocephalus can also occur with ICH complicated by IVH (Figure 17-2).

Most of the extravasation of contrast in the angiogram of a patient with ICH is seen within the first 3 to 6 hours of the onset of ictus.[2] Since the overall volume of the cranial vault cannot change, an increase in volume in one of its components (the brain parenchyma, cerebrospinal fluid [CSF], and blood, which are normally present at 80%, 10%, and 10%, respectively) leads to the displacement of other structures or an increase in intracranial pressure (ICP).[6-8] A disruption in the volume and compliance in one of the components of the intracranial vault and disruption of their relationship is known as the Monro doctrine.[6-8] The deterioration and resultant further rise in the ICP that occur later than 6 hours after ictus are thought to be caused by edema, hydrocephalus, or new ventricular hemorrhage. Perihematomal edema, hydrocephalus, and hemorrhagic enlargement worsen mass effect and elevate ICP. Strategies used to reduce hemorrhagic enlargement and edema are listed in Table 17-1.

PEARL

After the initial ictus, hematoma enlargement occurs in approximately 30% to 40% of patients with ICH and increases morbidity and mortality rates from 50% to 80%.[2]

FIGURE 17-1.

Hypertensive intraparenchymal hematoma with subfalcine herniation. Nonenhanced axial computed tomography (CT) demonstrates a large right basal ganglionic hypertensive bleed (*) with mass effect and midline shift or a subfalcine herniation to the left (black arrows). The frontal horns are part of the lateral ventricles. The right frontal horn is compressed so severely that it is almost completely obliterated. Dilation of the left frontal horn is the result of obstructive hydrocephalus, a consequence of compression of the third ventricle. Blood has also accumulated in the lateral ventricles (white arrows).

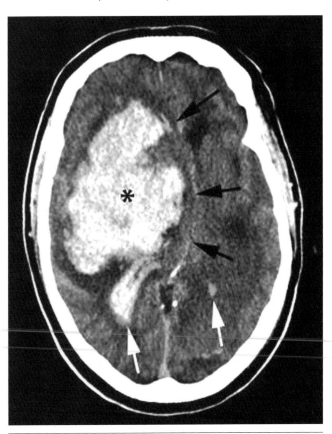

PEARL

If elevations in ICP are left untreated, uncal or central transtentorial, cerebellotonsillar, or upward posterior fossa herniation can occur.

Emergency Department Management

Essential to the emergency department treatment of ICH are rapid assessment, stabilization, and anticipation of the next steps in management (Table 17-2). In certain circumstances, rapid consultation with a neurosurgeon and transfer to an appropriate facility offer the best chance for survival.[3-5] A careful history and physical examination must be performed. Baseline laboratory studies should include a complete blood count, prothrombin time, partial thromboplastin time, liver and renal function tests, serum glucose, electrocardiography, and chest radiography, along with a toxicology screen for younger patients.[2-4]

Airway Assessment

On the patient's arrival, a rapid airway evaluation should be performed. The loss of airway protection should be immediately apparent in a patient who has sustained a significant ICH. Patients with difficulty handling secretions, difficulty swallowing, and hyperventilation or hypoventilation should be intubated. Following advanced trauma life support protocols, a rapid neurologic examination should be performed to deter-

FIGURE 17-2.

Massive ICH and IVH. Axial nonenhanced CT scan demonstrates a large bright or hyperattenuating dense hemorrhage throughout the left basal ganglia, extending intraventricularly. Clotted blood blocks the third ventricle, leading to marked hydrocephalus.

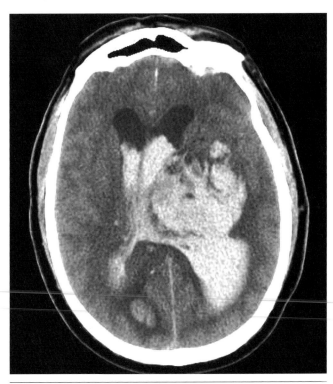

mine if the patient is alert, responsive to vocal or painful stimulus, or completely unresponsive (AVPU).

KEY POINT

Maintain a low threshold for intubating patients with an ICH because they are at high risk of neurologic deterioration and loss of airway protective reflexes.

Because etomidate and propofol have a rapid onset of action, allow quick recovery, and present minimal hemodynamic effects, they appear to be safe agents for induction prior to intubation. These agents are easy to titrate and allow the patient's neurologic status to be evaluated. Etomidate inhibits adrenal steroid production and is associated with increased mortality in critically ill patients.[8] Thus, its use for continued sedation in patients with ICH is not recommended.

Propofol appears to be the best agent for continued sedation. The most common side effects of propofol are hypotension, lactic acidosis, and hypercholesterolemia. The use of this agent for more than 48 hours has been associated with propofol infusion syndrome. This syndrome is characterized by severe metabolic acidosis, rhabdomyolysis, hyperkalemia, renal failure, and cardiovascular collapse, yet it does not appear to have an effect on mortality.[8,9]

Neuromuscular blocking drugs are used to facilitate airway control and prevent complications during intubation. Depolarizing neuromuscular blockade can cause muscle contractions and theoretically cause an increase in ICP; therefore, a nondepolarizing agent such as rocuronium or cisatracurium is preferred for those with ICH.[8,9] Of particular note and consistent with traditional teaching, the airway should be secured by the most experienced personnel and the physician should only use those medications with which he/she is most familiar in order to prevent errors.

Once the airway is secured, it is important to continue adequate analgesia and sedation to prevent the patient from hyperventilating, to facilitate imaging, and to continue the evaluation and management.

Continued neuromuscular blockade is sometimes employed to reduce ICP in patients who are not responsive to analgesics and sedation alone. Muscular activity can increase ICP by raising intrathoracic pressure and reducing cerebral venous outflow. The delicate balance of cerebral blood flow and ICP is described below. Simple measures to reduce ICP are also used at this time.[8,9]

TABLE 17-1.

Treatment strategies to reduce hemorrhagic enlargement and edema

Blood pressure reduction

Hemostatic therapy

Clot drainage

Decreasing intracranial pressure

Euvolemic resuscitation

PEARL

Elevate the head of the bed to 30° to improve venous return and aid in the reduction of ICP.

Breathing and Mechanical Ventilation

Implementation of a neuroprotective ventilatory strategy is important to maintain normocarbia and a target $Paco_2$ between 35 and 40 mm Hg.[3–5,8,9] Initial settings for mechanical ventilation are presented in Table 17-3.

KEY POINTS[3–5,8,9]

Maintain $Paco_2$ between 35 and 40 mm Hg.

Maintain plateau pressure <30 cm H_2O.

Maintain pH >7.15.

Circulation and Blood Pressure Control

Circulatory resuscitation and blood pressure management remain critical components in the management of patients who have sustained a devastating ICH. Unlike in ischemic stroke, in which medical complications are the most common cause of death, the keys to reducing death and disability caused by spontaneous intracerebral intraparenchymal hemorrhage are to act as rapidly as possible to identify the size and location of the initial bleeding and begin efforts to reduce hematoma enlargement.

KEY POINT

Large fluctuations in blood pressure can worsen neurologic injury and outcome.

Blood pressure and its management remain highly controversial in patients with ICH. It is currently unclear if elevations in blood pressure serve as the inciting event for ICH or are a reaction to the ICH in an effort to maintain cerebral perfusion pressure (CPP). The goal of circulatory resuscitation is to maintain adequate cerebral blood flow, especially to damaged areas of the brain.

The mean arterial pressure (MAP) minus the ICP is equal to the CPP. MAP is calculated as the diastolic blood pressure plus one third of the difference between the systolic and diastolic

TABLE 17-2.

Essentials of emergency department ICH management

Airway assessment

Early intubation and mechanical ventilation

Circulatory resuscitation

Hemostatic therapy

Blood pressure control

ICP monitoring

Supportive care—managing hyperglycemia, hyperthermia, and seizures

blood pressures. For example, a blood pressure of 120/80 mm Hg indicates a MAP of 93.3 (80 + 13.3). It is essential to maintain a CPP between 50 and 70 mm Hg.[3–5,8,9]

Cerebral blood flow is normally maintained at a relatively constant level by autoregulation of cerebrovascular resistance (CVR). Autoregulation of CVR becomes dysfunctional in ICH, and because of this the brain becomes exquisitely sensitive to even minor changes in CPP. With an acute reduction in blood pressure, CPP is reduced and ischemia results. Excessive elevations in the blood pressure elevate the CPP and can lead to cerebral edema and injury. Direct or worsening IVHs cause a rise in ICP and therefore result in diminished CPP. All treatment efforts are aimed at maintaining this delicate balance and homeostasis.

PEARL

A CPP between 50 and 70 mm Hg is thought to be neuroprotective.

The most recent guidelines from the American Heart Association state that "physicians must manage blood pressure on the basis of incomplete efficacy evidence."[4] Nevertheless, the blood pressure should be adjusted in an effort to maintain adequate CPP (Tables 17-4 and 17-5). The initial reduction of blood pressure should be no more than 15% in the first hour because many patients have accommodated to higher baseline blood pressures and rapid reductions could lead to worsening ischemia.[3–5,8,9] Recent studies indicate that for patients presenting with a systolic blood pressure of between 150 and 220 mm Hg, more aggressive lowering of blood pressure to 140/90 mm Hg is probably safe.[4,10]

The initial resuscitation fluid in ICH should be isotonic. Isotonic fluids such as normal saline offer the advantage of maintaining homeostasis by exerting little osmotic effect on surrounding tissues.[8–10] Dextrose-containing solutions (D_5W) and half normal saline introduce free water into the intravascular space, leading to increased capillary leakage and worsening perihematomal edema. Dextrose-containing solutions can also contribute to hyperglycemia, which can be detrimental to stroke patients.[4,8–10] The goal of fluid resuscitation should be to keep the patient euvolemic, not severely fluid restricted, and normal to hyperosmolar. Adequate resuscitation can be assessed by maintaining a urine output of 0.5 to 1 mL/kg/hr.

TABLE 17-3.

Initial mechanical ventilatory settings[3,8,9]

Mode: assist control
Tidal volume: 6 mL/kg of ideal body weight
Respiratory rate: 18–22 breaths/min
F_{IO_2}: 100%
PEEP: 5–7 cm H_2O

KEY POINT

The goal of fluid resuscitation should be to keep the patient euvolemic, not severely fluid restricted, and normal to hyperosmolar.

Hemostatic Therapy

For ICH patients who are taking an anticoagulant medication, who have an underlying factor deficiency, or who have received tissue plasminogen activator, it is critical to aggressively provide hemostatic therapy to prevent hematoma enlargement.[11–13] Importantly, therapy should not be delayed while awaiting the results of coagulation tests. ICH occurs with a frequency of approximately 0.3% to 0.6% per year in patients undergoing chronic warfarin anticoagulation. An elevated INR places the patient at risk for significant hematoma enlargement and death. The risk of ICH nearly doubles for each increase of 0.5 points in the INR above 4.5. Patients who develop an ICH while taking warfarin should receive vitamin K (10 mg via slow IV infusion over 10 minutes) and therapy to replace vitamin K-dependent factors.[4] In addition to vitamin K, these patients should receive either fresh frozen plasma (4-6 units) or prothrombin complex concentrates. In the most recent American Heart Association guidelines, prothrombin complex concentrates are considered a reasonable alternative to fresh frozen plasma.[4] Prothrombin complex concentrates demonstrate more rapid reversal of elevations in INR than do vitamin K and fresh frozen plasma. Some prothrombin complex concentrate preparations are available in the United States.

For patients who have been given intravenous tissue plasminogen activator for ischemic stroke, the risk of ICH is be-

TABLE 17-4.

Recommendations for treating elevated blood pressure in patients with spontaneous ICH. From: Broderick J, Connolly S, Feldmann E, et al. Guidelines for the management of spontaneous intracerebral hemorrhage in adults: 2007 updates: a guideline from the American Heart Association/American Stroke Association Stroke Council, High Blood Pressure Research Council, and the Quality of Care and Outcomes in Research Interdisciplinary Working Group. *Stroke*. 2007-38:2001-2023. Used with Permission.

If SBP is >200 mm Hg or MAP is >150 mm Hg, then consider aggressive reduction of blood pressure with continuous intravenous infusion and blood pressure monitoring every 5 minutes.
If SBP is >180 mm Hg or MAP is >130 mm Hg and there is evidence or suspicion of elevated ICP, then consider monitoring ICP and reducing blood pressure using intermittent or continuous intravenous medications to keep CPP >60 mm Hg.
If SBP is >180 mm Hg or MAP is >130 mm Hg and there is not evidence or suspicion of elevated ICP, then consider a modest reduction of blood pressure (eg, MAP of 110 mm Hg or target blood pressure of 160/90 mm Hg) using intermittent or continuous intravenous medications to control blood pressure, and clinically reexamine the patient every 15 minutes.

tween 3% and 9%. Interestingly, ICH occurs in 0.5% to 0.6% of patients treated with thrombolytic agents for other acute arterial and venous occlusions, with higher rates of hemorrhage in the elderly.[2–4] Patients with an ICH secondary to thrombolytic therapy should receive cryoprecipitate and platelet transfusions.

KEY POINT
Provide hemostatic therapy as soon as possible for patients with an ICH associated with the use of warfarin or a known factor deficiency.

Administer protamine sulfate (1 mg/100 units of heparin) to patients in whom ICH develops while they are receiving heparin therapy. Protamine sulfate is given by slow intravenous injection not to exceed 5 mg/min, with a total dose not to exceed 50 mg. The dose should be adjusted down from the last time heparin was given. Importantly, protamine sulfate can cause hypotension, nausea, vomiting, and anaphylaxis.

There was initial hope that recombinant activated factor VII (rFVIIa) would avoid hematoma enlargement, reduce mortality, and improve neurologic outcomes.[11,12] However, a phase III international trial of rFVIIa for ICH ended early because of increased mortality in the treated group. The complications and increased mortality rates associated with rFVIIa are thought to be related to arterial thromboembolic events.[11,12] These events include ischemic stroke, myocardial infarction, and vascular insufficiency and emphasize the fine balance between bleeding, perfusion, and ischemia. Currently, rFVIIa is not routinely recommended for the treatment of ICH.[4]

ICP Monitoring and Treatment

The treatment of elevated ICP begins with elevation of the head of the bed, fluid resuscitation, and sedation and analgesia.[4,5] Further treatment of elevated ICP in the setting of ICH is extrapolated from data on traumatic brain injury patients and consists of efforts to increase MAP and/or lower ICP to maintain an adequate CPP.[4,5,8,9] Normal ICP is less than 10 mm Hg; a pressure of more than 20 mm Hg is elevated.

The Lund protocol assumes a disruption of the blood–brain barrier and recommends manipulations to decrease the hydrostatic forces and increase the osmotic forces that favor the maintenance of fluid within the vascular compartment to reduce the ICP. Mannitol (Table 17-6) and hypertonic saline are two osmotic agents used to treat increased ICP. Hypertonic saline is being used increasingly in various settings as an alternative to mannitol to treat cerebral edema. Its theoretical advantages over mannitol are that the blood–brain barrier is less permeable to hypertonic saline and it may be a more effective osmotic agent. It is also a volume expander that does not appear to have any nephrotoxicity. It may be administered as boluses of 3% to 30% every 3 to 4 hours or as a continuous infusion. The goal is to maintain a serum sodium concentration of 145 to 155 mmol/liter.[9]

Another approach to treating increased ICP is CPP-guided therapy, which focuses on augmenting blood pressure to maintain a CPP between 50 and 70 mm Hg to minimize reflex vasodilation or ischemia. However, cerebral ischemia and hypoxia can still occur with CPP-guided therapy, and concern remains that blood pressure elevation to maintain CPP can advance intracranial hypertension.[4,8] A recent study concluded that most patients had increases in ICP when their MAP was elevated therapeutically.[4]

For the patient who is rapidly deteriorating, hyperventilation may be performed concurrently with osmolar therapy and additional neuromuscular blockade. In these cases, hyperventilation should be targeted to a $PaCO_2$ of 30 to 35 mm Hg.[3,5,8,9] Adequate sedation must continue, and it is of critical importance to work closely with a neurosurgeon, who may decide to place an internal intracranial monitoring device to directly measure the ICP (Table 17-7).

PEARL
Barbiturate anesthesia can be used if other mechanisms to reduce ICP fail. Barbiturate coma reduces cerebral metabolism, lowering cerebral blood flow and decreasing ICP.

TABLE 17-5.

Blood pressure medications used in ICH. From: Broderick J, Connolly S, Feldmann E, et al. Guidelines for the management of spontaneous intracerebral hemorrhage in adults: 2007 update: a guideline from the American Heart Association/American Stroke Association Stroke Council, High Blood Pressure Research Council, and the Quality of Care and Outcomes in Research Interdisciplinary Working Group. *Stroke.* 2007;38:2001-2023. Used with permission.

	Initial	Infusion
Labetalol	5–20 mg every 15 min	2 mg/min (maximum, 300 mg/day)
Nicardipine	N/A	5–15 mg/hr
Esmolol	250 mcg/kg IV push loading dose	25–300 mcg/kg/min
Enalapril	1.25–5 mg IV push every 6 hr[a]	N/A
Hydralazine	5–20 mg IV push every 30 min	1.5–5 mcg/kg/min
Nitroprusside	N/A	0.1–10 mcg/kg/min
Nitroglycerin	N/A	20–400 mcg/min

[a]Because of the risk of precipitous blood pressure lowering, the first dose of enalapril should be 0.625 mg.

TABLE 17-6.

Mannitol therapy for increased ICP

Initial dose: 1–1.5 g/kg of a 20% solution

Infusion: 0.25–0.5 g/kg every 6 hours

Goal: maintain serum osmolarity of 300–320 mOsm/kg

Therapy for presumed elevated ICP is unsatisfactory because CPP cannot be monitored reliably without an ICP monitoring device. Most therapies directed at lowering ICP are effective for only a limited time. The initial steps to control ICP may have to be taken without the benefit of an ICP monitor. An important early goal in the management of a patient with presumed elevated ICP is the placement of an ICP monitoring device.[2–5,8,9]

When an intraventricular catheter is used to monitor ICP, CSF drainage is an effective method of lowering the pressure, particularly in the setting of hydrocephalus. Ventriculostomy is typically performed in the neurologic ICU and can rapidly reduce ICP. The decision to undertake this procedure must be made by an experienced neurosurgical team that can carefully monitor the device and augment treatment.

Direct ICP monitoring allows one to accurately and reliably monitor and manage the ICP. CSF drainage carries the risks of infection and hemorrhage. Other methods used to directly measure ICP such as a subarachnoid or subdural bolt, a subdural catheter, or an intraparenchymal sensor can be placed directly into the brain tissue. These devices use micro- and fiberoptic transducers, which are easier to insert than a standard ventriculostomy catheter, but these devices cannot be reset to zero, so they are less accurate for monitoring ICP.[2]

Surgical Intervention

Several factors aid the neurosurgeon in deciding when to operate on a patient with ICH (Table 17-8). Craniotomy is typically performed for signs of increased ICP, as manifested by mass effect or midline shift and the absence of basal cisterns on the CT scan; age and level of function prior to the event must also be considered.[2–5] Young patients and those functioning at higher levels tend to fare better.

PEARL

The operative decision is made by combining clinical presentation and functional anatomy and takes into consideration the neurologic deficit, GCS score, age, CT data revealing midline shift, and the presence and site of hydrocephalus.[2–4,14]

TABLE 17-7.

Conditions for which ICP monitoring may be indicated

Clinical deterioration
Process merits aggressive medical care
Unilateral or bilateral posturing
SBP <90 mm Hg
At risk for increased ICP
Comatose and GCS score <8
Evidence of ICP by CT scan • Mass lesion • Midline shift • Effacement of the basilar cisterns

Open craniotomy and drainage of a hematoma by direct visualization remains the gold standard for the neurosurgical team, who can place a ventriculostomy catheter that can be used to drain CSF and lower ICP.[2] Other surgical techniques for the evacuation of hematomas are described below.

A burr hole can be made in the skull, allowing the hematoma to be aspirated with a needle. At this point, a 3- to 4-mm microsilicone catheter can be inserted to remove blood. Because the consistency of the hematoma is unpredictable, it can be difficult to aspirate the blood through these catheters. The procedure is not performed under direct visualization. To aid in the placement of catheters and devices, stereotactic surgery and aspiration with and without catheter placement may be performed.

Stereotactic surgery is an organized approach in three dimensions. In the past, the procedure was done with a frame; newer techniques are frameless. A special CT or MRI scan is used with a computer to perform computational analysis using a set of markers or fiducials that are affixed to the skull or scalp to obtain a detailed set of coordinates localizing specific anatomic sites in the brain. This approach permits precise targeting of the area to be drained.[2,8,9] Stereotactic aspiration has been combined with fibrinolysis to aid in clot removal.

Aspiration has also been combined with a mechanical assist device such as the Archimedes screw. The neuroendoscopic approach combines direct visualization and ultrasound guidance with a dual-channel drain and rinsing of the hematoma cavity with artificial CSF through a second catheter. Hemostasis can also be obtained by this technique using laser devices.[2,8,9]

The indications for surgery in supratentorial and infratentorial cerebral hemorrhage are different. The approach to the management of a patient with infratentorial cerebral hemorrhage has some unique features. When the ICH is located in the cerebellum and is larger than 3 cm, or if there is a cerebellar hemorrhage with brainstem compression or hydrocephalus, mortality rates approach 80% to 90%.[2] Emergent evacuation of the hemorrhage provides the only chance of survival; clinical outcome depends on prompt access to a qualified and experienced neurosurgeon (Figure 17-3). For these patients, medical management alone results in bad outcomes. Patients with smaller cerebellar hemorrhages without brainstem compression can be managed medically and do reasonably well.

There is no general agreement on the best time and indications for surgery in patients with supratentorial ICH. A landmark study advanced our understanding of the use of surgical evacuation for spontaneous ICH.[14] In the International Surgical Trial in Intracerebral Haemorrhage (STICH) study, Mendelow

TABLE 17-8.

Indications for surgical intervention for ICH[2,3,5,8,9,14,15]

Cerebellar hemorrhage >3 cm
Cerebellar hemorrhage with hydrocephalus
Clinically deteriorating status with signs of increased ICP
Lobar hemorrhages within 1 cm of the cranium

et al evaluated early surgery (within 30 hours) versus initial conservative treatment in patients with spontaneous, nontraumatic supratentorial ICH. The study demonstrated that early surgical intervention had no benefit over initial conservative management in terms of patient outcome.[14]

When the ICH is lobar and large and extends into the ventricles, mortality rates approach 80% to 90%.[2,14,15] Figure 17-4 represents a large left-sided intracerebral intraparenchymal hemorrhage in a 70-year-old man who was not taking anticoagulants and who presented obtunded (paralyzed and deeply comatose) with a large bleed in the dominant hemisphere, with midline shift. Despite the fact that the lesion was operatively approachable, it resided near eloquent (essential) brain. Based on this information, the neurosurgeon and family chose initial conservative management followed by admission and observation; unfortunately, the patient died.

Newer techniques are beginning to shape the management of patients with ICH. The international Clot Lysis Evaluating Accelerated Resolution of Intraventricular Hemorrhage (CLEAR–IVH) trial is an ongoing multicenter study evaluating the utility of intraventricular thrombolytics. It is showing improved outcomes for hemorrhagic stroke patients who have

intraventricular bleeding and hydrocephalus.[16] Small doses of thrombolytics are injected directly into the ventricles, and clotted blood in the ventricles is drained through a ventriculostomy, reducing hydrocephalus and ICP.

For contained deeper thalamic and putamen intracerebral intraparenchymal hemorrhage, mortality rates are significantly lower, at 20% to 40%.[2] Because these lesions are difficult to reach by standard craniotomy, less invasive methods to evacuate clots and monitor ICP are being explored. Stereotactic catheter placement with CSF drainage and monitoring along with microsurgery and endoscopic clot evacuation are two new alternatives to standard craniotomy. It appears that a less aggressive surgical technique causes less harm to eloquent brain but still allows blood drainage and monitoring of ICP. Stroke experts are anxiously awaiting the results of ongoing trials such as CLEAR-IVH.

Subcortical lobar ICHs that are located within 1 to 2 cm of the brain's surface and are smaller than 2 to 3 cm produce milder deficits, have the best prognosis, and are fatal in 10% of cases.[2] These lesions are easily accessible via standard craniotomy (Figure 17-5).

Supportive Care

Hyperglycemia in the first 24 hours after ICH is associated with adverse outcomes. Current guidelines recommend frequent monitoring and maintaining normoglycemia.[4]

Since fever increases metabolic demand in the brain, it can result in increased cerebral blood flow. By increasing the vol-

---

FIGURE 17-3.

Cerebellar/infratentorial bleed (*) in a child. Prognosis will be related to timely access to an operating room and an experienced neurosurgeon. Hematoma has extended extraaxially (arrow) and into fourth ventricle (arrowhead).

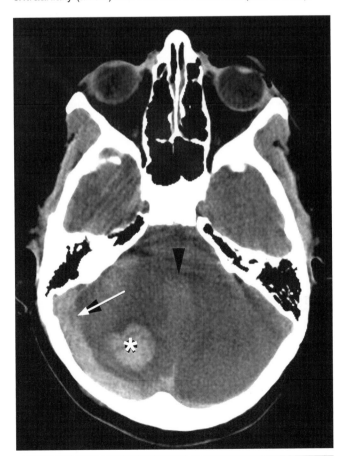

FIGURE 17-4.

Large intraparenchymal intracerebral hemorrhage

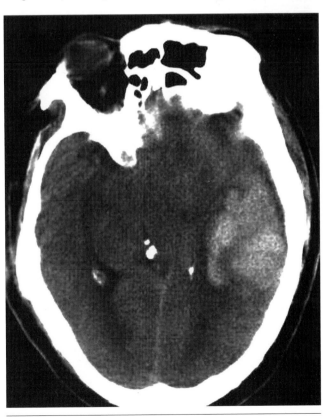

ume in the cranial vault, it contributes to elevated ICP. Acetaminophen and mechanical cooling may be used aggressively in patients with evidence of increased ICP. Caution should be taken to avoid over-cooling or rapid reversal of cooling to avoid rebound phenomena.[3–5,8,9]

Anticonvulsant drugs are indicated in patients with ICH who have exhibited convulsive seizures. Initial medications include lorazepam followed by direct administration of fosphenytoin or phenytoin.

Gastric prophylaxis with a proton pump inhibitor and sucralfate reduces morbidity.

ICH care should be delivered in a controlled, monitored setting with a focus on early mobilization and rehabilitation of stable patients.

Conclusion

Several aspects of the comprehensive management of patients with ICH have been discussed in order to aid in patient care and facilitate collaboration with our colleagues in neurology, neurosurgery, and interventional radiology.

FIGURE 17-5.

Moderate subcortical intracerebral hemorrhagic stroke. This moderately sized, right-sided intracerebral hemorrhagic stroke (*) occurred in a 40-year-old man who was awake but confused; there was no midline shift, no intraventricular extension, no hydrocephalus, and no clinical weakness. This bleed in the easily accessible frontal area of the brain in an awake patient was evacuated and treated by standard craniotomy without difficulty by a neurosurgeon.

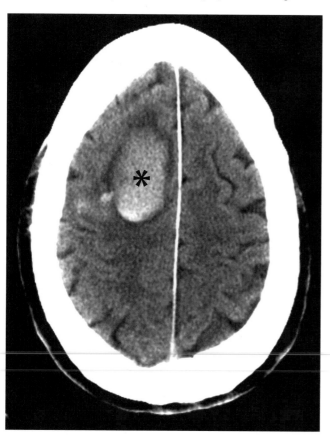

KEY POINTS
Anticipate that the patient will lose the airway.

Avoid rapid shifts and fluctuations in blood pressure.

Rapidly reverse coagulopathy.

Know the indications for surgery.

KEY POINTS
Maintain normoglycemia.

Give acetaminophen for fever.

Gastric prophylaxis reduces morbidity.

Encourage early mobilization and rehabilitation if the patient is stable.

KEY POINTS
Maintain $Paco_2$ between 35 and 40 mm Hg.

Administer anticonvulsant drugs to patients experiencing convulsive seizures.

Evacuate cerebellar hemorrhages.

References

1. Ropper AH, Samuels MA. *Adam's and Victor's Principles of Neurology*. 9th ed. New York, NY: McGraw-Hill; 2009.
2. Winn RH. *Youmans Neurological Surgery*. 4th ed. Philadelphia, PA: Saunders; 2004.
3. Broderick JP, Adams HP Jr, Barsan W, et al. Guidelines for management of spontaneous intracerebral hemorrhage: a statement for healthcare professionals from a special writing group of the Stroke Council, American Heart Association. *Stroke*. 1999;30:905-915.
4. Morgenstern LB, Hemphill JC, Anderson C, et al. Guidelines for the management of spontaneous intracerebral hemorrhage: a guideline for healthcare professionals from the American Heart Association/American Stroke Association. *Stroke*. 2010;41:2108-2129.
5. Juvela S, Kase CS. Advances in intracerebral hemorrhage management. *Stroke*. 2006;37:301-304.
6. Mokri B. The Monro-Kellie hypothesis: applications in CSF volume depletion. *Neurology*. 2001;56:1746-1748.
7. Neff S, Subramaniam RP. Monro-Kellie doctrine. *J Neurosurg*. 1996;85:1195.
8. Irwin RS, Rippe JM. *Irwin and Rippe's Intensive Care Medicine*. 6th ed. Philadelphia, PA: Lippincott Williams & Wilkins; 2008.
9. Gabrielli A, Layon AJ, Yu M. *Civetta, Taylor and Kirby's Critical Care*. 4th ed. Philadelphia, PA: Lippincott Williams & Wilkins; 2009.
10. Arima H, Wang JG, Huang Y, et al. Significance of perihematomal edema in acute intracerebral hemorrhage: the INTERACT trial. *Neurology*. 2009;73:1963-1968.
11. Mayer SA, Brun NC, Begtrup K, et al. Recombinant activated factor VII for acute intracerebral hemorrhage. *N Engl J Med*. 2006;352:777-785.
12. Mayer SA, Brun NC, Begtrup K, et al. Efficacy and safety of recombinant activated factor VII for acute intracerebral hemorrhage. *N Engl J Med*. 2008;358:2127-2137.
13. Aguilar MI, Hart RG, Kase CS, et al. Treatment of warfarin-associated intracerebral hemorrhage: literature review and expert opinion. *Mayo Clin Proc*. 2007;82:82-92.
14. Mendelow AD, Gregson BA, Fernandes HM, et al. STICH investigators. Early surgery versus initial conservative treatment in patients with spontaneous supratentorial intracerebral haematomas in the International Surgical Trial in Intracerebral Haemorrhage (STICH): a randomised trial. *Lancet*. 2005;365:387-397.
15. Gregson BA, Mendelow AD. STICH investigators. A tool for predicting outcome after spontaneous supratentorial intracerebral hemorrhage [abstract]. *Stroke*. 2006;37:624.
16. Morgan TA, Awad I, Keyl P. Preliminary report of the clot lysis evaluating accelerated resolution of intraventricular hemorrhage (CLEAR-IVH) clinical trial. *Acta Neurochir Suppl*. 2008;105:217-220.

CHAPTER 18

Status Epilepticus

Carl A. Germann and Andrew D. Perron

Introduction

Status epilepticus is a life-threatening neurologic disorder that describes any continuous seizure activity. Traditionally, generalized convulsive status epilepticus has been defined as either 30 minutes or more of continuous seizure activity or two or more seizures without returning to the baseline level of consciousness between seizures. This definition has recently evolved based on two key issues. First, evidence now indicates that neuronal injury likely occurs sooner than was first believed, and earlier treatment has a better chance of preventing the pathologic processes of status epilepticus.[1] Second, the vast majority of seizures that are going to self-terminate will do so within the first 5 minutes.[2] After this time, generalized convulsive activity has a significantly higher chance of continuing.[3] For the purposes of this chapter, status epilepticus is defined as continuous convulsive activity lasting longer than 5 minutes or recurrent seizures without return to the baseline mental status in the interictal period.

KEY POINTS

The vast majority of seizures self-terminate within 5 minutes.

Status epilepticus is defined as continuous convulsive activity lasting longer than 5 minutes or recurrent seizures without return to baseline mental status in the interictal period.

Background

Approximately 2 million people in the United States have epilepsy.[4] Three percent of the general population will have epilepsy at some point in their lives.[4] Status epilepticus accounts for about 7% of all epilepsy cases per year, with an overall incidence estimated at 50,000 to 200,000 cases annually in the United States.[5] In 12% to 30% of these patients, status epilepticus is the first epileptic event.[5,6]

Etiology, duration of the seizure, and patient age are important determinants of the outcome in status epilepticus. In prospective population-based studies, DeLorenzo et al found that the overall mortality rate was 22% for the entire population (13% for young adults, 38% for the elderly, and >50% for those older than 80 years).[6] Similar findings were reported by Hesdorffer and associates, who documented an overall mortality rate after status epilepticus of 21%.[7] Not surprisingly, seizure

FIGURE 18-1.

Status epilepticus: suggested medication algorithm

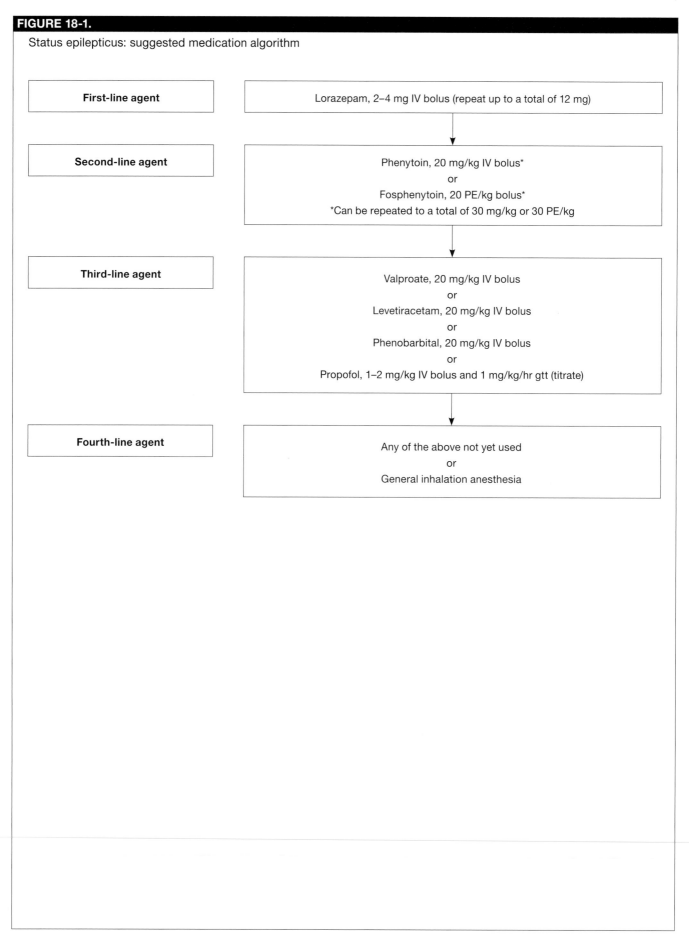

duration has a direct association with hypoxia, permanent neurologic injury, and increasing rates of mortality.[8]

Up to 70% of children with epilepsy presenting before 1 year of age will experience an episode of status epilepticus in their lifetime.[9] The estimated incidence of status epilepticus in childhood ranges from 10 to 38/100,000 per year.[7,10] Reported short-term mortality rates associated with pediatric status epilepticus (ie, death during hospital admission or within the first 30 to 60 days after the onset of childhood status epilepticus) in population-based studies are 2.7% to 5.2%.[5,11–14]

Etiology

In roughly one third of patients, an exacerbation of an idiopathic seizure disorder is thought to be the cause of status epilepticus.[15] However, in many patients with a preexisting seizure disorder, no obvious precipitating factor can be determined. Any condition that causes cortical structure damage can promote a seizure and status epilepticus. The most common causes of secondary seizure are listed in Table 18-1.[16] One large prospective, population-based study found status epilepticus to be associated with the following causes at the indicated frequencies: low blood concentrations of anticonvulsant drugs

TABLE 18-1.

Causes of secondary seizures

Anoxia/ischemic injury

Eclampsia

Infection
    Meningitis
    Encephalitis
    Abscess

Intracranial hemorrhage

Hypertensive encephalopathy

Metabolic disturbance
    Hypoglycemia
    Hypo/hypernatremia
    Uremia

Structural abnormality
    Aneurysm
    Mass lesion
    Congenital defect

Toxins
    Cocaine
    Ethanol withdrawal

Trauma

in patients with chronic epilepsy (34%); remote symptomatic causes (24%); acute cerebrovascular accidents (22%); anoxia or hypoxia (~10%); metabolic causes (~10%); and alcohol and drug withdrawal (~10%).[5] Remote symptomatic causes include patients with status epilepticus without an acute precipitating event but with a history of insults to the central nervous system (CNS) temporally distant from the first status epilepticus episode. These events and conditions include remote stroke, tumor, and intracranial hemorrhage.

There are very important differences in causes between the pediatric and adult populations. Status epilepticus related to infection is substantially more common in infants and children. Febrile status epilepticus, which occurs in 5% of patients experiencing febrile seizures, is the most common type of status epilepticus in childhood, accounting for at least one third to one half of all cases.[5,14] In children younger than 2 years, febrile childhood status epilepticus and acute symptomatic causes are most common, whereas chronic conditions are more common in older children.[17]

Pathophysiology

Failure of inhibitory neurotransmitters, most notably γ-aminobutyric acid (GABA), is thought to be the major mechanism leading to status epilepticus. Most focal seizures do not secondarily spread to produce a generalized event because local inhibitory GABA-mediated circuitry prevents enlargement of the ictus.[18] As a seizure continues, a breakdown occurs within this cortical "inhibitory surround," making it easier for seizure activity to spread. Recurrent or prolonged seizures thereby induce a positive feedback loop that helps sustain, rather than inhibit, further ictal activity. In essence, "seizures beget seizures."[19] In addition to GABA-mediated seizure inhibition, activation of the N-methyl-D aspartate (NMDA) receptor by the excitatory neurotransmitter glutamate can be required for the propagation of seizure activity. Despite this knowledge, our understanding of the cellular and molecular mechanisms by which epilepsy develops or persists is still incomplete.

Neuronal injury begins to occur within several minutes of seizure onset.[20] Neuronal death can occur under certain circumstances after as little as 30 to 60 minutes of continuous seizure activity.[21-23] Neuronal injury is thought to be caused by an influx of calcium caused by the release of excitatory neurotransmitters, specifically glutamate via NMDA receptor activation.[20] It has been postulated that this can occur because of a mechanistic shift from inadequate GABAergic inhibitory receptor-mediated transmission to excessive NMDA excitatory receptor-mediated transmission.[24]

Clinical Presentation

There are three main types of status epilepticus—generalized convulsive, focal motor, and nonconvulsive; the most common is generalized convulsive status epilepticus. These seizures can be overt or have subtle motor manifestations, especially if the episode is prolonged. Much rarer forms of status epilepticus are focal motor status epilepticus (eg, simple and complex partial seizures) and nonconvulsive status epilepticus (absence seizure). Simple partial seizures are characterized by continuous or repeated focal motor seizures (eg, twitching of a digit), focal sensory symptoms (eg, the sensation of flashing lights in one visual field), or cognitive symptoms (eg, aphasia) without impaired consciousness. Complex partial seizures are characterized by continuous or repeated episodes of focal motor, sensory, or cognitive symptoms with impaired consciousness. Absence (petit mal) epilepsy is characterized by altered mental status. This can present as confusion or stupor. Associated symptoms of absence seizures include myoclonus, eye blinking, perseveration, and language difficulty. Any type of seizure can occur continuously or in rapid succession and thus fulfill the criteria for status epilepticus.

The acute phase of status epilepticus is dominated by signs and symptoms of sympathetic overdrive. Systemic responses include hypertension, hyperthermia, tachycardia, cardiac arrhythmias, hyperglycemia, and metabolic acidosis. The initial phase of status epilepticus results in an increased systemic blood pressure with an increase in peripheral vascular resistance. As the status becomes prolonged, the blood pressure will normalize or even begin to fall, with resultant hypotension.[25] In a study of 21 patients, White et al found a mean elevation of systolic pressure of 85 mm Hg and an elevation of diastolic pressure of 42 mm Hg.[26] Hyperthermia frequently occurs in status epilepticus and is usually caused by motor activity and central sympathetic drive. Aminoff and Simon reported that 75 of 90 patients with status epilepticus had hyperthermia, with temperatures reaching 42°C.[25] Although vigorous muscle activity can lead to hyperthermia, an infectious source must also be considered. Hyperthermia can worsen neuronal damage and should be treated aggressively with cooling.

Boggs and associates reported new specific electrocardiographic abnormalities in 58.3% of patients in status epilepticus.[27] The most frequently observed abnormalities were ischemic changes. The authors also found that patients with electrocardiographic abnormalities had a higher mortality rate (37% versus 12%) than patients without electrocardiographic changes.[27]

Hyperglycemia often results from increased catecholamines, but with prolonged status epilepticus, increased insulin secretion can result in hypoglycemia. Although rare, a massive release of insulin can lead to hypoglycemia, which critically restricts glucose delivery to the brain. This is particularly dangerous in infants and should be corrected immediately.[28,29] If the physician cannot check for hypoglycemia or if there is any doubt, glucose should be administered empirically.

Severe metabolic acidosis can occur secondary to excess anaerobic metabolic activity. In a study of 70 spontaneously ventilating patients with status epilepticus, 23 had a pH of less than 7.0.[25] The acidosis has both a respiratory and a metabolic component but usually should not be treated. Induced acidosis has not been correlated with the degree of neuronal injury, and acidosis is known to be an anticonvulsant.

The mortality associated with status epilepticus is largely related to the metabolic stress and complications associated with repeated muscular convulsions. For example, rhabdomyolysis, aspiration pneumonitis, neurogenic pulmonary edema, and respiratory failure can result from convulsions. If there is a possibility of rhabdomyolysis from prolonged muscle contractions, succinylcholine chloride should be avoided because of potential hyperkalemia-induced cardiac arrhythmias. Peripheral intravenous access is needed to provide fluid resuscitation and help prevent renal damage. Loss of protective airway reflexes is common in patients who have prolonged or recurrent seizures and promotes the likelihood of pulmonary aspiration. In addition, the development of pulmonary edema during status epilepticus is well documented.[30,31] In animal studies, pulmonary vascular pressure has been found to be elevated in status epilepticus and may contribute to this phenomenon.[26]

Emergency Department Evaluation

Initial evaluation requires a detailed inquiry, but it should not delay treatment. Even though laboratory or radiographic studies generally have a low yield for patients presenting with a single seizure, status epilepticus should prompt a workup for the cause and potentially reversible conditions. The first step includes a determination of whether the patient has a history of epilepsy or a condition that predisposes him or her to a seizure. A search for secondary causes of status epilepticus includes eliciting a history of or suspicion of drug or alcohol abuse, metabolic derangement or other active systemic illness, or recent traumatic injury.

Rapid bedside testing for glucose is indicated in all patients. Hypoglycemia can induce cortical hyperexcitability, either through an osmotic effect or by increasing glutamate and decreasing the GABA concentration.[18] Measurement of electrolyte levels, particularly sodium, calcium, and magnesium, is recommended. In patients taking anticonvulsant medications, medication levels should be tested. Elevation of creatine kinase levels resulting from rhabdomyolysis can be seen after prolonged convulsions and can lead to acute renal failure. Blood culture, urinalysis, and lumbar puncture are indicated if an infectious source is suspected. There is hope that laboratory tests will eventually provide the means for detecting and defining the critical factors that distinguish a single epileptic seizure from status epilepticus.[16]

If head trauma is suspected by history or physical examination, emergent computed tomography (CT) scan of the head is indicated. For patients presenting with a first episode of epilepsy, a noncontrast head CT is the imaging modality of choice for detecting hemorrhage. Urgent head CTs should also be considered in patients who have focally abnormal examinations, persistently impaired consciousness, headaches, fever, or a history of trauma. Patients who have a higher likelihood of structural abnormalities, such as those with HIV infection and other immunocompromised states, cancer, alcohol abuse, anticoagulation, vascular disease, or a demographic risk of cysticercosis, should also be imaged. A recent consensus statement from the American Academy of Neurology recommends that patients who have new seizures without obvious causes (eg, hypoglycemia or exposure to certain toxins) should have brain imaging.[32] Although magnetic resonance imaging (MRI) provides more information than CT, it is rarely indicated in the acute phase of evaluation, but it is the preferred modality in nonemergency or elective situations.[32] In the acute setting, MRI can be indicated in patients who fail to return to baseline mental status or neurologic function.

Although electroencephalographic (EEG) monitoring is not routinely performed in the emergency department, it may be required to evaluate for subtle generalized convulsant or nonconvulsant status epilepticus. Likewise, if a seizure does not fully resolve or the patient fails to return to an alert, cognitive baseline, an electroencephalogram is recommended to exclude ongoing ictal activity. For inpatients, EEG monitoring is commonly performed to confirm the diagnosis, document a possible epileptic focus, and evaluate for residual nonclinical epileptiform activity.

KEY POINTS

Routine laboratory tests are generally not recommended for a single seizure; however, patients in status epilepticus should have their creatine kinase, electrolyte, and anticonvulsant medication levels checked.

The American Academy of Neurology recommends brain imaging for patients who have new seizures without obvious causes (eg, hypoglycemia or exposure to certain toxins).

Management

Given the new definition of status epilepticus and the understanding that neuronal injury occurs much earlier in the process than was originally believed, the approach to and management of patients with status epilepticus have evolved toward more rapid and aggressive treatment in the emergency department[33] (Figure 18-1). There are many pharmacologic approaches to choose from for treatment of status epilepticus, yet there is a paucity of randomized trials to indicate whether one is superior to another.[2,34,35] Regardless of the medication regimen, it is important to recognize that all these medications can result in a further decline in mental status and ventilation. Therefore, throughout treatment, clinicians must be prepared to manage the patient's airway and provide hemodynamic support.

Although opinions differ on the best sequence of medications, benzodiazepines are considered the first-line treatment for status epilepticus. All benzodiazepines work by increasing the effects of GABA, the primary inhibitory neurotransmitter in the brain. There is no consensus as to which benzodiazepine is the most effective in terminating seizures.[36] Lorazepam, diazepam, and midazolam are all possible choices.

First-Line Agents

Lorazepam is very effective at terminating seizures (equal to diazepam) but takes slightly longer to reach peak effect when given intravenously (1–2 minutes for lorazepam versus 20–30 seconds for diazepam). Lorazepam alone will terminate seizures in 50% to 70% of patients.[37] The advantage of lorazepam is that its antiseizure properties will last 4 to 6 hours; diazepam's effects can be as short as 20 minutes. The primary downside to lorazepam is its lack of stability at room temperature, making it less likely to be available in the prehospital setting. For efficacy and antiseizure duration, however, it is unparalleled, so it is the first drug of choice for most clinicians. A Cochrane review supports lorazepam as the drug of choice for seizure termination[38] (Table 18-2).

Diazepam has a high lipid solubility and can therefore easily cross the blood–brain barrier, making it highly effective in rapidly terminating seizures when administered at dosages of 0.1 to 0.3 mg/kg IV. However, due to the same lipid solubility, the drug will quickly redistribute into adipose tissue throughout the body, resulting in a drop in CNS levels within 20 minutes. Diazepam is reported to initially terminate seizures in 50% to 80% of patients. However, if no anticonvulsant drug is administered, status epilepticus will recur in 50% of patients within the next 2 hours.[39] One of the primary advantages to diazepam is that it remains stable in liquid form at room temperature for long periods, unlike other common benzodiazepines. This stability makes diazepam common in the prehospital arena. Diazepam is also available in a rectal gel formulation that is useful for nonhospitalized patients and those without ready intravenous access.[40]

Midazolam is the most water-soluble of the benzodiazepines. This makes it the slowest to cross the blood–brain barrier and hence to reach peak effects in the CNS. The primary advantage of midazolam over the other benzodiazepines is that it can be used in continuous infusion for refractory status epilepticus and is associated with the fewest cardiovascular side effects.[41]

Lorazepam has a longer duration of action than diazepam.

Diazepam is commonly used by emergency medical services personnel since it can be stored at room temperature.

Second-Line Agents

Following initial treatment of status epilepticus with a benzodiazepine, the anticonvulsant medication phenytoin (or its prodrug, fosphenytoin) is usually added to the pharmacologic regimen. The primary advantage of these drugs is their efficacy in preventing recurrence of seizures for much longer periods than the benzodiazepines. These medications act in the motor cortex as well as the brainstem to suppress seizure activity.

Phenytoin has a long track record of effectiveness in treating seizures and status epilepticus. It is loaded intravenously, with a goal of 18 to 20 mg/kg. The speed of the infusion is usually limited to 50 mg/min because of the propylene glycol in which the drug is solubilized. Infusing phenytoin faster than this can cause hypotension and cardiac arrhythmias. Because of these side effects, patients must be on a cardiac monitor during intravenous loading. If status epilepticus continues after the initial loading dose of 18 to 20 mg/kg, the clinician can increase the total dose up to 30 mg/kg. Beyond this dose, phenytoin is unlikely to terminate status epilepticus (Table 18-3).

Fosphenytoin is a water-soluble prodrug of phenytoin. Following administration, plasma esterases will convert fosphenytoin into phosphate, formaldehyde, and phenytoin. Because fosphenytoin does not require propylene glycol for suspension, it can be infused much faster than phenytoin (up to 150 mg/min). It is dosed in phenytoin equivalents (PE) (ie, 18–20 PE/kg load). If status epilepticus persists after the initial load, as with phenytoin, the clinician may give additional drug, up to a total of 30 PE/kg. Beyond this dose, there is unlikely to be any additional benefit (Table 18-4).

Fosphenytoin, a prodrug of phenytoin, can be intravenously loaded faster than phenytoin without the risk of hypotension or cardiac arrhythmias.

Third-Line Agents

If a patient has received an adequate dose of benzodiazepines as well as phenytoin/fosphenytoin and is still seizing, he or she is now considered to have "refractory status epilepticus," and the clinician will need to try a third-line (and potentially fourth-line) agent. Status epilepticus refractory to two agents is a demarcation line where morbidity and mortality clearly begin a steep rise and even more rapid treatment is needed. The clinician should be prepared at this point to definitively manage the airway if hypoventilation occurs and may need to start addressing the metabolic acidosis associated with prolonged seizure.

Controversy persists as to which medication is the best third-line agent. There are very few studies to guide the clinician and none that demonstrates clear superiority of one treatment over another. Phenobarbital has traditionally been used, but several other medications appear to have roughly equal efficacy. Given this, the clinician should become familiar with one or two third-line medications and be prepared to use them if a patient develops refractory status.

Valproic acid (Table 18-5) is a potential choice that has gained popularity as a third-line agent in refractory status. Some authors have advocated it as a potential alternative to phenytoin as a second-line agent.[42] It is dosed to achieve a load of 20 mg/kg. It is approved by the US Food and Drug Administration (FDA) for this indication, but its use is limited by the recommended slow infusion rate (20 mg/min maximum). A growing number of reports support faster intravenous loading of the agent (eg, 10 mg/kg/min).[43,44] These small studies found no significantly increased risk of hypotension or cardiac arrhythmias at these

---

TABLE 18-3.

Phenytoin dosing in status epilepticus

Bolus: 20 mg/kg

Maximum rate: 50 mg/min

Watch for cardiovascular effects (patient must be monitored).

Example:
  70-kg patient
  Bolus = 1,400 mg
  28 min required for bolus (minimum)
  CNS level reached in 10–15 min after bolus
  Total time to clinical effect = 40 min

TABLE 18-4.

Fosphenytoin dosing in status epilepticus

Bolus: 20 PE/kg

Maximum rate: 150 PE/min

Example:
  70-kg patient
  Bolus = 1,400 PE
  10 min required for bolus
  CNS level reached in 10 min after bolus
  Total time to clinical effect = 20 min

TABLE 18-2.

Lorazepam dosing in status epilepticus

Children
  0.1 mg/kg IV bolus
  May repeat × 2

Adults
  2–4 mg IV bolus
  Once 8–12 mg has been administered, the ceiling effect has been reached.

higher loading rates. Preexisting liver disease is a concern with this agent because hyperammonemic encephalopathy can result.[45]

Levetiracetam (Table 18-6) is one of the newer agents available for refractory status (approved by the FDA in 2006). It has multiple sites of action in the CNS but ultimately works to enhance the action of GABA. The intravenous formulation of this medication is approved for refractory status in adults but not in children. The dosing for status epilepticus is 20 mg/kg, and it can be loaded at a rate of 5 mg/kg/min. Small studies have shown at least equal effectiveness with the other third-line agents, but more extensive data are lacking.[46,47]

The barbiturates have been the traditional third-line agent in the treatment of refractory status. They also bind to GABA receptors and amplify their neuroinhibitory effects. The downside to all the barbiturates is their tendency to cause hypoventilation and hypotension. Once they are used, the clinician should be ready for airway management as well as hemodynamic support of the patient.

Phenobarbital (Table 18-7) has a long track record of being used for refractory status epilepticus. An initial dose of 20 mg/kg is used, and the drug can be infused at a rate of 30 to 50 mg/min. As noted above, once infusion has begun, careful monitoring of ventilatory and cardiac status is mandatory. Due to its extremely long half-life (80–100 hours), prolonged sedation is expected.

Pentobarbital is used less frequently in the treatment of refractory status epilepticus. At doses of 10 mg/kg, its efficacy is similar to that of phenobarbital, but, because of the drug's negative inotropic effects combined with its vasodilatory effects, vasopressors are almost always necessary. Administration rates start at 100 mg/min but usually need to be titrated down because of the issues mentioned above.

Propofol is a phenolic compound with anticonvulsive properties unrelated to any of the other anticonvulsants. When administered intravenously at general anesthetic doses, it has shown anecdotal evidence of being effective in seizure termination.[48–50] It is loaded at a dose of 2 mg/kg and is maintained at 0.1 to 0.2 mg/kg/min. Intubation and ventilation are required. It should be noted that propofol can cause a propofol infusion syndrome in some patients, characterized by metabolic acidosis, rhabdomyolysis, renal failure, and cardiac dysfunction.[51] It is generally thought that the risk of this syndrome is greatest when high doses are used for more than 2 days.

KEY POINTS

There is no consensus on the preferred third-line agent for the treatment of status epilepticus.

The use of barbiturates (phenobarbital and pentobarbital) requires monitoring for respiratory depression and hypotension.

The intravenous formulation of levetiracetam is not FDA approved for use in children.

Valproic acid use can result in hyperammonemic encephalopathy in individuals with preexisting liver disease.

Fourth-Line Agents

When all treatment fails to stop refractory status epilepticus, general inhalational anesthesia becomes the treatment of last resort. The goal is to induce burst suppression on continuous electroencephalography. Once this point is reached, morbidity and mortality rates are extremely high.

Nonconvulsive Status Epilepticus and Subtle Status Epilepticus

Nonconvulsive and minimally convulsive status epilepticus are two entities that clinicians should be alert for in the appropriate patient population.[52] Subtle status epilepticus should be suspected in any patient who does not regain consciousness within 20 or 30 minutes after cessation of generalized seizure activity. Extremely subtle motor activity, such as eyelid twitching, can indicate ongoing seizure activity in this population. Both nonconvulsive and subtle status epilepticus represent continuing seizure activity without recognizable motor activ-

---

TABLE 18-5.

Valproic acid dosing in status epilepticus

20-mg/kg load
FDA-approved maximum rate: 20 mg/min
Many studies demonstrate safety of 300 mg/min
Example: 　70-kg patient 　1,400-mg load 　FDA bolus = 70-min load 　High bolus = 5–10-min load

---

TABLE 18-6.

Levetiracetam dosing in status epilepticus

20-mg/kg load
Maximum rate: 5 mg/kg/min
Example: 　70-kg patient 　1,400-mg load 　5–10 min required for load

---

TABLE 18-7.

Phenobarbital dosing in status epilepticus

20-mg/kg load
Maximum rate: 1–2 mg/kg/min
Example: 　70-kg patient 　1,400-mg load 　At intermediate rate (1.5 mg/kg/min), 15–20-min load

ity. With subtle status epilepticus, the motor activity is either fragmentary or so subtle as to be easily missed. The electrical seizure activity in the brain, however, is persistent. Patients with subtle status epilepticus have an extremely grave prognosis. It is considered the end stage of generalized convulsive status, characterized by complete dissociation between electrical activity in the brain and motor response in the body. It must be considered in the comatose patient who has had or is suspected to have had refractory status. An electroencephalogram is required to identify this entity once motor activity ceases.

Nonconvulsive status does not necessarily carry the same grave prognosis as subtle status epilepticus.[53] It can be a manifestation of absence seizures or partial seizures (simple or complex). Patients with nonconvulsive absence seizures will present with a clear change in level of consciousness but are generally not comatose. Typically they are described as lethargic and confused, with slowed speech. No deaths or long-term morbidity have been described with nonconvulsive status in absence seizures. Confirmation with electroencephalography is recommended, and treatment is with benzodiazepines as a first-line agent, followed by valproic acid as a second-line agent.

Partial seizures (simple or complex) can result in status epilepticus but, as with absence seizures, the morbidity and mortality rates are much lower than with subtle status epilepticus. Aggressive treatment is rarely required. Standard agents used for convulsive status epilepticus will usually terminate these seizures.

KEY POINTS

Both nonconvulsive and subtle status epilepticus represent continuing seizure activity without recognizable motor activity.

Patients with subtle status epilepticus (considered the complete dissociation between electrical activity in the brain and motor response in the body) have an extremely grave prognosis.

Partial seizures (simple or complex) can result in status epilepticus; however, the morbidity and mortality rates are much lower than with subtle status epilepticus.

Toxicologic and Pharmaceutical-Induced Seizures

A number of substances have been reported to cause seizures as a side effect of a therapeutic dosage or a manifestation of toxic overdose or withdrawal. Commonly encountered toxins and medications that can precipitate status epilepticus are listed in Table 18-8.

Alcohol-related seizures usually occur 6 to 48 hours after a significant reduction in the serum alcohol level. The diagnosis of alcohol-withdrawal seizures is primarily based on information from the patient's history. The clinician must also consider other causes; alcoholic patients are also at risk for cerebrovascular insults, metabolic disorders, trauma, and infection. In the acute setting, benzodiazepines are usually sufficient in treating and preventing successive withdrawal seizures by providing a GABA-enhancing effect similar to that of ethanol.

Cocaine-related seizures can result from direct CNS toxicity or as a product of hypoxemia related to cardiac toxicity. Patients with this toxic reaction can also have hyperthermia, rhabdomyolysis, and cardiac arrhythmias. Benzodiazepines are an appropriate first-line agent for treating seizure and sympathetic stimulation.

Isoniazid is a first-line agent in the chemoprophylaxis and treatment of tuberculosis. It can cause nausea, altered mental status, ataxia, and seizures when toxic amounts are ingested. Isoniazid is believed to cause seizures by depleting vitamin B_6, which leads to impaired synthesis of GABA. Unlike most toxin-associated seizures, isoniazid toxicity has a specific antidote. A dose of 1 mg of vitamin B_6 (pyridoxine) intravenously should be given for each 1 mg of isoniazid recently ingested. If the ingested amount is unknown, 5 mg should be given.

Conclusion

Status epilepticus is defined as any seizure lasting longer than 5 minutes or any recurrent seizure without return to baseline mental status in the interictal period. This relatively new definition resulted from the realization that neuronal injury occurs much earlier in the process than was originally believed. Prompt administration of anticonvulsants may decrease neuronal injury and further seizure activity. Supportive care and early use of benzodiazepines are the initial treatments of choice for status epilepticus.

References

1. Donaire A, Carreno M, Gomez B, et al. Cortical laminar necrosis related to prolonged focal status epilepticus. *J Neurol Neurosurg Psychiatry.* 2006;77:104-106.
2. Lowenstein DH, Alldredge BK. Status epilepticus. *N Engl J Med.* 1998;338:970-976.
3. Lowenstein DH, Cloyd J. Out of hospital treatment of status epilepticus and prolonged seizures. *Epilepsia.* 2007;48(suppl 8):96-98.
4. Annegers JF. The epidemiology of epilepsy. In: Wyllie E, ed. *The Treatment of Epilepsy: Principles and Practice.* 3rd ed. Philadelphia, PA: Lippincott Williams & Wilkins; 2001:131-138.
5. Shorvon S. *Status Epilepticus: Its Clinical Features and Treatment in Children and Adults.* Cambridge, UK: Cambridge University Press; 1994.
6. DeLorenzo RJ, Hauser WA, Towne AR, et al. A prospective, population-based epidemiologic study of status epilepticus in Richmond, Virginia. *Neurology.* 1996;46:1029-1035.

TABLE 18-8.

Medications and toxins that can induce status epilepticus

Medications
- Analgesics (eg, local anesthetics, meperidine, tramadol)
- Antibiotics (eg, β-lactam antibiotics, isoniazid, quinolones)
- Immunomodulators (eg, cyclosporine, tacrolimus)
- Psychotropics (eg, cyclic antidepressants, antipsychotics, lithium)
- Salicylates
- Theophylline

Toxins/Illicit Drugs
- Amphetamines
- Cocaine
- Ethanol (withdrawal)
- Hydrocarbons
- Insecticides and rodenticides
- Phencyclidine

7. Hesdorffer DC, Logroscino G, Cascino G, et al. Incidence of status epilepticus in Rochester, Minnesota, 1965–1984. *Neurology.* 1998;50:735-741.

8. DeLorenzo RJ, Towne AR, Pellock JM, et al. Status epilepticus in children, adults and the elderly. *Epilepsia.* 1992;33(suppl 4):S15-S25.

9. Hauser WA. Status epilepticus: epidemiological considerations. *Neurology.* 1990;40(suppl 2):9-13.

10. Vignatelli L, Tonon C, D'Alessandro R. Incidence and short-term prognosis of status epilepticus in adults in Bologna, Italy. *Epilepsia.* 2003;44:964-968.

11. Verity CM, Ross EM, Golding J. Outcome of childhood status epilepticus and lengthy febrile convulsions: findings of national cohort study. *BMJ.* 1993;307:225-228.

12. Waterhouse EJ, Garnett LK, Towne AR, et al. Prospective population-based study of intermittent and continuous convulsive status epilepticus in Richmond, Virginia. *Epilepsia.* 1999;40:752-758.

13. Chin RF, Neville BG, Peckham C, et al. Incidence, cause, and short-term outcome of convulsive status epilepticus in childhood: prospective population-based study. *Lancet.* 2006;368(9531):222-229.

14. DeLorenzo RJ, Pellock JM, Towne AR, et al. Epidemiology of status epilepticus. *J Clin Neurophysiol.* 1995;12:316-325.

15. Huff JS. Seizures and status epilepticus in adults: part II. *Emerg Med Rep.* 2007;28:281-288.

16. Lowenstein DH. Status epilepticus: an overview of the clinical problem. *Epilepsia.* 1999;40:s3-s8.

17. Shinnar S, Pellock JM, Moshe SL, et al. In whom does status epilepticus occur: age-related differences in children. *Epilepsia.* 1997;38:907-914.

18. Mirski MA, Varelas PN. Seizures and status epilepticus in the critically ill. *Crit Care Clin.* 2008;24:115-147.

19. Towne AR, Waterhouse EJ, Boggs JG, et al. Prevalence of nonconvulsive status epilepticus in comatose patients. *Neurology.* 2000;54:340-345.

20. Marik PE, Varon J. The management of status epilepticus. *Chest.* 2004;126:582-591.

21. Fountain NB, Lothman EW. Pathophysiology of status epilepticus. *J Clin Neurophysiol.* 1995;12:326-342.

22. Payne TA, Bleck TP. Status epilepticus. *Crit Care Clin.* 1997;13:17.

23. Chapman MG, Smith M, Hirsch NP. Status epilepticus. *Anaesthesia.* 2001;56:648-659.

24. Bleck TP. Refractory status epilepticus in 2001. *Arch Neurol.* 2002;59:188-189.

25. Aminoff MJ, Simon RP. Status epilepticus: causes, clinical features and consequences in 98 patients. *Am J Med.* 1980;69:657-666.

26. White PT, Grant P, Mosier J, et al. Changes in cerebral dynamics associated with seizures. *Neurology.* 1961;11:354-361.

27. Boggs JG, Painter JA, DeLorenzo RJ. Analysis of electrocardiographic changes in status epilepticus. *Epilepsy Res.* 1993;14:87-94.

28. Meldrum BS. Endocrine consequences of status epilepticus. *Adv Neurol.* 1983;34:399-403.

29. Dwyer BE, Wasterlain CG. Neonatal seizures in monkeys and rabbits: brain glucose depletion in the face of normoglycemia, prevention by glucose loads. *Pediatr Res.* 1985;19:992-995.

30. Terrence CF, Rao GR, Pepper JA. Neurogenic pulmonary edema in unexpected death of epileptic patients. *Ann Neurol.* 1981;9:458-464.

31. Simon RP. Physiologic consequences of status epilepticus. *Epilepsia.* 1985;26(suppl 1):S58-S66.

32. Greenberg MK, Barsan WG, Starkman S. Neuroimaging in the emergency patient presenting with seizure. *Neurology.* 1996;47:26-32.

33. Rosetti AO, Logoroscino G, Bromfield EB. Refractory status epilepticus: effect of treatment aggressiveness on prognosis. *Arch Neurol.* 2005;62:1698-1702.

34. Beren RG. An alternative perspective on the management of status epilepticus. *Epilepsy Behavior.* 2008;12:349-353.

35. Abend NS, Dlugos DJ. Treatment of refractory status epilepticus: literature review and a proposed protocol. *Pediatr Neurol.* 2008;38:377-390.

36. Cock HR, Schapira AH. A comparison of lorazepam and diazepam as initial therapy in convulsive status epilepticus. *Q J Med.* 2002;95:225-231.

37. Alldredge BK, Gelb AM, Isaacs SM, et al. A comparison of lorazepam, diazepam, and placebo for the treatment of out-of-hospital status epilepticus. *N Engl J Med.* 2001;345:631-637.

38. Prasad, K, Al-Roomi, K, Krishnan, P, et al. Anticonvulsant therapy for status epilepticus. *Cochrane Database Syst Rev.* 2005;CD003723.

39. Walker M. Status epilepticus: an evidence based guide. *BMJ.* 2005;331:673-677.

40. Fakhoury T, Chumley A, Bensalem-Owen M. Effectiveness of diazepam rectal gel in adults with acute repetitive seizures and prolonged seizures: a single-center experience. *Epilepsy Behav.* 2007;11:357-360.

41. Kumar A, Bleck TP. Intravenous midazolam for the treatment of refractory status epilepticus. *Crit Care Med.* 1992;20:483-488.

42. Misra UK, Kalita J, Patel R. Sodium valproate vs. phenytoin in status epilepticus: a pilot study. *Neurology.* 2006;67:340-342.

43. Wheless JW, Vazquez BR, Kanner AM, et al. Rapid infusion with valproate sodium is well tolerated in patients with epilepsy. *Neurology.* 2004;63:1507-1508.

44. Limdi NA, Knowlton RK, Cofield SS, et al. Safety of rapid intravenous loading of valproate. *Epilepsia.* 2007;48:478-483.

45. Rossetti AO, Bromfield EB. Efficacy of rapid IV administration of valproic acid for status epilepticus. *Neurology.* 2005;65:500-501.

46. Knake S, Gruener J, Hattemer K, et al. Intravenous levetiracetam in the treatment of benzodiazepine refractory status epilepticus. *J Neurol Neurosurg Psych.* 2008;79:588-589.

47. Eue S, Grumbt M, Muller M, et al. Two years of experience in the treatment of status epilepticus with intravenous levetiracetam. *Epilepsy Behav.* 2009;15:467-469.

48. Prasad A, Worrall BB, Bertram EH, et al. Propofol and midazolam in the treatment of refractory status epilepticus. *Epilepsia.* 2001;42:380-386.

49. Rossetti AO, Reichhart MD, Schaller MD, et al. Propofol treatment of refractory status epilepticus: a study of 31 episodes. *Epilepsia.* 2004;45:757-763.

50. Paravanian I, Uusaro A, Kalvanian R, et al. Propofol in the treatment of refractory status epilepticus. *Intensive Care Med.* 2006;32:1075-1079.

51. Zarovnaya EL, Jobst BC, Harris BT. Propofol-associated fatal myocardial failure and rhabdomyolysis in an adult with status epilepticus. *Epilepsia.* 2007;48:1002-1006.

52. Meierkord H, Holtkamp M. Non-convulsive status epilepticus in adults: clinical forms and treatment. *Lancet Neurol.* 2007;6:329-339.

53. Shovron S. What is nonconvulsive status epilepticus, and what are its subtypes? *Epilepsia.* 2007;48(suppl 8):35-38.

CHAPTER 19

The Crashing Anaphylaxis Patient

Jonathan E. Davis and Robert L. Norris

IN THIS CHAPTER

Airway management in anaphylaxis

Epinephrine in allergic emergencies—which patients, by what route, and when to avoid

Second-line pharmacotherapy in allergic emergencies—antihistamines, corticosteroids

Special situations—β-blockers, pregnancy, bradykinin-mediated angioedema

Disposition of patients with severe allergic reactions

Introduction

Perhaps no other diagnostic entity embodies the true essence of emergency care better than anaphylaxis: the rapid and often unpredictable onset of potentially lethal symptoms, the propensity for significant morbidity and mortality if not treated swiftly and aggressively, and the wide availability of highly effective treatment modalities—all frequently occurring in people who are young and otherwise healthy. Anaphylaxis is a severe, life-threatening, systemic reaction that affects all ages. It results from the sudden release of active mediators from mast cells, which are located in tissues, and basophils, which are located in the bloodstream. The clinical syndrome is variable and can involve multiple target organs, including the skin and the respiratory, gastrointestinal (GI), and cardiovascular systems (Table 19-1).

Respiratory and cardiovascular symptoms cause the greatest concern because they carry the greatest potential for morbidity or mortality. During the second National Institute of Allergy and Infectious Diseases (NIAID)/Food Allergy and Anaphylaxis (FAAN) symposium, a panel of experts agreed on a broad definition of anaphylaxis that would be useful to both the medical and lay communities: "a serious allergic reaction that is rapid in onset and may cause death."[1]

The signs and symptoms of an acute allergic reaction are best viewed as a continuum (Figure 19-1). It is useful to define a point along this spectrum that distinguishes anaphylaxis from milder allergic phenomena because anaphylaxis necessitates more aggressive treatment.

A reasonable *working* definition of anaphylaxis involves allergic signs/symptoms with one or both of the following features: respiratory compromise and hemodynamic instability, ranging anywhere from presyncope to cardiovascular collapse. Experts participating in the second NIAID/FAAN symposium proposed clinical criteria for diagnosing anaphylaxis (Table 19-2).[1]

Pathophysiology

A classic IgE-mediated allergic response (Gell and Coombs type I, immediate hypersensitivity) consists of three steps:

1) Sensitization (allergen exposure leads to the production of IgE antibodies)
2) An early phase reaction (subsequent allergen exposure causes IgE-mediated release of preformed substances from mast cells and basophils)
3) A late phase reaction (immune cells produce additional inflammatory mediators)

Treatment is aimed at halting preformed mediator release

and shutting down the intracellular machinery that produces new mediators.

An anaphylactoid reaction (also known as "nonallergic anaphylaxis") is an immediate systemic reaction resulting from the release of identical mediators from mast cells and basophils; it differs from anaphylaxis in that it is not IgE mediated.[2] Therefore, unlike in allergic anaphylaxis, adverse anaphylactoid reactions can occur on first exposure to the inciting agent since prior sensitization is not required. The clinical presentation and management of anaphylactoid reactions are exactly the same as for anaphylaxis.

Etiology

Anaphylaxis has multiple etiologic culprits, including foods, medications, stinging insects, latex, and exercise (Table 19-3). Food-induced anaphylaxis is now generally regarded as the single most common cause of anaphylaxis treated in emergency departments in the United States.[3,4] Many infants outgrow their allergies to eggs, milk, and soy products. On the other hand, the most prevalent food allergies in adults (to peanuts, tree nuts, fish, and shellfish) are usually not outgrown and can remain problematic for the individual throughout life, even if they first develop during childhood.

PEARL

Food-induced anaphylaxis is generally regarded as the most common cause of anaphylaxis treated in the emergency department.

Mortality

Certain factors are associated with especially severe or fatal anaphylaxis. In particular, asthma has been shown to be an independent risk factor for death from anaphylaxis.[5,6] Peanuts and tree nuts have also been associated with severe reactions, accounting for most fatal or near-fatal food reactions in the United States.[7] Adolescents appear to be at increased risk for severe or fatal anaphylaxis: they are more prone to engage in risky behaviors despite known allergy, they are less likely to recognize allergic triggers, they may "deny" symptoms, and they may not carry or use their epinephrine self-administration device.[8]

KEY POINT

Risk factors for fatal anaphylaxis include a history of bronchospasm, nut allergies (peanut, tree nut), and adolescent age.

PEARL

Asthma is an independent risk factor for death from anaphylaxis.

Differential Diagnosis

Anaphylaxis must be considered in the differential diagnosis for any patient with an acute onset of respiratory distress, bronchospasm, hypotension, or cardiac arrest (Table 19-4).

Emergency Department Evaluation

The emergency department evaluation begins with rapid triage and stabilization of the symptomatic patient. Patients with rapidly progressive symptoms or abnormal vital signs should be taken immediately to an area fully equipped with advanced airway equipment and critical care capabilities. Anaphylaxis is a dynamic process; frequent reassessments are crucial. It should also be appreciated that patients who present with initially mild symptoms and who appear stable have the potential for rapid deterioration. The clinical presentation of anaphylaxis can vary

TABLE 19-1.

Target organs and symptoms in anaphylaxis

Cardiovascular — Hypotension, lightheadedness, near syncope, syncope, arrhythmias, angina

Respiratory — Upper airway—oropharyngeal, hypopharyngeal, or laryngeal edema

Lower airway—bronchospasm

Gastrointestinal — Nausea, vomiting, diarrhea, cramping

Skin — Flushing, erythema, pruritus, urticaria, angioedema

Central nervous system — Headache, confusion, altered level of consciousness

FIGURE 19-1.

The clinical spectrum of allergic manifestations. The arrow denotes a reasonable point along the spectrum of allergic signs and symptoms at which to classify a reaction as anaphylaxis.

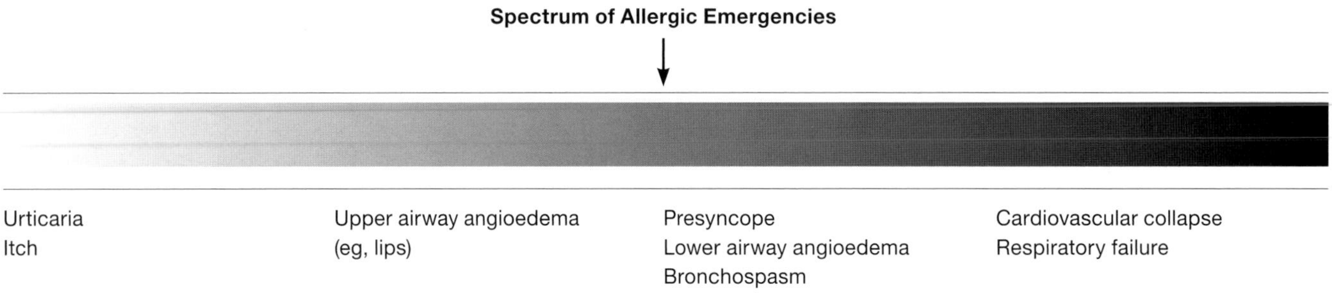

Spectrum of Allergic Emergencies

Urticaria	Upper airway angioedema	Presyncope	Cardiovascular collapse
Itch	(eg, lips)	Lower airway angioedema	Respiratory failure
		Bronchospasm	

between children and adults, with respiratory symptoms predominating in children and cardiovascular manifestations predominating in adults.[4,9]

PEARL

Patients who present with initially mild symptoms and who appear stable have the potential for rapid deterioration.

History and Physical Examination

In many cases, the most valuable information comes from those who observed an allergic event from its onset. Take the time to interview caretakers, bystanders, friends, family members, emergency medical services (EMS) personnel, and anyone else who may have witnessed an out-of-hospital episode to elicit specific information regarding the initial signs and symptoms. Although there is great variability, one study in children determined that the mean latency period between allergen exposure and symptom onset was about 15 minutes.[10] Obtain the patient's medical history, focusing on a history of allergy, asthma, or any other preexisting atopic conditions. Maintain a particularly high level of vigilance in patients with a history of asthma or reactive airway disease, especially if the condition is poorly controlled, because fatal anaphylactic reactions are more likely to occur in such individuals.[11,12]

TABLE 19-2.

Clinical criteria for diagnosing anaphylaxis. Adapted from: Sampson HA, Munoz-Furlong A, Campbell RL, et al. Second symposium on the definition and management of anaphylaxis: summary report – Second National Institute of Allergy and Infectious Disease/Food Allergy and Anaphylaxis Network Symposium. *J Allergy Clin Immunol.* 2006;117(2):393. Copyright 2006. Used with permission from American Academy of Allergy, Asthma, and Immunology.

Anaphylaxis is highly likely when any *one* of the following three criteria is fulfilled:

1. Acute onset of an illness (minutes to several hours), with involvement of the skin, mucosal tissue, or both (eg, generalized hives; pruritus or flushing; swollen lips, tongue, uvula) *and at least* one of the following:
   a. Respiratory compromise
   b. Reduced blood pressure (BP) or associated symptoms of end-organ dysfunction

2. Two (or more) of the following, occurring rapidly (minutes to several hours) after exposure to a *likely allergen* for that patient:
   a. Involvement of the skin or mucosal tissue
   b. Respiratory compromise
   c. Reduced blood pressure (BP) or associated symptoms
   d. Persistent GI symptoms

3. Reduced BP after exposure to a *known allergen* for that patient (minutes to several hours):
   a. Infants and children: low systolic BP (age specific) or >30% decrease in systolic BP
   b. Adults: systolic BP <90 mm Hg or >30% decrease from baseline

PEARL

Be particularly vigilant in patients with a history of bronchospasm (eg, asthma, reactive airway disease) because fatal anaphylactic reactions are more likely in these patients.

The various signs and symptoms of anaphylaxis and their frequencies, based on a compilation of nearly 1,900 patients representing all ages and reactions resulting from a wide variety of allergens, are presented in Table 19-5.[13] Respiratory failure and cardiovascular collapse represent the major threats to life. Losses of up to 35% of circulating blood volume can occur within 10 minutes after the onset of symptoms, primarily from third spacing.[14] The absence of cutaneous findings speaks against the diagnosis of anaphylaxis in general; however, it by no means excludes it. In fact, cutaneous findings are absent entirely in up to 10% of cases.[13] Severe anaphylaxis can occur with no cutaneous manifestations whatsoever.[15,16]

KEY POINTS

Anaphylaxis, including severe reactions, can occur in the absence of cutaneous findings such as urticaria or flushing.

Involvement of the respiratory or cardiovascular system distinguishes anaphylaxis from other allergic phenomena.

Up to 35% of the circulating blood volume can be lost within 10 minutes after the onset of anaphylaxis, primarily from third spacing.

TABLE 19-3.

Causes of anaphylaxis

Category	Example(s)
Foods	Children: eggs, milk, soy
	Adults: peanuts, tree nuts, fish, shellfish
Medications	Antimicrobials, anesthetics, insulin
Hymenoptera	Apidae family (honeybee, bumblebee)
	Vespid family (yellow jacket, hornet, wasp)
	Formicid family (fire ant)
Latex	Proteins in natural rubber latex; additives used in processing latex
Vaccines	Proteins cross-reactive with egg; hydrolyzed gelatin, sorbitol, neomycin
Blood components	Packed red blood cells
Biologic fluids	Human seminal fluid
Exercise	Ingestion of certain foods prior to exercise
Idiopathic	Diagnosis of exclusion

Emergency Department Treatment

As with any emergency condition, initial attention must focus on the ABCs—airway, breathing, and circulation. Definitive airway management is of paramount importance as the window for effective intervention can dwindle rapidly if decisions are not made swiftly and decisively. Administering supplemental oxygen, establishing large-bore vascular access, and infusing crystalloid are essential in most cases of anaphylaxis. Remain vigilant for early clinical signs of shock. Compensated pediatric shock can present with tachycardia alone; hypotension can be a late finding. The recommended initial pediatric fluid infusion (crystalloid or colloid) is 10 to 20 mL/kg, titrated to response.[1] In certain cases, fluid administration of 80 to 100 mL/kg or more may be necessary.

Common medications used in the treatment of anaphylaxis are listed in Table 19-6.

TABLE 19-4.

Differential diagnosis of anaphylaxis. Adapted from: Lieberman P. Anaphylaxis and anaphylactoid reactions. In: Adkinson NF Jr, Yunginer JW, Busse WW, et al, eds. *Middleton's Allergic Principles and Practice.* 6th ed. St Louis, MO: Mosby-Yearbook; 2003:1510. Copyright 2003. Used with permission from Elsevier.

Category	Example(s)
Anaphylactic and anaphylactoid reactions	Reactions to exogenously administered agents
	Related to physical factors (exercise, cold, heat, sunlight)
	Idiopathic
Vasopressor reactions	Neurocardiogenic reaction
Other forms of shock	Hemorrhagic
	Cardiogenic
	Endotoxic
"Flush" syndromes	Carcinoid
	Postmenopausal
	Medullary carcinoma of the thyroid
"Restaurant" syndromes	Monosodium glutamate (MSG) reaction
	Scombroid poisoning
Excess endogenous production of histamine syndromes	Systemic mastocytosis
	Urticaria pigmentosa
	Basophilic leukemia
	Acute promyelocytic leukemia
Nonorganic disease	Panic attack
	Munchausen stridor
	Vocal cord dysfunction syndrome
	Globus hystericus
Miscellaneous	Angiotensin-converting enzyme (ACE) inhibitor/angiotensin receptor blocker (ARB) associated angioedema
	Hereditary angioedema
	Pheochromocytoma

TABLE 19-5.

Frequency of signs and symptoms of anaphylaxis. Adapted from: Joint Task Force on Practice Parameters for the American Academy of Allergy, Asthma and Immunology; the American College of Allergy, Asthma and Immunology; and the Joint Council of Allergy, Asthma and Immunology. The diagnosis and management of anaphylaxis: an updated practice parameter. *J Allergy Clin Immunol.* 2005:115:S497. Copyright 2005. Used with permission from American Academy of Allergy, Asthma, and Immunology.

	Sign/Symptom	Frequency (%)*
Cutaneous	Overall	90
	Urticaria and angioedema	85–90
	Flushing	45–55
	Pruritus without rash	2–5
Respiratory	Overall	40–60
	Dyspnea, wheeze	45–50
	Upper airway angioedema	50–60
	Rhinitis	15–20
Cardiovascular	Dizziness, syncope, hypotension	30–35
Abdominal	Nausea, vomiting, diarrhea, cramping	25–30
Miscellaneous	Headache	5–8
	Substernal pain	4–6
	Seizure	1–2

Data based on a compilation of the records of 1,865 patients.
*Percentages are approximate.

Epinephrine

Epinephrine therapy should be considered a second "A" ("adrenaline") in the ABCs prioritization of anaphylaxis management. Guidelines uniformly recommend epinephrine as the first-line treatment for severe allergic reactions, albeit on the basis of less-than-optimal evidence.[13,17] Epinephrine has numerous identifiable physiologic benefits in the treatment of anaphylaxis (Table 19-7), although its particular indications and dosing regimens are a frequent source of confusion.[18]

Current guidelines recommend prompt administration of epinephrine to any patient with anaphylaxis.[13] However, the issue of what precisely constitutes anaphylaxis arises repeatedly, fueling uncertainty regarding the appropriateness of epinephrine use. Aggressive management with appropriate doses and routes of epinephrine is universally recommended as first-line therapy. Indeed, anecdotal consensus, as well as evidence from the literature, suggests that poor outcomes are most often associated with either failure to give or delays in administering epinephrine.[5] Practitioners should err on the side of injecting epinephrine sooner, except, possibly, in the case of patients with clearly mild allergic symptoms that do not appear to be progressing.

KEY POINT

Epinephrine is the single most important and sole first-line pharmacologic agent for the treatment of anaphylaxis. Current guidelines recommend its prompt administration to any patient with anaphylaxis.

Recent evidence suggests that intramuscular administration of epinephrine is preferred over subcutaneous, regardless of patient age.[17] Subcutaneous absorption is highly dependent on cutaneous blood flow, which can be compromised in anaphylaxis, and can be further aggravated by epinephrine's potent local vasoconstrictor activity, leading to slow and erratic absorption.[19,20] The typical dose for intramuscular administration is 0.01 mg/kg, up to a maximum of 0.2 to 0.5 mg (maximum 0.3 mg for children) of a 1:1,000 dilution, repeated every 5 minutes as needed.[21]

KEY POINT

Current guidelines recommend intramuscular epinephrine administration. In the crashing patient, consider the use of intramuscular epinephrine from an autoinjector unit (eg, EpiPen) if one is readily available. This can save vital time in the management of a rapidly decompensating patient.

Virtually all reported adverse outcomes related to epinephrine result from intravenous administration. Major adverse events have been reported when intravenous epinephrine is administered too rapidly, as an inadequately diluted solution, or in excessive dosage.[22] Intravenous epinephrine has been associated with the induction of fatal cardiac arrhythmias, myocardial infarction, and intracranial hemorrhage.[23-26] However, published reports on the dangers of intravenous epinephrine consistently fail to emphasize that other factors related to the underlying pathophysiologic process (hypoxia, acidosis, effects of inflammatory mediators) may be responsible for the observed complications.[27] Based on these points, intravenous epinephrine should be reserved for patients with severe cardiovascular compromise (ie, a profound decrease in peripheral perfusion that would significantly hamper intramuscular absorption) or when repeated intramuscular dosing fails to alleviate symptoms.

A firm intravenous dose cannot be recommended. The amount of intravenous epinephrine that should be administered depends on the severity of the episode and should be titrated to response. A frequently recommended adult intravenous dosing regimen uses a 1:100,000 epinephrine solution, slowly infusing 100 mcg (0.1 mg) over 5 to 10 minutes (Table 19-8).[13,21,28]

Other authors have suggested 5- to 10-mcg IV bolus doses for treatment of hypotension, and 100- to 500-mcg IV bolus doses in adults with severe cardiovascular collapse.[29] For chil-

TABLE 19-6.

Common medications used in the treatment of anaphylaxis

	Pediatric		Adult	
	Route	Dosage	Route	Dosage
Epinephrine	IM	0.01 mg/kg, maximum 0.3 mg per dose	IM	0.2–0.5 mg every 5 min as needed
	IV	0.1–2 mcg/kg/min infusion	IV	100 mcg of 1:100,000 dilution over 5–10 min
H$_1$ antihistamine	IV/IM	Diphenhydramine, 1 mg/kg (maximum 50 mg)	IV/IM	Diphenhydramine, 25–50 mg
H$_2$ antihistamine	IV	Ranitidine, 1 mg/kg	IV	Ranitidine, 50 mg (maximum 50 mg)
Corticosteroid	IV	Methylprednisolone, 1–2 mg/kg (maximum 125 mg)	IV	Methylprednisolone, 125 mg
Bronchodilator	Nebulized	Albuterol, 1.25–2.5 mg per dose, repeat as needed	Nebulized	Albuterol, 2.5 mg per dose, repeat as needed

dren, use continuous intravenous epinephrine infusion (range, 0.1–2 mcg/kg/min) titrated to response.[30] Intravenous administration of epinephrine to a child should be done cautiously, and it is paramount that the weight-based dosages are double-checked to avoid a medication error catastrophe. Continuous low-dose epinephrine infusion may, in fact, represent the safest and most effective form of intravenous delivery in patients of any age, as the dose can be titrated to desired effect while minimizing the potential for accidental administration of large or concentrated bolus doses of epinephrine.[1] There are very few controlled studies to support any of these recommendations.[31]

KEY POINT

Reserve intravenous epinephrine for patients with severe cardiovascular compromise or for situations in which repeated intramuscular epinephrine has failed to bring about clinical improvement.

PEARL

In the pediatric patient, it is prudent to double-check weight-based dosages of intravenous epinephrine to avoid a medication error catastrophe.

Although there is a paucity of controlled data to adequately address safety concerns, some lessons can be gleaned from experience with the use of epinephrine for asthma.[22,23] These data should not be overly generalized, but they suggest a more favorable safety profile for epinephrine than is routinely acknowledged, particularly when it is administered by routes other than the intravenous. Younger patients have an even more attractive risk-benefit profile for epinephrine in general, as they are likely to tolerate most of the potential complications better than adults.

Of concern to many practitioners is the administration of epinephrine to higher-risk patients, particularly those who are elderly or have a comorbid condition such as hypertension, coronary artery disease, or cerebrovascular disease. The decision to administer epinephrine must be evaluated on a case-by-case basis, with a rapid analysis of benefits weighed against potential risks. Critical to this equation is the fact that anaphylaxis is a life-threatening emergency and, as such, is associated with morbidity and mortality in these higher-risk patients. The potential risks associated with epinephrine need to be balanced against the risks associated with withholding the most critical therapy in anaphylaxis management.

KEY POINT

Anaphylaxis is a life-threatening emergency with inherent morbidity and mortality. Therefore, the risks of epinephrine use need to be balanced against the risks of withholding the most critical pharmacotherapy in anaphylaxis management.

Antihistamines

The role of H_1 antihistamines in allergic emergencies is well documented, although a recent Cochrane review was unable to establish any evidence supporting their benefit.[32] Less sedating H_1 antagonists such as cetirizine (Zyrtec) and loratadine (Claritin) may be used as a substitute for oral diphenhydramine in patients with milder allergic symptoms. However, they have no role in the crashing patient because they are not available for intravenous use in the United States.

Although the precise role of H_1 antagonists in the treatment of allergic emergencies remains to be completely elucidated, their potential benefit, combined with a low propensity for adverse events, makes their use advisable.[32-34] There is no specific evidence regarding the superiority of a particular H_2 antihistamine, but agents other than cimetidine may be preferable to avoid effects on the cytochrome P450 system.[35]

Corticosteroids

Although corticosteroids have traditionally been used in the management of anaphylaxis, their effects have never been validated in controlled trials. However, based on their known beneficial effects in asthma and other allergic diseases, their administration is warranted in allergic emergencies, particularly

TABLE 19-7.

Physiologic effects of epinephrine in anaphylaxis

Receptor	Physiologic Effect
α	Increased peripheral vascular resistance
	Reversal of peripheral vasodilation
	Decreased angioedema and urticaria
β₁	Positive cardiac inotropic effects
	Positive cardiac chronotropic effects
β₂	Bronchodilation
	Increased intracellular cAMP production – reduces inflammatory mediator production/release from mast cells and basophils

TABLE 19-8.

Recommended dilution of epinephrine for intravenous use in adult patients with anaphylaxis[28]

1)	Create 10 mL of a 1:100,000 epinephrine dilution
	Add 0.1 mg (0.1 mL) of a 1:1,000 epinephrine solution to 9.9 mL normal saline
	or
	Add 0.1 mg (1 mL) of 1:10,000 epinephrine solution to 9 mL normal saline
	Resulting solution = 0.1 mg of epinephrine (100 mcg) in 10 mL = 10 mcg/mL
2)	Then administer 10 mL of a 1:100,000 epinephrine solution over 5–10 minutes
	100 mcg over 5–10 minutes = 10–20 mcg/min

in severe reactions. The theoretic objective of the administration of corticosteroids is to temper the continued intracellular synthesis and release of potent pro-inflammatory mediators and to possibly blunt, although not necessarily completely prevent, biphasic or multiphasic anaphylaxis. Practice guidelines suggest that the intravenous route is the preferred method of administration, but there is no evidence supporting any specific dose, route of administration, or particular formulation.

Inhaled Bronchodilators

Nebulized inhaled bronchodilators (such as albuterol sulfate) may be used continuously or intermittently for the treatment of anaphylaxis-induced bronchospasm.

Glucagon; Alternative Vasopressors

Glucagon may have a role in treating anaphylaxis refractory to standard therapy, especially in the case of coexisting β-adrenergic receptor blockade.[36] Epinephrine stimulates intracellular cyclic AMP (cAMP) production through interactions with β-adrenergic receptors. Glucagon exerts its intracellular effects by mediating cAMP production entirely independently of the adrenergic system.[37] A recent evidence-based review of the role of glucagon in refractory anaphylaxis concluded that, despite the limited quality of the evidence, glucagon may benefit patients who are taking β-blockers when all other treatments have failed.[38] The initial pediatric bolus dose is 20 to 30 mcg/kg (maximum dose of 1 mg); the recommended adult dose is 1 to 5 mg IV over 5 minutes, followed by a continuous infusion of 5 to 15 mcg/min titrated to clinical response.[13] Airway protection should be considered prior to infusion as glucagon can cause significant emesis.

Alternative vasopressor agents should be considered in the event that epinephrine and volume expansion fail to maintain adequate blood pressure or perfusion. In this case, norepinephrine (initial 0.05–0.1 mcg/kg/min, titrate to effect; maximum dose 2 mcg/kg/min) or dopamine (initial 2–5 mcg/kg/min, titrate to effect; maximum dose 20 mcg/kg/min) should be administered.

KEY POINTS

Epinephrine

- Undisputed first-line agent and treatment of choice for anaphylaxis; despite this status, the drug remains underutilized.

- Intramuscular administration is preferred. Reserve intravenous administration for patients in extremis and unresponsive to repeated intramuscular dosages and those in profound shock.

- There are no absolute contraindications; exercise caution in patients taking β-adrenergic blockers and in pregnant patients.

Antihistamines

- Adjunctive therapy for anaphylaxis

- $H_1 + H_2$ blockade combination is preferable.

Corticosteroids

- Adjunctive therapy for anaphylaxis

- May have a role in mitigating recurrent anaphylaxis.

Disposition

One of the most difficult decisions in treating patients with allergic emergencies is determining appropriate disposition from the emergency department. Patients with severe reactions (eg, hypotension or airway involvement) or a slow response to standard therapies require admission for continued monitoring. On the other end of the spectrum, patients with clearly mild reactions may be discharged home safely. Most patients fall somewhere in between, making disposition more challenging. Critical to these decisions is recognizing the potential for recurrent

TABLE 19-9.

High-risk features of anaphylaxis to consider when determining patient disposition

Factor	High-Risk Features
Presenting symptom severity	Initially severe symptoms are an important consideration, even if symptoms have improved (or resolved) following initiation of treatment
Anaphylaxis history	Any history of severe, protracted, or recurrent anaphylaxis
Particular allergen	Nut (peanut or tree nut) reactions are associated with particularly high morbidity and mortality rates
Medical comorbidities	Conditions such as asthma (particularly high morbidity and mortality rates in the setting of anaphylaxis), congestive heart failure, renal disease (at risk for fluid overload with volume resuscitation)
Baseline medications	Particularly, use of β-adrenergic blocker (including ophthalmic preparations)
Access to medical care	Distant from or having reduced access to medical care
Age	Patients at extremes of age have reduced compensatory abilities; adolescents may be at risk for severe/fatal anaphylaxis because of compliance issues
Home situation	Patients who live alone; barriers to understanding discharge instructions and self-care education

anaphylaxis. Recurrent (biphasic or multiphasic) anaphylaxis is defined as the reappearance of allergic phenomena following the complete resolution of the original reaction, without reexposure to the inciting allergen. Recurrence could involve only nuisance-level symptoms or more ominous physiologic derangements, including respiratory compromise and hemodynamic instability. Recurrence has been reported to be as high as 20% and to occur as long as 72 hours following the inciting event.[39] Corticosteroid administration does not eliminate the possibility of recurrence. Factors to consider in determining which patients are at greater risk for rapid decompensation initially or in the event of recurrent anaphylaxis are presented in Table 19-9.

Protracted (prolonged or refractory) anaphylaxis has also been reported.[40] Patients with this condition may present with refractory hypotension or bronchospasm, which may present unique challenges in terms of circulatory support and ventilator management, respectively.

There is no firmly established observation time for patients following an episode of anaphylaxis. A minimum of several hours following treatment appears reasonable for mild episodes, whereas at least 24 hours of observation appears prudent for severe episodes or patients with high-risk or otherwise troubling features. A recent consensus statement recommended 4 to 6 hours of observation for most patients, with more prolonged observation or admission for those with severe or refractory symptoms and those with reactive airway disease.[1] Overall, practitioners should have a low threshold for prolonged observation, particularly when high-risk features (such as asthma or nut allergy) are present.

KEY POINTS

There is no firmly established observation period for patients following an episode of anaphylaxis.

A low threshold for prolonged observation in patients with severe reactions or high-risk features is advised. Exercise particular caution in asthmatics and patients with "nut" allergies, as they are at risk for severe symptoms or fatal outcome.

Post-Reaction Treatment

There is little disagreement that epinephrine self-administration devices should be given to individuals who have a history of anaphylaxis involving respiratory distress or shock and who cannot strictly and reliably avoid the triggering allergen. The immediate availability of self-injectable epinephrine is im-

portant in the initial 72-hour period for the treatment of recurrent anaphylaxis induced by *any* allergen. A more difficult decision involves patients who experienced only mild symptoms after exposure to an allergic trigger.[41] An initial episode, no matter how mild, may not predict the severity of future events, particularly in the case of food-induced allergy.[42] Between 44% and 59% of patients with initially mild symptoms exhibit life-threatening anaphylaxis after a second exposure to the same allergic trigger.[43] In recurrent anaphylaxis, in a small percentage of patients, the symptoms on recurrence are more severe than during the initial reaction.[44]

PEARL

Many patients with initially mild symptoms can exhibit life-threatening anaphylaxis after a second exposure to the same allergic trigger.

Patients and caretakers should be instructed on the indications for epinephrine administration and proper device use. Epinephrine device formulations currently available in the United States include EpiPen (Dey Pharma, L.P., Basking Ridge, NJ) (0.3 mg), Twinject (Paladin Labs, Quebec, Canada) (0.3 mg), EpiPen Jr (0.15 mg), and Twinject Jr (0.15 mg). Weight-based guidelines for the use of these devices in children are summarized in Table 19-10.[8] Great care must be exercised if the decision is made to teach parents how to draw up a dose of epinephrine for children weighing less than 10 kg. Evidence has demonstrated that caretakers have significant difficulty doing so and often draw up inappropriate doses (too low or too high).[45]

Other recommended post-reaction treatments include oral H_1/H_2 antihistamines and corticosteroids. Many authors recommend continuation of oral medications for at least 72 hours, although there is no specific evidence to support a firm recommendation.[46]

Conclusion

Anaphylactic reactions are life threatening and almost always unanticipated. Any delay in the recognition of initial signs and symptoms may result in a poor outcome. Even when the symptoms are mild initially, the potential for progression to airway obstruction or vascular collapse must be appreciated, and treatment must be initiated swiftly and aggressively. Epinephrine is the cornerstone of therapy. Second-line pharmacotherapies include H_1/H_2 antihistamines and corticosteroids. Disposition from the emergency department is fraught with potential dangers. Prolonged observation is prudent following significant reactions and for patients with other high-risk features, particularly asthma or a "nut" allergy. Ensuring that patients have continuous access to and familiarity with their epinephrine self-administration device is critical to preventing morbidity and mortality. Fortunately, with such widely available and highly effective treatment modalities, the battle against our own immune system can be won more often than not.

TABLE 19-10.

Weight-based epinephrine self-administration device selection

Weight (kg)	Epinephrine Dose/Device
<10	Ampule/needle/syringe administration
10–25	0.15-mg EpiPen Jr or Twinject Jr
>25	0.3-mg EpiPen or Twinject

References

1. Sampson HA, Munoz-Furlong A, Campbell RL, et al. Second symposium on the definition and management of anaphylaxis: summary report – Second National Institute of Allergy and Infectious Disease/Food Allergy and Anaphylaxis Network symposium. *J Allergy Clin Immunol.* 2006;117(2):391-397.

2. Johansson SG, Bieber T, Dahl R, et al. Revised nomenclature for allergy for global use: report of the Nomenclature Review Committee of the World Allergy Organization, October 2003. *J Allergy Clin Immunol.* 2004;113(5):832-836.

3. Sampson HA. Anaphylaxis and emergency treatment. *Pediatrics.* 2003;111:1601-1608.

4. Braganza SC, Acworth JP, Mckinnon DRL, et al. Paediatric emergency department anaphylaxis: different patterns from adults. *Arch Dis Child.* 2006;91:159-163.

5. Sampson HA, Mendelson L, Rosen JP. Fatal and near-fatal anaphylactic reactions to food in children and adolescents. *N Engl J Med.* 1992;327:380-384.

6. Roberts G, Patel N, Levi-Schaffer F, et al. Food allergy as a risk factor for life-threatening asthma in childhood: a case-controlled study. *J Allergy Clin Immunol.* 2003;112:1:168-174.

7. American College of Allergy, Asthma and Immunology. Food allergy: a practice parameter. *Ann Allergy Asthma Immunol,* 2006;96(3 suppl 2):S1-S68.

8. Sicherer SH, Simons FER, Section on Allergy and Immunology, American Academy of Pediatrics. Self-injectable epinephrine for first-aid management of anaphylaxis. *Pediatrics.* 2007;119(3):638-646.

9. Sampson HA. Anaphylaxis: persistent enigma. *Emerg Med Australas.* 2006;18:101-102.

10. Novembre E, Cianferoni A, Bernardini R, et al. Anaphylaxis in children: clinical and allergologic features. *Pediatrics.* 1998;101:e8.

11. Bock SA, Munoz-Furlong A, Sampson HA. Fatalities due to anaphylactic reactions to foods. *J Allergy Clin Immunol.* 2001;107:191-193.

12. Sampson HA, Munoz-Furlong A, Bock SA, et al. Symposium on the definition and management of anaphylaxis: summary report. *J Allergy Clin Immunol.* 2005;115(3):584-591.

13. Joint Task Force on Practice Parameters for the American Academy of Allergy, Asthma and Immunology; the American College of Allergy, Asthma and Immunology; and the Joint Council of Allergy and Immunology. The diagnosis and management of anaphylaxis: an updated practice parameter. *J Allergy Clin Immunol.* 2005;115:S483-S523.

14. Fisher MM. Clinical observations on the pathophysiology and treatment of anaphylactic cardiovascular collapse. *Anaesth Intensive Care.* 1986;14:17-21.

15. Viner NA, Rhamy RK. Anaphylaxis manifested by hypotension alone. *J Urol.* 1975;113:108-110.

16. Soreide E, Buxrud T, Harboe S. Severe anaphylactic reactions outside hospital: etiology, symptoms and treatment. *Acta Anaesthesiol Scand.* 1988;32:339-342.

17. Sheikh A, Shehata A, Brown SGA, et al. Adrenaline for the treatment of anaphylaxis: Cochrane systematic review. *Allergy.* 2009;64:204-212.

18. Lieberman P. Use of epinephrine in the treatment of anaphylaxis. *Curr Opin Allergy Clin Immunol.* 2003;3:313-318.

19. Simons FER, Roberts JR, Gu X, et al. Epinephrine absorption in children with a history of anaphylaxis. *J Allergy Clin Immunol.* 1998;101:33-37.

20. Simons FER, Gu X, Simons KJ. Epinephrine absorption in adults: intramuscular versus subcutaneous injection. *J Allergy Clin Immunol.* 2001;108:871-873.

21. Soar J, Deakin CD, Nolan JP, et al. European Resuscitation Council Guidelines for Resuscitation 2005: Section 7. Cardiac arrest in special circumstances. *Resuscitation.* 2005;67(suppl 1):S135-S170.

22. McLean-Tooke APC, Bethune CA, Fay AC, et al. Adrenaline in the treatment of anaphylaxis: what is the evidence? *BMJ.* 2003;327:1332-1335.

23. Johnston SL, Unsworth J, Gompels MM. Adrenaline given outside the context of life threatening allergic reactions. *BMJ.* 2003;326:589-590.

24. Douglass JA, O'Hehir RE. Adrenaline and non-life threatening allergic reactions. *BMJ.* 2003;327:226-227.

25. Karch SB. Coronary artery spasm induced by intravenous epinephrine overdose. *Ann Emerg Med.* 1989;7:485-488.

26. Ellis AK, Day JH. The role of epinephrine in the treatment of anaphylaxis. *Curr Allergy Asthma Rep.* 2003;3:11-14.

27. Brown AF. Intramuscular or intravenous adrenaline in acute, severe anaphylaxis? *J Accid Emerg Med.* 2000;17:152-155.

28. Barach EM, Nowak RM, Lee TG, et al. Epinephrine for treatment of anaphylactic shock. *JAMA.* 1984;251:2118-2122.

29. Hepner DL, Castells MC. Anaphylaxis during the perioperative period. *Anesth Analg.* 2003;97:1381-1395.

30. Liberman DB, Teach SJ. Management of anaphylaxis in children. *Pediatr Emerg Care.* 2008;24:861-866.

31. Brown SGA, Blackman KE, Stenlake V, et al. Insect sting anaphylaxis; prospective evaluation of treatment with intravenous adrenaline and volume resuscitation. *Emerg Med J.* 2004;21:149-154.

32. Sheikh A, Ten Broek V, Brown SG, et al. H$_1$-antihistamines for the treatment of anaphylaxis: Cochrane systematic review. *Allergy.* 2007;62:830-837.

33. Lin RY, Curry A, Pesola G, et al. Improved outcomes in patients with acute allergic syndromes who are treated with combined H$_1$ and H$_2$ antagonists. *Ann Emerg Med.* 2000;36:462-468.

34. Runge JW, Martinez JC, Caravati EM, et al. Histamine antagonists in the treatment of allergic reactions. *Ann Emerg Med.* 1992;21:237-242.

35. Shannon M. Drug-drug interactions and the cytochrome P450 system: an update. *Pediatr Emerg Care.* 1997;13:350-353.

36. Pollack CV. Utility of glucagon in the emergency department. *J Emerg Med.* 1993;11:195-205.

37. Sherman MS, Lazar EJ, Eichacker P. A bronchodilator action of glucagon. *J Allergy Clin Immunol.* 1988;81:908-911.

38. Thomas M, Crawford I. Best evidence topic reports: glucagon infusion in refractory anaphylactic shock in patients on beta-blockers. *Emerg Med J.* 2005;22:272-276.

39. Lieberman P. Biphasic anaphylaxis. *Ann Allergy Asthma Immunol.* 2005;95:217-226.

40. Stark BJ, Sullivan TJ. Biphasic and protracted anaphylaxis. *J Allergy Clin Immunol.* 1986;78(1 Part 1):76-83.

41. Sicherer SH, Simons ER. Quandaries in prescribing an emergency action plan and self-injectable epinephrine for first-aid management of anaphylaxis in the community. *J Allergy Clin Immunol.* 2005;115:575-583.

42. Kumar A, Teuber SS, Gershwin ME. Why do people die of anaphylaxis? A clinical review. *Clin Devel Immunol.* 2005;12:281-287.

43. Vander Leek TK, Liu AH, Stefanski K, et al. The natural history of peanut allergy in young children and its association with serum peanut-specific IgE. *J Pediatr.* 2000;137:749-755.

44. Smit DV, Cameron PA, Rainer TH. Anaphylaxis presentations to an emergency department in Hong Kong: incidence and predictors of biphasic reactions. *J Emerg Med.* 2005;28:381-388.

45. Simons FER, Chan ES, Cu X, et al. Epinephrine for out-of-hospital (first-aid) treatment of anaphylaxis in infants: is the ampule/needle/syringe method practical? *J Allergy Clin Immunol.* 2001;108:1040-1044.

46. Brown AFT. Therapeutic controversies in the management of acute anaphylaxis. *J Accid Emerg Med.* 1998;15:89-95.

CHAPTER 20

Bedside Ultrasonography in the Critically Ill Patient

Justin O. Cook, Lisa D. Mills, and Daniel R. Mantuani

IN THIS CHAPTER

Cardiac examination
Pericardial effusion
Ejection fraction
Right ventricular strain
Wall motion assessment

Inferior vena cava examination

Lung examination
Pneumothorax
Pleural effusion

Abdominal aorta examination

Cardiac arrest evaluation

Introduction

In the assessment of the undifferentiated, critically ill patient, bedside ultrasonography contributes a wealth of clinical information for use by emergency physicians. Beyond ultrasonography's immediate diagnostic capabilities, serial ultrasonographic examinations allow physicians to evaluate a patient's response to resuscitation; ultrasound is an increasingly essential adjunct in critical procedures.

Specifically, bedside ultrasonography increases the accuracy of the final diagnosis and speeds the time to diagnosis in the undifferentiated, critically ill patient.[1] To this end, several approaches to goal-directed ultrasonography in the critical patient have been proposed, most notably the Undifferentiated Hypotension Protocol (UHP) and the Rapid Ultrasound in SHock (RUSH) protocol.[2,3] These protocols merit review by emergency department sonographers because they contribute pragmatic and conceptually novel approaches to the evaluation of critically ill patients in the emergency department or ICU. In the realm of pediatric critical care ultrasonography, Pershad and colleagues have elaborated the delightfully titled BLEEP protocol (Bedside Limited Echocardiography by Emergency Physicians).[4]

The Cardiac Examination

Echocardiography, although the most technically challenging bedside ultrasound application, may be the most valuable in the immediate evaluation and management of a critically ill patient. The emergency physician's immediate goals should be to detect pericardial tamponade and estimate left ventricular contractility. Abundant literature supports the accuracy of these assessments by emergency physicians with focused training.[5–8] An experienced sonographer can discern echocardiographic findings of tamponade, right ventricular dysfunction, wall motion abnormalities, and thoracic aortic pathology.

Echocardiographic Technique

For the purposes of rapid bedside echocardiography, the examination consists of any of three basic views, as follows: the parasternal views, the subxiphoid view (familiar to most as the cardiac view traditionally employed in the focused assessment with sonography for trauma [FAST] exam), and the apical or four-chamber view. The parasternal views are further divided into the parasternal long-axis (PSLAX) and the parasternal short-axis (PSSAX) views. In many patients, a single view may provide only limited information. For this reason, physicians should be familiar with the use of multiple echocardiographic windows. All basic echocardiography can be performed with a microconvex or curvilinear transducer. The microconvex transducer offers the advantages of fitting between rib spaces and being supported by more cardiac-specific software.

Begin with the patient supine or in the left lateral decubitus position. Employ a curvilinear or microconvex transducer. The PSLAX view is obtained by placing the transducer in the left parasternal area at approximately the fourth rib interspace, with the transducer marker pointing toward the patient's right shoulder and the on-screen transducer indicator on the left side of the screen; this is the most common positioning in emergency medicine ultrasound. Oriented in this manner, this window reveals the left ventricle deep to the smaller right ventricle, with the aortic outflow tract to the left side of the screen and the mitral valve at center of the image (Figure 20-1). The bright white (hyperechoic) stripe seen beneath the wall of the left ventricle is the pericardium. The round, dark structure beneath the pericardium is the descending thoracic aorta, a key landmark for determining the location of a fluid collection (Figures 20-1 and 20-2).

From here, the PSSAX view is obtained by rotating the probe 90° clockwise, so the transducer marker is pointed toward the left shoulder. This gives a view of the left ventricle in cross-section.

The subxiphoid or subcostal view (Figure 20-3) uses the liver as a window to visualize the heart, with the transducer aimed at the patient's left shoulder, as in the FAST exam. This view has limited utility in estimation of ejection fraction, but it is particularly valuable in assessing for pericardial effusion, as discussed below.

The apical view, while it yields a rather complete and anatomically familiar representation of the heart, can be the most difficult of the three primary windows to visualize consistently.[9] Place the transducer at the point of maximal impulse (often slightly inferolateral to the left nipple) with the patient in the left lateral decubitus position to obtain the apical four-chamber view (Figure 20-4). Direct the indicator toward the bed, rotating toward the left axilla to sharpen the image. The entire transducer is angled to about 45°, with the cord toward the patient's feet, to align it in the long axis of the left ventricle.

Pericardial Effusion

The detection of a hemodynamically significant pericardial effusion (by definition, tamponade) may be the single most important and timely diagnostic appraisal to be made in a critically ill patient. Clearly, tamponade can cause sudden cardiac collapse, yet it can be managed promptly by an emergency physician (a procedure best performed with ultrasound guidance) to great benefit of the patient.

KEY POINT

Echocardiographic evaluation of critically ill patients, especially those who are hypotensive or dyspneic, should begin with the goal of immediately excluding pericardial effusion.

The signs and symptoms of pericardial effusion (and even tamponade) may be clinically occult. In a study by Blaivas,[10] the incidence of pericardial effusion in patients presenting to the emergency department with dyspnea was found to be as high as 14%. Four percent of patients with dyspnea had symptomatic effusions.[10] The finding of a pericardial effusion of any size in a dyspneic or hemodynamically compromised patient must immediately raise consideration of cardiac tamponade, especially as the sonographic findings of tamponade can be difficult to appreciate. The physician must synthesize the clinical picture with echocardiographic findings to determine the significance of a pericardial effusion.

Effusions are likely to be dependent. In the PSLAX view, they manifest as a black (anechoic) stripe posterior (far field) to

FIGURE 20-1.

PSLAX long-axis view with probe marker *(PM)* at upper left side of screen, the emergency physician's convention. *LV*, left ventricle; *RV*, right ventricle; *PS*, pericardial stripe; *Ao*, aortic outflow tract; *MV*, mitral valve; *DTA*, descending thoracic aorta.

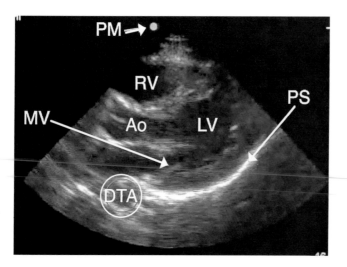

FIGURE 20-2.

Another PSLAX view showing a rather dilated left ventricle in a patient with poor contractility, clinically with pulseless electrical activity at the time of the examination. The *arrow* points to the descending thoracic aorta, which is seen in cross-section in this window.

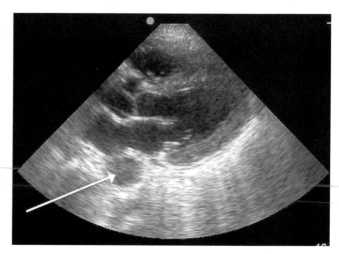

the left ventricle but anterior (near field) to the bright, hyperechoic stripe of the pericardium. Such a dark fluid collection *posterior* (far field) to the pericardial stripe indicates a pleural effusion, a "masquerader" of pericardial effusion. In the subxiphoid view, an effusion often appears as an anechoic stripe anterior (near field) between the liver and the left ventricle and surrounded by the bright white of the pericardium. Larger effusions can be seen in both the near and far fields surrounding the myocardium in the parasternal (Figures 20-5 and 20-6) or subxiphoid view (Figure 20-7).

PEARL

Beware of a potential false-positive result: in both the PSLAX and subxiphoid views, an anterior hazy stripe may be a fat pad, which is a normal finding. Generally, an effusion is dark if it is fresh blood or has a mixed density if it contains clotted blood.

Tamponade is most readily seen as right ventricular collapse in diastole, often appearing as a "bowing" or inward concavity of the right ventricular free wall; this can be appreciated in the PSLAX view (Figure 20-8). In other views, right atrial collapse in systole can also indicate tamponade. Impending tamponade is suggested by a "plethoric" inferior vena cava (IVC) (an IVC that shows no change in caliber with spontaneous respiration), a finding that is expected in situations of elevated right-sided filling pressures. This underscores the importance of pairing the cardiac and IVC examinations, which is discussed in more detail in the section on IVC examination.

KEY POINTS

Employ multiple cardiac views to increase the sensitivity of the examination.

The finding of a pericardial effusion in a dyspneic or hemodynamically impaired patient immediately raises consideration of cardiac tamponade.

Visual assessment reliably and sufficiently estimates ejection fraction.

Image the heart and IVC: these views often provide complementary information.

Ejection Fraction

The PSLAX view is the most commonly used window for estimation of left ventricular function. With real-time visualization of the contracting ventricle in the PSLAX view, the physician can make a reasonable estimation of ejection fraction, categorizing its function among three general appearances—normal, depressed, or hyperdynamic—while also noting ventricular filling.

Consensus among emergency physician sonographers holds

FIGURE 20-3.

Subxiphoid view of heart

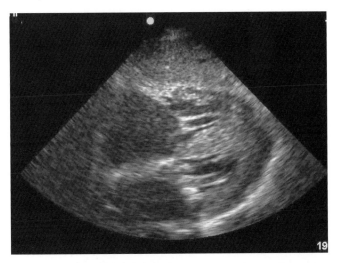

FIGURE 20-4.

Apical view of the heart, showing all four chambers

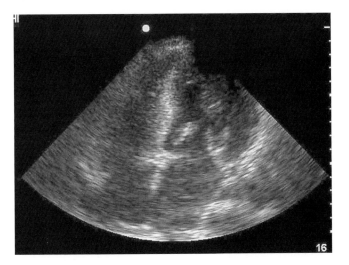

FIGURE 20-5.

Pericardial effusion (labeled as PE) seen in PSLAX view. Note that fluid collects posteriorly here, the dependent area, where effusions are most commonly found in this window. Also note that the effusion appears *anterior* to the dark circle (unlabeled), which is the descending thoracic aorta, a clue that this is a pericardial and not a pleural effusion. Image courtesy of Ralph Wang, MD, University of California, San Francisco.

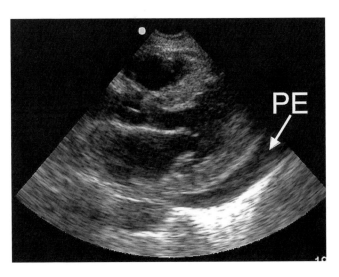

that ejection fraction is estimated by visual assessment of the left ventricle rather than a more time-consuming series of measurements from static images or "cine" extrapolations. Ejection fraction is normal when the septal and posterior walls (the walls seen most readily in the PSLAX view) contract at least 50% in systole relative to their position in diastole. (This is to say, the black cavity within the gray walls of the left ventricle decreases in size approximately 50%.) In a depressed heart, the walls of the left ventricle close significantly less than 50% during systole. This is called a "hypodynamic heart." The left ventricle is described as hyperdynamic when the walls of the ventricle appear to nearly touch in systole and are relatively small compared to the ventricle (indicating poor ventricular filling).

Additional information about contractility and specific wall motion abnormalities can be obtained in the PSSAX view. The left ventricle is seen in cross-section (Figure 20-9).

Optimal views can be hindered by the patient's habitus or pathology. In such instances, if the physician can obtain a limited PSLAX view, the movement of the mitral valve can be used to roughly rule-in a normal ejection fraction. An anterior mitral valve leaflet that "slaps" up against the septum usually indicates normal left ventricular function.

Assess cardiac function early in the resuscitation of the hypotensive patient; the results will tailor the resuscitation. A significantly depressed ejection fraction, especially when pulmonary edema is clinically evident, may be the rare instance in which aggressive fluid resuscitation should be withheld or applied with close observation. Consider vasopressor or inotropic agents, cardiology consultation, and other interventions (eg, balloon pump, emergent cardiac catheterization), as indicated by the clinical features and ECG. The finding of a hyperdynamic heart is particularly valuable as it suggests that the patient may derive great benefit from volume resuscitation.

Right Ventricular Strain as a Marker of Pulmonary Embolism

Echocardiography cannot be considered a substitute for formal imaging in the diagnosis of pulmonary embolism because no sonographic finding is sufficiently specific for it. However, definitive imaging is difficult to obtain in an unstable patient. Moreover, clues from a bedside echocardiogram, after excluding tamponade and more readily assessed causes of circulatory compromise such as tension pneumothorax, can provide evidence to suggest a hemodynamically compromising pulmonary embolism.

A massive pulmonary embolus can cause right ventricular strain. This manifests in several ways, including right ventricular size and wall motion changes. Normally, the right ventricle is about 50% to 60% of the size of the left ventricle. In the setting of acute right ventricular strain, the right ventricle enlarges and may equal or exceed the size of the left ventricle. The echocardiographic windows most valuable for this comparison are the apical, subxiphoid, and the parasternal views. Excessive right ventricular strain causes dilation and hypokinesis of the right ventricle. In the setting of pulmonary embolism, the classic finding of right ventricle free-wall hypokinesis with sparing of the right ventricle apex (McConnell sign) may be more suggestive of acute pulmonary embolism as distinct from other causes of chronic right ventricular strain.[11]

In the PSSAX view, the "D sign," or flattening of the septum (caused by increased right-sided pressures with concomitant decreased left-sided filling pressures), can also suggest acute pulmonary embolus.[12] A right atrial or right ventricular clot might be seen, offering an additional, but rare, clue[13] (Figure 20-10).

FIGURE 20-6.

Pericardial effusion (labeled as *PE*) seen in PSSAX view. The black, or hypoechoic, stripe appears to encircle the left ventricle, prominent both deep and anterior to the myocardium. The bright white, hyperechoic, pericardium can be seen deep (unlabeled). Image courtesy of Ralph Wang, MD, University of California, San Francisco.

FIGURE 20-7.

Pericardial effusion seen in subxiphoid view. Effusion is present in both near and far fields, as indicated by *arrows*. Image courtesy of Arun Nagdev, MD, ACMC-Highland.

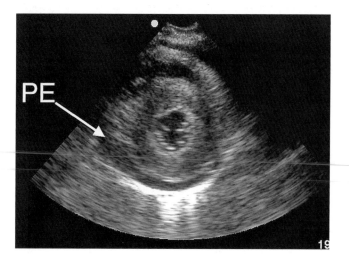

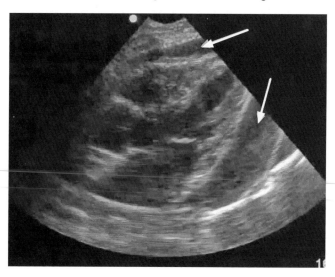

PEARL

Echocardiographic findings that suggest pulmonary embolism:

- Right ventricular size equal to left ventricular size with right ventricular hypokinesis

- McConnell sign: right ventricle hypokinesis with sparing of right ventricle apex

- D sign: flattening of the septum into the left ventricle, as seen in the PSSAX view (Figure 20-10)

Caveat: An enlarged, thick-walled right ventricle suggests long-standing right ventricular strain rather than acute strain.

The finding of right ventricular strain in a patient with acute pulmonary embolism can be of prognostic value as a mode of risk stratification and in consideration of thrombolytic therapy. Even normotensive patients with pulmonary embolism who show signs of right ventricular strain have a significantly higher inpatient mortality rate and risk of shock related to the embolism.[14]

Wall Motion Abnormalities

In patients with acute coronary syndrome, the detection of wall motion abnormalities on echocardiography illuminates acute cardiac dysfunction, which is of value if the ECG is ambiguous or if the patient has a left bundle-branch block of unknown age.

To assess wall motion defects, look for thickening within the ventricular muscle. Normally, the myocardium thickens in early systole. An ischemic myocardium can have a variety of appearances, described as hypokinetic (decreased systolic thickening), akinetic (no systolic thickening), or dyskinetic (outward bowing of the wall in systole). These findings can occur globally, as in diffuse cardiomyopathy, or segmentally, as in the case of a singularly compromised vascular territory.

The PSLAX view allows rapid gestalt of left ventricular

FIGURE 20-8.

In this PSLAX view, there is a large anterior pericardial effusion (the *arrow* is located within the effusion), with "bowing" of the right ventricular wall (to which the *arrow* points). This "bowing" is suggestive of pericardial tamponade. Ventricular chambers are labeled as *RV* (right) and *LV* (left). Normally, a posterior effusion is seen in tamponade but is interestingly absent in this static image. Image courtesy of Arun Nagdev, MD, ACMH-Highlands.

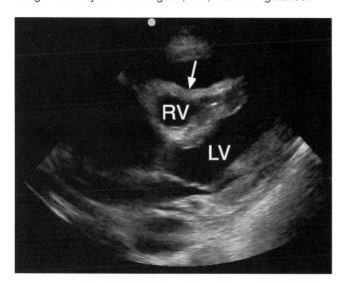

FIGURE 20-9.

PSSAX view near the apex of the heart (probe is angled toward patient's hip), showing the left ventricle in cross-section. The *arrow* points to the interventricular septum. A wisp of pericardial effusion can be seen in the far field. Image courtesy of Arun Nagdev, MD, ACMC-Highland.

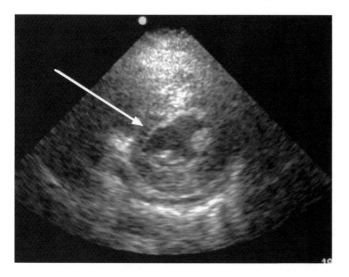

FIGURE 20-10.

This PSSAX view shows septal "bowing" of the interventricular septum (*arrow*) into the left ventricle (*LV*). The left ventricle has assumed a D shape in response to the pressure differential between the right and left ventricles, the so-called D sign. Notice the very dilated right ventricle (*RV*) compared with the relatively small and underfilled left ventricle. Image courtesy of Michael Stone, MD, RDMS, ACMC-Highland.

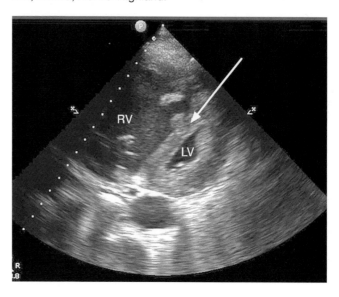

function. However, only the interventricular and lateral walls are seen. When imaging the left ventricle for wall motion abnormalities, the PSSAX view, which demonstrates the entire circumference of the left ventricle, provides the most data. The physician can get his or her bearings by first locating the interventricular septum, using this landmark to discern other areas of the myocardium. From here, rock the transducer toward the right shoulder and then toward the left hip, panning through the entire left ventricle. This allows the entire left ventricle to be imaged from apex to aortic valve.

Thoracic Aorta Examination

Close inspection of the descending thoracic aorta can enable the physician to rapidly identify a thoracic aortic dissection. Such "clutch" bedside diagnoses have been described in an increasing number of case reports and have been experienced by the authors (who are emergency physicians).[15-18] Transthoracic echocardiography provides three key views of the thoracic aorta: the aortic root, the aortic arch, and a single limited image of the descending aorta. The aortic root is well visualized via the PSLAX window, which also captures a single slice of the descending aorta.

The suprasternal window allows imaging of the aortic arch. The transducer is placed in the sternal notch and directed toward the feet. When this view is successfully obtained, this window shows the aortic arch with some detail (Figure 20-11). The addition of color flow allows study of blood flow relative to the flap.

Features suggestive of aortic dissection include an intimal flap or dilation of the aortic root. A dilated aortic root is more than 3.8 cm in diameter (which can be identified in the PSLAX view [Figure 20-12]).

FIGURE 20-11.

Suprasternal view of a normal aortic arch, with *arrow* indicating the arch. This image was taken in a very thin patient using the linear probe. Image courtesy of Arun Nagdev, MD, ACMC-Highland.

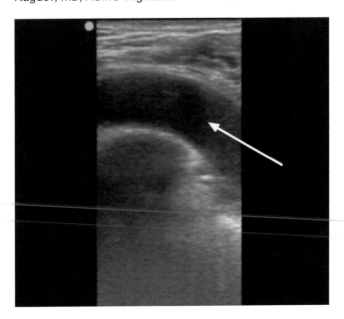

In the right clinical setting, the presence of a pericardial effusion should prompt the physician to consider aortic dissection because tamponade is often the immediate cause of sudden cardiac collapse in type A dissections. In such cases, pericardiocentesis may have only transient benefit.

Inferior Vena Cava Examination

One of the most challenging tasks in any resuscitation is the determination of a patient's volume status. Recent debate, especially in the sepsis literature, has elaborated the concept of "fluid responsiveness"—defined as the likelihood that an increase in cardiac output (and therefore perfusion) will result from volume infusion. The usefulness of the most widely accepted marker of volume status, central venous pressure (CVP), has recently been called into question,[19] tarnishing its role as the centerpiece marker in early goal-directed therapy and sepsis management.

The case against CVP concerns its inability to reasonably determine the likelihood of fluid responsiveness beyond the accuracy of a coin flip. Dynamic markers of fluid responsiveness, such as pulse-pressure variation (PPV) and passive leg raising (PLR), have gained broader acceptance as reliable markers of fluid responsiveness. In addition to PPV and PLR, sonographic evaluation of the IVC has gained recognition as a valuable tool for volume status assessment, or an assessment of the "tank."[3]

Less obvious in the emergency medicine literature is ultrasound's ability to predict volume responsiveness, although evidence in the intensive care literature suggests a useful relationship.[20,21] Being noninvasive and easily repeated (serial assessments of response to therapy are the cornerstone of critical

FIGURE 20-12.

PSLAX view showing descending thoracic aorta (circled hypoechoic area) with hyperechoic, mobile, linear dissection flap (*arrow*). Its appearance is much more striking in motion. The *boxed area* includes the aortic outflow tract and aortic root. The root is somewhat dilated, although difficult to appreciate in this static image.

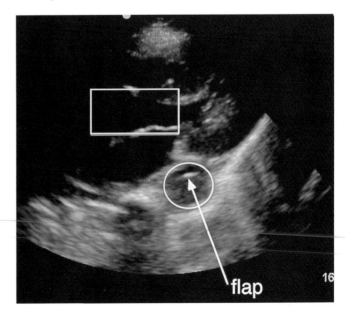

care), ultrasonography of the IVC offers clear advantages over invasive measures of CVP. Emergency medicine literature on this subject is emerging, most notably a recent study by Nagdev et al, which found that emergency physicians were able to accurately predict which patients had a CVP lower than 8 mm Hg based on a bedside sonographic assessment (using visual estimation) with sensitivity of 91% (95% CI, 71%–99%) and specificity of 94% (95% CI, 84%–99%).[22]

In order to visualize the IVC, place a curvilinear or microconvex transducer in the subxiphoid area, directed perpendicular to the floor. As is the convention in emergency medicine

FIGURE 20-13.

Longitudinal view of the IVC, showing the right atrial border to the left side of the image. The diameter of the IVC should be assessed at a point about 3 cm caudal to the right atrial junction. Image courtesy of Arun Nagdev, MD, ACMC-Highland.

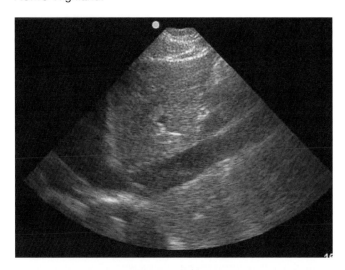

FIGURE 20-14.

Longitudinal view showing a very narrow IVC, defined as "flat"—suggestive of a volume-depleted patient. Image courtesy of Arun Nagdev, MD, ACMC-Highland.

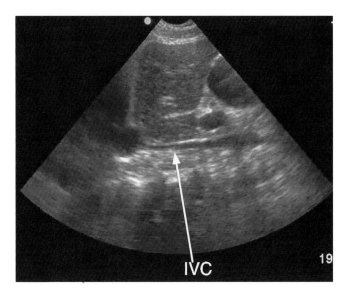

ultrasonography, the transducer indicator should point to the patient's right. Identify the round, hypoechoic (dark) aorta to the left of the patient's spine, the eccentrically shaped hypoechoic IVC to the right of the spine, and the bright thoracic spine deep relative to those structures in this transverse/axial plane.

Next, tilt the cable end of the transducer to the patient's left, centering the IVC in the image field. With the IVC at the center of the screen, rotate the transducer clockwise 90° to view the IVC longitudinally. Visualize the right atrium contracting at the cephalic termination of the IVC (Figure 20-13).

From here, the goal is to visually estimate the change in IVC diameter (collapse of near field wall toward far field wall) with normal respiration (or with positive-pressure ventilation) at a point approximately 3 cm distal to the junction with the right atrium, or at about the level of the right renal vein takeoff.[23] The degree to which the IVC collapses is believed to correlate with intravascular volume status. The degree of collapse of the IVC has been described as the "caval index"—that is, a collapse of the IVC of more than 50% of its normal size would indicate a caval index above 0.5. The relationship of IVC collapse to CVP is as follows:

- IVC collapse of more than 50% (caval index above 0.5) suggests a CVP of less than 8 cm H_2O, a hypovolemic state;
- IVC collapse of less than 50% (caval index below 0.5) suggests a CVP of less than 10 cm H_2O, a hypervolemic state.

A particularly dehydrated patient can show a frankly "flat" appearing IVC, which is demonstrative of volume depletion

FIGURE 20-15.

Normal lung, showing two comet tails (*arrows*) visible on this static image. Lung sliding and comet tails, being dynamic findings, are difficult to appreciate in static images.

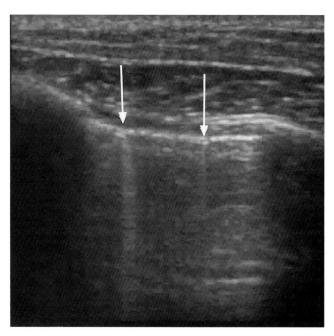

(Figure 20-14). Treatment hinges on clinical presentation and desired clinical endpoint.

KEY POINT

Physiology of IVC collapse: In a spontaneously breathing patient, the relatively negative intrathoracic pressure of inspiration draws blood from the IVC into the thorax, resulting in a transient decrease in the caliber of the IVC.

In some cases, the IVC may not appear to change with the respiratory cycle. A so-called plethoric IVC suggests elevated right atrial pressure. The differential diagnosis includes massive pulmonary embolus, tamponade, significant pulmonary hypertension, volume overload with cardiac dysfunction, restrictive heart disease, intrinsic positive end-expiratory pressure, tension pneumothorax, or any cause of elevated intrathoracic pressure. (This finding should prompt the physician to obtain a bedside echocardiogram if it has not been done already.)

Note, however, that patients on positive-pressure ventilation have a reversed relationship of IVC diameter to inspiration because positive pressure during inflation/inspiration of lungs results in IVC *distention*. Critical care studies have shown a somewhat more complex relationship of IVC diameter to respiration because of chest wall mechanics and intraabdominal pressure changes with the positive-pressure respiratory cycle. In short, an IVC that distends more than 15% with positive-pressure ventilation represents a patient who is likely to be fluid responsive. A patient who has no significant increase in IVC diameter with positive pressure is less likely to benefit from fluids.[24] Given these small tolerances, this time-consuming determination must be measured with screen calipers using static images. The literature supporting this approach is sparse.[21,22,24]

Volume-overloaded patients who have had previous treatment with vasodilators or diuretics may demonstrate significant

IVC collapse (despite having significant fluid volume), yielding a false-positive interpretation.

KEY POINT

Reassess the IVC after interventions to assess response to therapy.

Lung Examination

Increasingly, emergency physicians are using ultrasonography to evaluate lung pathology. The most established applications include detecting the presence or absence of pleural sliding, identifying pneumothorax or unventilated lung (as with mainstem intubation), and imaging the costophrenic angles to reveal pleural effusion.

Routinely, pneumothorax is diagnosed with plain radiographs of the chest, which can be time-consuming and insensitive. Interestingly, the sensitivity of ultrasonography for detection of pneumothorax appears to rival that of standard chest radiographs, while computed tomography remains the gold standard.[25] Patient positioning (such as a supine trauma patient) can obfuscate the radiographic findings of pneumothorax. Although radiographic imaging is the best means for determining pneumothorax size, ultrasonography can offer a suggestion of pneumothorax size if the "lung point" can be seen.

Pneumothorax Evaluation

Begin by using the linear transducer (a microconvex transducer can also be used). Orient the transducer longitudinally on the patient. Beginning at the second or third intercostal space, visualize the bright, hyperechoic pleura between the ribs (the

FIGURE 20-17.

Lung ultrasound image showing no lung sliding. Ribs (R), seen in transverse section, display distal shadowing. The bright white line (*arrow*) is the pleura without comet tails or signs of sliding.

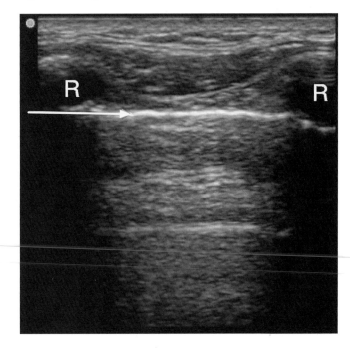

FIGURE 20-16.

Another "lung point" sign. The *arrow* indicates the point at the pleural interface where sliding lung is seen on the left side of the screen (with three comet tails), with adjacent absence of lung to the right of this point. Image courtesy of Seric Cusick, MD, University of California, Davis.

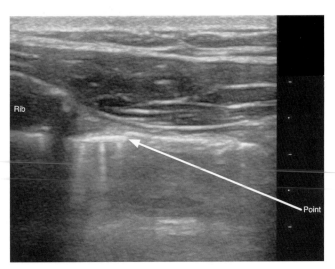

ribs appear as bright, semicircular surfaces with shadowing distally). Compare the affected with the unaffected side. Image the lung in two or three different interspaces.

Lungs, being air filled, show very poorly on ultrasound; the pleura, however, is easily appreciated as hyperechoic lines between rib shadows. Once the pleura has been identified, look for "lung sliding"—the appearance, at the interface of the pleural layers, of the visceral pleura sliding back and forth with respiration. The presence of lung sliding is a normal finding, as the pleural surfaces slide freely against one another. An additional finding in the normal lung, although it is subtle in some patients, is the appearance of brightly hyperechoic, round "beads," with linear far-field artifacts that slide side-to-side with respiration; these are called comet tails (Figures 20-15 and 20-16).

The absence of lung sliding (that is, the pleura appears as a stationary hyperechoic line during respiration) suggests pneumothorax (Figure 20-17). However, this finding lacks some specificity, as the absence of sliding also can be noted in a nonventilated lung. Additionally, the absence of sliding can be seen occasionally in patients with severe bullous lung disease and has been reported in cases of severe infiltrate and acute respiratory distress syndrome.[26,27]

Lung sliding can be difficult to discern in some cases; employing "movement mode" (abbreviated "M-mode") on the ultrasound machine can increase sensitivity. In M-mode, data from a single vertical slice of the image (usually displayed as a vertical green line on first press of the M-mode button) are displayed in the y-axis over time (time = x-axis). Represented in this way, the normal finding is "the beach" or "the seashore sign"—a linear appearance in the upper part of the image ("waves") with granularity ("sand") below the level of pleura. Such a linear finding in M-mode represents a structure with no significant movement relative to the y-axis, as one would expect with the soft tissues of chest wall, assuming the operator is holding the transducer immobile against the chest. In a normal lung, however, side-to-side motion at the pleural interface and below results in a grainy artifact deep to the level of the pleura, representing a sand-like artifact (Figure 20-18). Hence, the seashore—the normal finding, and a good place to be.

Linearity below as well as above the pleural interface suggests the absence of pleural movement on the side being examined—"waves" but no "sand." This has been called the "stratosphere sign" (Figure 20-19).

Be sure to image both sides of the chest in all patients—both to increase sensitivity and to make a reasonable comparison to discern what may appear to be a vaguely abnormal finding. The absence of sliding will be seen only in the interspaces where the pneumothorax is located. Consequently, small pneumothoraces—or those in locations difficult to image (apical or medial in particular)—are poorly detected by ultrasound.[25] The overall sensitivity of ultrasonography for pneumothorax appears to be better than 90%.[25]

Increase specificity with the "lung point" sign. Finding the interface of sliding lung and absence of sliding in a single interspace, the so-called lung point, is a highly specific finding for pneumothorax (reportedly with specificity as high as 100%)[28] and suggests the "edge" of the pneumothorax—the point at which the pleura separates at the chest wall. This information can help the physician estimate the size of the pneumothorax as well (Figures 20-16 and 20-20).

Pleural Effusion

In the critically ill patient, pleural effusion or hemothorax can also be readily identified. With the patient supine, place the transducer in the midaxillary to posterior axillary line within the 8th to 11th interspaces. Fluid will appear black (hypoechoic) between the white (hyperechoic) pleura. The physician can quickly image the pleural interface to assess for an intrathoracic collection of fluid (Figure 20-21).

FIGURE 20-18.

Normal lung seen on M-mode: the "seashore sign." Note *linearity* above the bright, white pleural interface, with *granularity* deep to this line. Life is good on the beach.

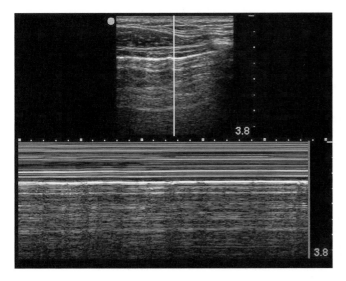

FIGURE 20-19.

The appearance of pneumothorax on M-mode: the "stratosphere sign." Linearity predominates, giving an appearance of "waves" without any "beach." No one wants to be lost at sea.

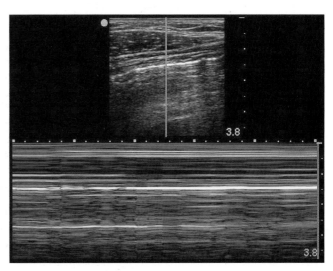

Abdominal Aorta Examination

This examination is similar to the IVC examination. Select a curved abdominal-type or microconvex transducer. With the patient supine, place the transducer in the epigastric area, aiming perpendicular to the floor. Turn your attention to the aorta at this level, imaging it in the transverse plane. Interposed bowel markedly decreases image quality, such that you may initially see nothing. Apply steady pressure (this may take some time, and patience will be rewarded) to displace bowel from between the transducer and the aorta. Follow the aorta down to the level of the aortic bifurcation (at about the umbilicus), paying attention to the size of the aorta and its appearance. Then rotate the transducer 90° to view the aorta in its longitudinal plane. In obese patients, it may be easier to start imaging from the umbilicus as the aorta may be more superficial here, contrary to what one might expect.

Measure the aorta from outer wall to outer wall. An aortic diameter larger than 3 cm is technically aneurysmal, and a diameter wider than 5 cm should cause more immediate concern, especially if the patient is symptomatic. There may be a mural thrombus in the vessel, which appears gray, in contrast to black blood. If the vessel is not aneurysmal, and if clinical suspicion is suggestive, look for an intimal flap. Color-flow technology may elucidate flow on either side of the flap and can demonstrate perfusion to branching vessels, which can contribute to prognostic considerations in the management of a patient with an acute dissection.

KEY POINT

A frequent misconception is that aortic rupture can be detected by ultrasonography. In fact, most ruptures occur into the retroperitoneum, an area that cannot be visualized with ultrasonography.

Cardiac Arrest Evaluation

In a patient without palpable pulses, echocardiography may suggest a cause of circulatory collapse (such as pericardial effusion with tamponade or hypovolemia), just as in patients with pulses. A key consideration is that detection of pulses during a cardiac arrest is difficult. In fact, physicians often incorrectly detect the presence or absence of pulses during cardiac arrest.[29] By visualizing the contractile function of the heart, the physician may find organized cardiac activity in a pulseless patient, which should prompt aggressive resuscitative efforts in appropriate clinical instances. Cardiac standstill, defined as complete absence of cardiac activity, indicates a more dismal prognosis, which can bolster the decision to discontinue resuscitative measures.[30] M-mode can be used to better discern subtle cardiac movement and in patients in whom cardiac windows are somewhat limited.

The examination may be performed using the parasternal or subxiphoid view during pulse checks in CPR.[31] The subxiphoid view may be useful (particularly for detecting pericardial effusion) during chest compressions, especially as recent advanced cardiovascular life support advances have stressed the importance of minimizing interruptions. An algorithm for such an approach to bedside ultrasonography in non-arrhythmogenic cardiac arrest has been proposed.[32]

FIGURE 20-20.

The "lung point" sign. *Long arrow* indicates the point at the pleural interface where sliding lung is seen on the right side, with adjacent absence of lung to the left of this point. *Short arrows* indicate the movement of this interface when seen in real time. Image courtesy of Zareth Irwin, MD, University of California, Irvine.

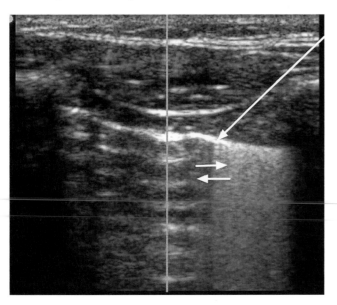

FIGURE 20-21.

Image of the right costophrenic angle, showing the superior edge of the liver with an adjacent hypoechoic pleural effusion. Note the dark appearance of the effusion in contrast to the more heterogeneous echogenicity of the lung parenchyma, seen to the left of the screen (unlabeled). Image courtesy of Arun Nagdev, MD, ACMC-Highland.

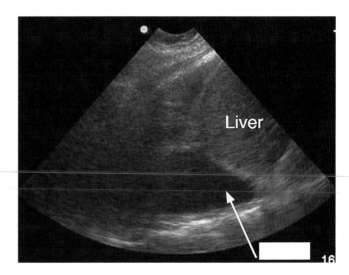

Conclusion

Ultrasonography allows rapid identification of pathology and provides a means of reassessment after therapeutic interventions in critically ill patients. Applications for critical care ultrasonography continue to be discovered and investigated. As skill with ultrasonography in the emergency department increases, so will the sophistication of our studies and the quality of our instruments.

References

1. Jones AE, Tayal VS, Sullivan DM, et al. Randomized, controlled trial of immediate versus delayed goal-directed ultrasound to identify the cause of nontraumatic hypotension in emergency department patients. *Crit Care Med.* 2004;32:1703-1708.

2. Rose J, Bair A, Mandavia D, et al. The UHP ultrasound protocol: a novel ultrasound approach to the empiric evaluation of the undifferentiated hypotensive patient. *Am J Emerg Med.* 2001;19:299-302.

3. Perera P, Mailhot T, Riley D, et al. The RUSH exam: Rapid Ultrasound in SHock in the evaluation of the critically ill. *Emerg Med Clin North Am.* 2010;28:29-56.

4. Pershad J, Myers S, Plouman C, et al. Bedside limited echocardiography by the emergency physician is accurate during evaluation of the critically ill patient. *Pediatrics.* 2004;114:e667–e671.

5. Randazzo MR, Snoey ER, Levitt MA, et al. Accuracy of emergency physician assessment of left ventricular ejection fraction and central venous pressure using echocardiography. *Acad Emerg Med.* 2003;10:973-977.

6. Moore CL, Rose GA, Tayal VS, et al. Determination of left ventricular function by emergency physician echocardiography of hypotensive patients. *Acad Emerg Med.* 2002;9:186-193.

7. Jones AE, Craddock PA, Tayal VS, et al. Diagnostic accuracy of identification of left ventricular function among emergency department patients with nontraumatic symptomatic undifferentiated hypotension. *Shock.* 2005;24:513-517.

8. Mandavia DP, Hoffner RJ, Mahaney K, et al. Bedside echocardiography by emergency physicians. *Ann Emerg Med.* 2001;38:377-382.

9. Moore CM. Current issues with emergency cardiac ultrasound probe and image conventions. *Acad Emerg Med.* 2008;15:278-284.

10. Blaivas M. Incidence of pericardial effusions in patients presenting to the emergency department with unexplained dyspnea. *Acad Emerg Med.* 2001;8:1143-1146.

11. McConnell MV, Solomon SD, Rayan ME, et al. Regional right ventricular dysfunction detected by echocardiography in acute pulmonary embolism. *Am J Cardiol.* 1996;78:469-473.

12. Come PC. Echocardiographic evaluation of pulmonary embolism and its response to therapeutic interventions. *Chest.* 1992;101:151S-162S.

13. Goldhaber SZ. Echocardiography in the management of pulmonary embolism. *Ann Intern Med.* 2002;136:691-700.

14. Grifoni S, Olivotto I, Cecchini P, et al. Short-term clinical outcome of patients with acute pulmonary embolism, normal blood pressure, and echocardiographic right ventricular dysfunction. *Circulation.* 2000;101:2817-2822.

15. Budhram G, Reardon R. Diagnosis of ascending aortic dissection using emergency department bedside echocardiogram. *Acad Emerg Med.* 2008;15:58.

16. Fojtik JP, Costantino TG, Dean AJ. The diagnosis of aortic dissection by emergency medicine ultrasound. *J Emerg Med.* 2007;32:191-196.

17. Blaivas M, Sierzenski PR. Dissection of the proximal thoracic aorta: a new ultrasonographic sign in the subxiphoid view. *Am J Emerg Med.* 2002;20:344-348.

18. Barrett C, Stone MB. Emergency ultrasound diagnosis of type A aortic dissection and apical pleural cap. *Acad Emerg Med.* 2010;17:e23-e24.

19. Marik PE, Baram M, Vahid B. Does central venous pressure predict fluid responsiveness? A systematic review of the literature and the tale of seven mares. *Chest.* 2008;134:172-178.

20. Feissel M, Michard F. The respiratory variation in inferior vena cava diameter as a guide to fluid therapy. *Intensive Care Med.* 2004;30:1834-1837.

21. Vignon P. Evaluation of fluid responsiveness in ventilated septic patients: back to venous return. *Intensive Care Med.* 2004;30:1699-1701.

22. Nagdev AD, Merchant RC, Tirado-Gonzalez A, et al. Emergency department bedside ultrasonographic measurement of caval index for non-invasive determination of low central venous pressure. *Ann Emerg Med.* 2010;55:290-295.

23. Wallace DJ, Allison M, Stone MB. Inferior vena cava percentage collapse during respiration is affected by the sampling location: an ultrasound study in healthy volunteers. *Acad Emerg Med.* 2010;17:96-99.

24. Barbier C, Loubieres Y, Schmit C, et al. Respiratory changes in inferior vena cava diameter are helpful in predicting fluid responsiveness in ventilated septic patients. *Intensive Care Med.* 2004;30:1740-1746.

25. Wilkerson RG, Stone MB. Sensitivity of bedside ultrasound and supine anteroposterior chest radiographs for the identification of pneumothorax after blunt trauma. *Acad Emerg Med.* 2010;17:11-17.

26. Lichtenstein DA, Menu Y. A bedside ultrasound sign ruling out pneumothorax in the critically ill: lung sliding. *Chest.* 1995;108:1345-1348.

27. Simon BC, Paolinetti L. Two cases where bedside ultrasound was able to distinguish pulmonary bleb from pneumothorax. *J Emerg Med.* 2005;29:201-205.

28. Lichtenstein D, Meziere G, Biderman P, et al. The "lung point": an ultrasound sign specific to pneumothorax. *Intensive Care Med.* 2000;26:1434-1440.

29. Andrew H, Travers, Thomas D, et al. Part 4: CPR overview: 2010 American Heart Association Guidelines for Cardiopulmonary Resuscitation and Emergency Cardiovascular Care. *Circulation.* 2010;122(suppl 3):S676-S684.

30. Salen P, Melniker L, Chooljian C, et al. Does the presence or absence of sonographically identified cardiac activity predict resuscitation outcomes of cardiac arrest patients? *Am J Emerg Med.* 2005;23:459-462.

31. Tsung JW, Blaivas M. Feasibility of correlating the pulse check with focused point-of-care echocardiography during pediatric cardiac arrest: a case series. *Resuscitation.* 2008;77:264-269.

32. Hernandez C, Shuler K, Hannan H, et al. C.A.U.S.E.: cardiac arrest ultra-sound exam—a better approach to managing patients in primary non-arrhythmogenic cardiac arrest. *Resuscitation.* 2008;76:198-206.

Acknowledgment

The authors would like to thank Arun Nagdev, MD, Michael Stone, MD, and Ralph Wang, MD, for their teaching contributions in the creation of this chapter.

CHAPTER 21

The Difficult Emergency Delivery

Jennifer V. Pope and Carrie D. Tibbles

IN THIS CHAPTER

Assessment of the laboring patient

Preparing for precipitous delivery

Management of delivery complications

The perimortem cesarean delivery

Introduction

The arrival of a woman in labor in an emergency department is an anxiety-provoking event for all involved. Many women who present to the emergency department in labor have had little or no prenatal care, increasing the risk of complications to both mother and fetus.[1,2] The goal of this chapter is to review the assessment of a woman in labor, the steps in a precipitous delivery, and the management of complications associated with a vaginal delivery.

Triage of the Pregnant Patient in Labor

Because the emergency department is a suboptimal place for a delivery, interhospital transfer of patients in labor should be considered carefully. The Emergency Medical Treatment and Labor Act (EMTALA) requires that all patients have a medical screening examination. Although labor can be an emergency medical condition, stabilization does not necessarily mean delivery in each case. As is the case for other emergency medical conditions, the transferring physician must certify that the benefits of transfer outweigh the risks. Emergency physicians must be aware of their hospitals' policies and resources for laboring patients. The triage of pregnant patients in labor is summarized in Figure 21-1.

PEARLS

The physician who initiates an interhospital transfer must certify that the benefits of transport outweigh the risks.

Under EMTALA guidelines, stabilization of a pregnant woman who is having contractions does not automatically mean delivery of the baby.

Assessment of the Laboring Patient

After 20 weeks' gestation, any woman with complaints of abdominal pain, back pain, or vaginal bleeding or discharge should be assessed for active labor.[3,4] Methods for assessing the laboring patient are described in Figure 21-2. Perform a focused history and physical, including information about gestational age and parity. If the patient does not know the gestational age, it can be estimated based on the date of her last menstrual period (Nägele rule[5]), fundal height, and ultrasonography.

PEARLS

Nägele rule = first day of last menstrual period + 9 months + 7 days[5]

Measure the fundal height with a tape measure from the pubic symphysis to the top of the fundus. The measurement in centimeters roughly estimates the gestational age in weeks. Fundal height at the umbilicus represents about 20 weeks' gestation.

FIGURE 21-1.

Triage of the pregnant patient in labor

```
                  ┌─────────────────────────────────┐
                  │ Can this patient be safely       │
                  │ transported to labor and         │
                  │ delivery?                        │
                  └─────────────────────────────────┘
        ┌──────────────────┼──────────────────┐
        ▼                  ▼                  ▼
┌───────────────┐  ┌───────────────┐  ┌───────────────┐
│  Early labor  │  │  Delivery is  │  │  High risk    │
│               │  │  imminent     │  │               │
└───────────────┘  └───────────────┘  └───────────────┘
        │                  │                  │
        ▼                  ▼                  ▼
┌───────────────┐  ┌───────────────┐  ┌───────────────┐
│ Transfer to   │  │ Prepare for   │  │ Stat          │
│ labor and     │  │ emergency     │  │ transport     │
│ delivery      │  │ department    │  │ (if possible) │
│               │  │ delivery      │  │               │
└───────────────┘  └───────────────┘  └───────────────┘
```

FIGURE 21-2.

Assessment of the pregnant patient in labor

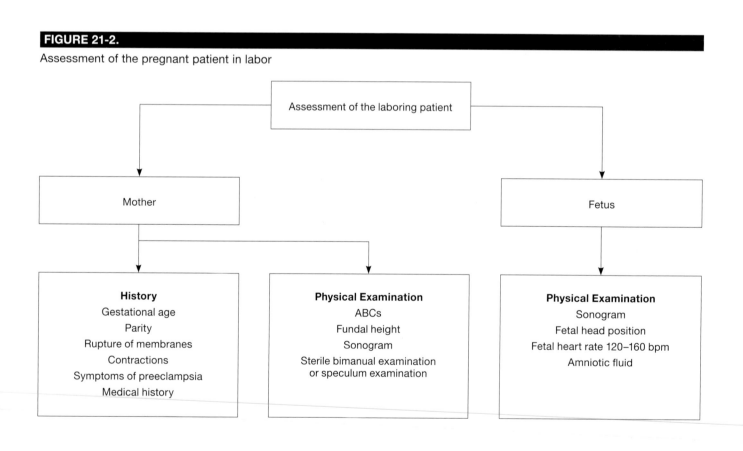

History	Physical Examination	Physical Examination
Gestational age	ABCs	Sonogram
Parity	Fundal height	Fetal head position
Rupture of membranes	Sonogram	Fetal heart rate 120–160 bpm
Contractions	Sterile bimanual examination or speculum examination	Amniotic fluid
Symptoms of preeclampsia		
Medical history		

To differentiate between true and false labor, ask specific questions regarding possible rupture of membranes, vaginal bleeding or mucus plug, timing of contractions, and the urge to push. In the brief review of systems, it is also important to ask about fevers, headache, visual changes, significant edema, and right upper quadrant pain in order to assess for potential complications from infection or eclampsia. Obtain a medical and surgical history, information about use of medications, and an allergy history.

Perform a physical examination, starting with vital signs, airway, breathing, and circulation. Next, measure the fundal height and determine the position of the fetus. It is estimated that the frequency of malpresentation at 32 weeks is as high as 15% and decreases to 4% at term.[6] If time permits, Leopold maneuvers may be attempted to determine fetal lie. These maneuvers are sensitive and specific when performed by an experienced clinician.[6] For emergency physicians who do not routinely perform Leopold maneuvers, ultrasonography is a more useful tool to determine the position of the head, location of the placenta, presence of amniotic fluid, and fetal heart rate.

If there is no reported significant vaginal bleeding and the patient appears to be in active labor, perform a sterile bimanual examination to determine cervical dilation, effacement, and fetal station. Cervical dilation refers to the diameter of the cervix. Cervical effacement, or thinning of the cervix, is described as a percentage of normal length of the cervix (about 2 cm)—from 0% to 100%. Fetal station refers to the level of the presenting part compared with the maternal ischial spine. Presentation above the ischial spine is referred to as –1 station. Presentation at the ischial spine is 0 station. If the presenting part is below the ischial spine, the scenario is a +1, +2, or +3 station.[7] A patient who is 10 cm dilated, 100% effaced, and at +3 station has an impending delivery. If there is significant vaginal bleeding, do not perform a bimanual examination because bleeding might indicate placenta previa or abruption. If either is suspected, immediately transfer the patient to labor and delivery for a possible cesarean delivery.[3]

A sterile speculum examination can be performed to visualize the cervix and determine if amniotic fluid is leaking. Amniotic fluid will turn nitrazine paper yellow to blue and, when smeared on a glass slide, will form crystals in a ferning pattern.[3] If amniotic fluid is present, the presence or absence of brown staining is important to note: meconium contamination occurs in 20% of vaginal deliveries, and fetal aspiration of meconium can cause severe neonatal distress.[3,8]

PEARLS

When examining the cervix, recognize that the cervix can lie inferior to the head when the head is engaged, making the assessment more challenging. Run your hand along the head until you reach the cervix.

If meconium is present, prepare for potential respiratory distress in the newborn.

KEY POINTS

Perform a focused history and physical examination.

Determine fetal position and fetal heart beat.

Look for the presence of amniotic fluid.

Perform a sterile bimanual examination or sterile speculum examination.

Preparation for Delivery

Emergency physicians should know where their department's delivery kit is located. The equipment needed for delivery is listed in Table 21-1. A neonatal warmer and resuscitation equipment should be available. If the hospital has an obstetric and neonatal team, the team should be contacted immediately when the department is notified by EMS of an impending precipitous delivery.

PEARL

When a delivery is imminent, turn on the neonatal warmer so that it can warm up.

Normal Delivery

Normal labor is divided into three stages: 1) the start of regular contractions to full cervical dilation, 2) delivery of the infant, and 3) delivery of the placenta.[9] This chapter focuses on the second and third stages.

During the second stage of labor, the patient should be placed in the dorsal lithotomy position. Physicians must know the cardinal movements of labor (Figure 21-3) in order to guide the delivery. The head engages at the end of pregnancy (during the first stage of labor). Flexion, descent, and internal rotation result in the sagittal suture (crown) moving into the anterior/posterior diameter of the pelvis.[9] The second stage typically proceeds as follows:

- Most women have the urge to push.
- If time permits, clean the perineal area and drape it with sterile towels.
- As extension of the head occurs, the perineum will start to bulge and crowning will occur.
- If necessary, a mediolateral episiotomy can be performed at this time. In general, an episiotomy should be performed only if absolutely necessary because it is

TABLE 21-1.
Equipment for emergency delivery

Sterile gloves and gown
Cleaning solution
Two hemostat clamps
Scissors
Bulb syringe
Red-topped blood collection tube (cord blood)
Infant warmer
Neonatal resuscitation equipment

associated with increased maternal blood loss, risk of disruption of the anal sphincter, and delay in return of sexual activity.[9]

- To minimize injury to the perineum, apply gentle pressure on the draped perineum with one hand and place the other hand on the presenting head to minimize uncontrolled head movements, which can tear the perineum.[3,4]
- With an index finger, sweep the neck to check for a nuchal cord. If the cord is present, attempt to gently slip it over the infant's head. If the cord is too tight, apply two clamps and cut the cord between them and continue with a rapid delivery.[4,9]
- With the next contraction, external rotation of the head occurs and the shoulder should follow the path of the head. The anterior shoulder rotates under the pubic arch. Apply gentle downward traction to deliver the anterior shoulder.
- The posterior shoulder is then delivered with gentle upward traction on the head.
- Finally, the body and legs are delivered.
- Use a bulb syringe to clear the infant's airway.
- Place two clamps on the cord 3 or 4 cm from the infant and cut between them. Place cord blood in a sterile vacuum blood-collection tube.[3]
- Stimulate and warm the infant while placing him or her in the mother's arms or a warmer.

- Obtain Apgar scores at 1, 5, and 10 minutes.

The third stage of delivery involves delivery of the placenta, which can take 2 to 30 minutes. Signs of placental separation include a gush of fresh blood, cord lengthening, and the uterus becoming firm.[9] At this time, it is acceptable to apply gentle traction on the cord while applying counterpressure just above the symphysis to prevent uterine inversion.[9] Once the placenta is delivered, inspect it to ensure complete removal. To decrease the risk of postpartum hemorrhage from uterine atony, transabdominally massage the uterus and start 20 units of oxytocin in 1 liter of normal saline at 200 mL/hr.[9,10] Inspect the perineum, vagina, and cervix for lacerations that need to be repaired.

KEY POINTS

Steps in normal delivery:

- Clean the perineum.
- Apply gentle pressure to the perineum with one hand and control delivery of the head with the other hand.
- Sweep the neck to check for a nuchal cord.
- Deliver the anterior shoulder.
- Deliver the posterior shoulder.
- Deliver the body.
- Suction the airway.
- Clamp and cut the cord.
- Document Apgar score at 1, 5, and 10 minutes.

FIGURE 21-3.

Movements of normal delivery. Mechanism of labor and delivery for vertex presentations. A. Engagement, flexion, and descent. B. Internal rotation. C. Extension and delivery of the head. After delivery of the head, check the neck for encirclement by the umbilical cord. D. External rotation, bringing the thorax into the anteroposterior diameter of the pelvis. E. Delivery of the anterior shoulder. F. Delivery of the posterior shoulder. Note that after delivery, the head is supported and used to gently guide delivery of the shoulder. Traction should be minimized. From: Tintinalli J, Stapczynski J, Ma OJ, et al, eds. *Tintinalli's Emergency Medicine: A Comprehensive Study Guide.* 7th ed. New York, NY: McGraw-Hill; 2010:707. Copyright McGraw-Hill, 2010. Used with permission.

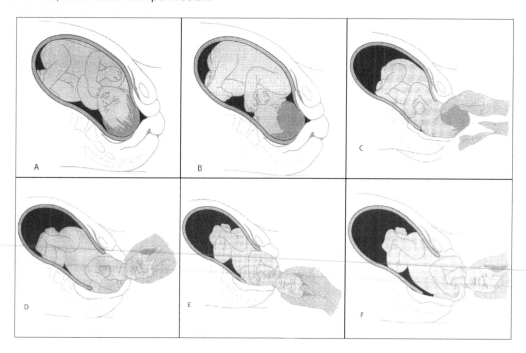

Complications of Delivery

Shoulder Dystocia

Shoulder dystocia, an obstetric emergency, occurs in 0.13% to 2% of vaginal deliveries.[11] It is the inability to deliver the shoulder, often when the fetal head recoils back toward the perineum (the turtle sign).[11] It occurs because the shoulder girdle is in the anteroposterior position instead of the oblique position, causing the anterior shoulder to become lodged behind the pubic symphysis.[11] Risk factors include macrosomia, maternal obesity, and prolonged second stage of labor.[11] One large study reported the complications of neonatal brachial plexus injury in 20% of cases of shoulder dystocia, clavicle and humerus fracture in 10.6%, and neonatal asphyxia in 8.6%.[12]

As soon as dystocia is identified, stop the mother from pushing and call for help. Consider draining the bladder to make more room anteriorly; episiotomy may be warranted.[4] As demonstrated in Figure 21-4, immediately have two assistants flex the mother's thighs back to her chest wall (McRoberts maneuver) to rotate the pubic symphysis cephalad and dislodge the anterior shoulder. The McRoberts maneuver has been reported to be successful in 42% of cases.[13] If this does not work, have an assistant apply suprapubic pressure to attempt to dislodge the anterior shoulder from behind the symphysis. Success rates of these two maneuvers have been reported between 54% and 90%.[11,13] If the shoulders are still not deliverable, a Woods or corkscrew maneuver can be performed by pushing the posterior shoulder 180° clockwise to make it the anterior shoulder (Figure 21-5). If this is not successful, attempt to deliver the posterior arm by inserting a hand posteriorly and applying gentle pressure at the antecubital fossa to flex the arm and sweep it over the chest to deliver it. If none of these maneuvers is successful, the clavicle may be fractured to diminish the width of the shoulder girdle and deliver the infant.[13]

FIGURE 21-4.

McRoberts maneuver. The maneuver consists of removing the legs from the stirrups and sharply flexing the thighs up onto the abdomen, as shown by the horizontal arrow. The assistant is simultaneously providing suprapubic pressure (vertical arrow). From: Cunningham FG, Leveno KL, Bloom SL, et al, eds. *Williams Obstetrics.* 22nd ed. New York, NY: McGraw-Hill; 2005:515. Copyright McGraw-Hill, 2005. Used with permission.

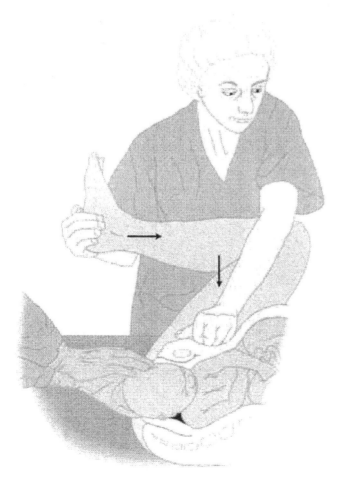

KEY POINTS

Shoulder dystocia:

Step 1: Stop pushing. Consider draining the bladder and performing an episiotomy.

Step 2: Perform a McRoberts maneuver and apply suprapubic pressure.

Step 3: Attempt a Woods maneuver.

Step 4: Deliver the posterior arm.

Step 5: Fracture the clavicle.

FIGURE 21-5.

Woods corkscrew maneuver. The hand is placed behind the posterior shoulder of the fetus. The shoulder is then rotated progressively 180° in a corkscrew manner so that the impacted anterior shoulder is released. From: Cunningham FG, Leveno KL, Bloom SL, et al, eds. *Williams Obstetrics.* 23rd ed. New York, NY: McGraw-Hill; 2010:484. Copyright McGraw-Hill, 2010. Used with permission.

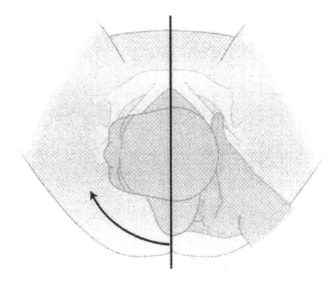

Umbilical Cord Prolapse

Umbilical cord prolapse occurs when the cord passes through the cervix with or without the presenting part. The incidence of overt prolapse (displacement of the cord into the vagina after rupture of the membranes) in cephalic presentations is about 0.5% and higher with malpresentation.[13] This is a life-threatening emergency for the fetus since the presenting part compresses the cord and cuts off all blood flow and oxygen. If a cord is felt or seen, immediately tell the mother to stop pushing and lift the presenting part off the cord. Wrap any exposed cord in moist sterile gauze. If obstetric support is available, call for immediate cesarean section. Filling the bladder with 500 mL of saline to elevate the presenting part has also been described.[13] When obstetric support is not available and delivery is imminent, manually reduce the cord and rapidly complete a vaginal delivery.[3,13] In the obstetric literature, perinatal mortality rates from umbilical cord prolapse have decreased to less than 10% as a result of increased use of cesarean section and improved neonatal resuscitation skills.[14]

KEY POINTS

Umbilical cord prolapse:

- Lift the presenting part off the cord and wait for obstetric backup.

- Fill the bladder with 500 mL of saline to elevate the presenting part.

Breech Presentation

Breech presentation complicates 3% to 4% of all pregnancies.[11,13] These presentations have a high rate of perinatal morbidity and mortality from congenital abnormalities as well as from complications of cord prolapse and birth trauma.[11] Three types of breech presentation occur: complete breech (thighs and knees flexed), footling breech (one or both legs extended), and frank breech (thighs flexed and knees extended)(Figure 21-6).[11] The difficulty with these presentations is that delivery of the legs and torso does not dilate the vaginal canal enough for the passage of the fetal head, so the head becomes stuck. Breech presentation is identified by vaginal examination or ultrasonog-

---

FIGURE 21-6.

Management of the vaginal frank breech delivery. A. The Pinard maneuver. The operator's hand is placed behind the fetal thigh, putting gentle pressure at the knee and allowing delivery of the leg. B. A similar maneuver of the opposite leg. C. The feet are grasped with the thumb and third finger over the lateral malleolus, and the second finger is placed between the two ankles. D. With maternal expulsive efforts, the breech is delivered to the level of the umbilicus. The sacrum should be kept anterior. E. Again, with maternal expulsive efforts, the infant is delivered to the level of the clavicles, with the sacrum kept anterior. F. The fetus is rotated 90°, which allows visualization of the now anterior right arm. G. The arm is well visualized, and a single digit is used to deliver it. Delivery of the opposite arm is accomplished by rotating the fetus 180° in a clockwise direction and repeating the maneuver. H. Delivery of the fetal vertex is accomplished by placing the operator's fingers over the maxillary processes of the fetus, with the body kept parallel to the floor. The body should never be lifted above parallel to prevent hyperextension of the neck. An assistant applies suprapubic pressure, aiding flexion of the fetal head and accomplishing delivery. From: Tintinalli J, Stapczynski J, Ma OJ, et al, eds. *Tintinalli's Emergency Medicine: A Comprehensive Study Guide.* 7th ed. New York, NY: McGraw-Hill; 2010:710. Copyright McGraw-Hill, 2010. Used with permission.

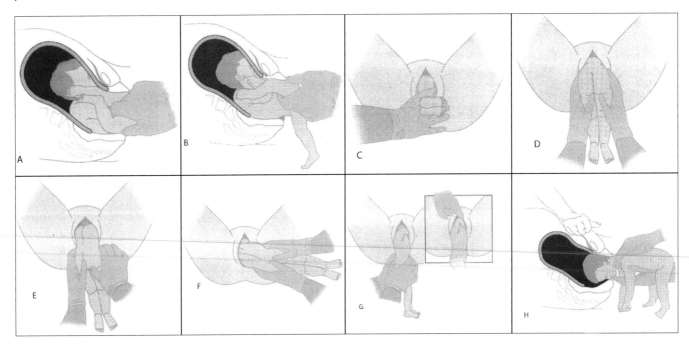

raphy. Cesarean section is the preferred method of delivery of these infants, but this procedure is not always feasible. Avoid applying traction on the legs or body until the infant has delivered to the level of the umbilicus.

- Deliver one leg, followed by the other leg.
- With the sacrum anterior, place thumbs over the sacrum and fingers over the iliac crests and allow delivery of the torso.
- Rotate the infant 90° and deliver the anterior arm, then rotate the infant 180° to deliver the other arm.
- Finally, with the sacrum anterior, have an assistant apply transabdominal pressure over the head while keeping the fingers over the maxillary process to keep the infant's head flexed. Hook the fingers of the other hand over the shoulder while applying gentle downward traction over the shoulders.[11,13]
- If the head cannot be delivered through the cervix, incisions can be made at the 6-o'clock or the 2- and 10-o'clock positions of the cervix, but this results in significant maternal hemorrhage.[11,13]

KEY POINTS

Breech presentation:

- Deliver the legs.
- Keep the sacrum anterior.
- Deliver the torso.
- With the sacrum anterior, keep the infant's head flexed and apply downward traction over the shoulders.
- Clamp and cut the cord.

Postpartum Hemorrhage

Postpartum hemorrhage is the second most common cause of pregnancy-related death in the United States.[15] It is classified as immediate (ie, within the first 24 hours) or delayed (ie, after the first 24 hours and then up to 6 weeks).[10] Causes of immediate postpartum hemorrhage, defined as blood loss greater than 500 mL during a vaginal delivery, are listed in Table 21-2. The management of delayed postpartum hemorrhage is beyond the scope of this chapter but is described in emergency medicine textbooks.

Uterine atony is the most common cause of postpartum hemorrhage and occurs more frequently if the uterus has been overextended (macrosomia), in association with a precipitous delivery, or if the uterus is fatigued from prolonged labor.[10] Management consists of manual massage, with one hand placed externally on the abdomen and the other placed internally, massaging the uterus upward.[10] Simultaneously, medications may be started to increase uterine muscle tone (Table 21-3).[16] If this fails, the birth canal should be inspected for lacerations or hematomas of the perineum, vagina, or cervix. Retained placental parts can cause bleeding and can be found by digital examination of the uterus. If the placental parts cannot be removed easily, wait for obstetric backup and consider packing the uterus if hemorrhage is significant.[10]

Uterine Inversion/Uterine Rupture

The incidence of uterine inversion is about 1 in 2,500 pregnancies. The cause is unclear, but the complication is often described in association with cord traction and excessive fundal pressure.[17] Recognition and immediate action are crucial. Im-

TABLE 21-2.

Causes of immediate postpartum hemorrhage

Uterine atony
Genital lacerations
Retained placenta
Hematoma
Coagulopathy
Uterine inversion
Uterine rupture

TABLE 21-3.

Medical management of uterine atony

Medication	Dose	Side Effects
Oxytocin	20 units in 500 mL normal saline at 10 mL/min until uterus is firm or 10 units IM	Hypotension, nausea, vomiting
Methylergonovine maleate	0.2 mg IM; may repeat every 2–4 hours	Hypertension, nausea, vomiting
Carboprost tromethamine	250 mcg IM	Nausea, vomiting, diarrhea
Dinoprostone	20 mg suppository vaginally or rectally	Abdominal pain, nausea, vomiting

FIGURE 21-7.

Procedure for perimortem cesarean section. A. Make a midline vertical abdominal incision. B. Incise through the fascia and muscles into the peritoneum. C. Make a vertical uterine incision. D. Deliver the infant. E. Remove the placenta and membranes. From: Katz VL. Cardiopulmonary resuscitation during pregnancy and perimortem cesarean section. In: Pearlman MD, Tintinalli JE, eds. *Emergency Care of the Woman.* New York, NY: McGraw-Hill; 1998:378. Copyright McGraw-Hill, 1998. Used with permission.

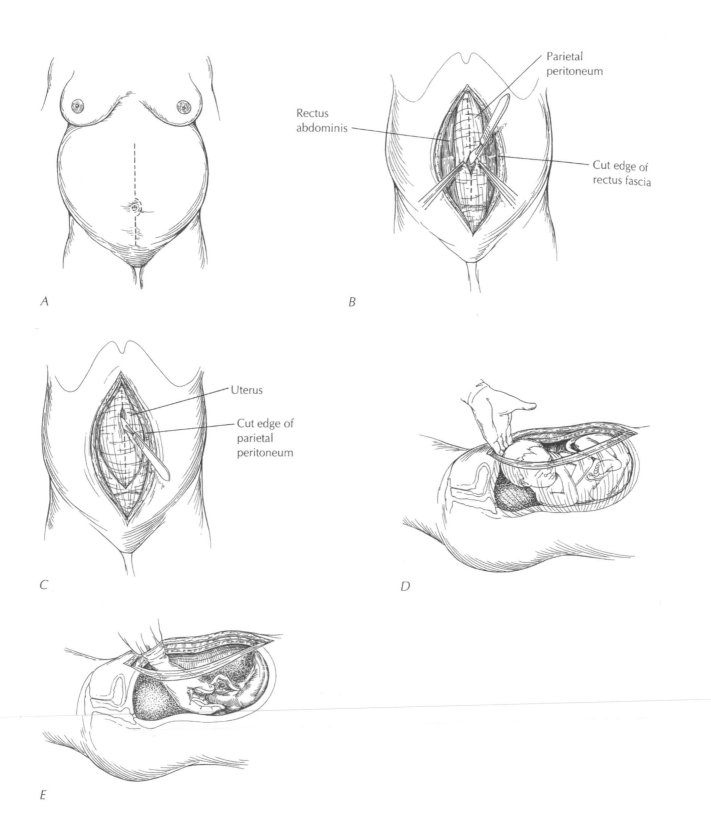

mediately stop all uterotonic medications. Manually reduce the uterus by applying pressure on the fundus with a hand directed inward toward the umbilicus.[17] If the placenta is still attached, do not attempt to remove it before the uterus is reduced. Pharmacologic relaxation of the uterus with terbutaline, magnesium, or nitroglycerin can be required for reduction.[17] Once the uterus is reduced, uterotonic medications can be restarted.

With an incidence of about 0.1%, uterine rupture is a rare but life-threatening obstetric emergency.[17] Risk factors include previous cesarean delivery, use of labor-induction medications, and trauma.[17] The clinical presentation can vary from uterine tenderness to maternal shock.[17] If this condition is suspected, surgical intervention is required. The emergency physician should continue standard hypovolemic resuscitation practices until surgical support is available.

PEARL

Oxytocin should not be given as an intravenous push because it causes hypotension. The uterus has limited receptors for oxytocin, so it cannot respond to increased doses. Additional medications should be tried if bleeding persists.

KEY POINT

Uterine atony is the most common cause of postpartum hemorrhage. Treatment includes manual massage of the uterus and administration of uterotonic medications.

Perimortem Cesarean Section

Perimortem cesarean section should be considered in any pregnant woman in cardiac arrest with a viable gestation of greater than 24 weeks.[3,4] Based on limited data, the recommendation is that the procedure should be performed within 4 minutes after maternal cardiac arrest.[18] Through a literature search, Katz and associates found reports of 38 perimortem cesarean sections performed between 1985 and 2004; most of the surviving infants reported as normal were delivered within 5 minutes, but others reported as normal were delivered more than 15 minutes after the death of the mother.[19] In fact, one case report describes a child who was delivered 30 minutes after maternal cardiac arrest and who, 4 years later, is developing normally.[20]

The cesarean section procedure is described below:

- Cardiopulmonary resuscitation (CPR) should be continued throughout the procedure.
- If gestational age is unknown, fundal height can be measured while CPR is ongoing.
- Make a midline vertical incision from the epigastric area to the pubic symphysis (Figure 21-7).
- Penetrate all abdominal layers and find the uterus.
- Use retractors or assistants to hold back the abdominal wall. Drain the bladder if time permits.
- Make an incision at the fundus of the uterus. Insert two fingers to lift the uterine wall away from the fetus.
- Using a scalpel or scissors, incise from the fundus to the bladder reflection.[3]
- Remove the infant, suction the mouth, and clamp the cord.

- The incision made on the mother should be closed based on the resuscitation efforts and in conjunction with a surgical team.

Undertaking a perimortem cesarean section is a difficult decision for any emergency physician to make. Physicians need to be aware of the indications for this procedure and its sequence. Time to delivery is a crucial factor. In some cases, cesarean section will improve the mother's hemodynamics to the extent that resuscitation may be successful.[19] Physicians are likely to fear litigation in these dire scenarios, but, to date, no lawsuits have been filed against anyone who has performed a perimortem cesarean section.

KEY POINTS

Start perimortem cesarean section within 4 minutes after maternal cardiac arrest or as soon as possible.

Most experts believe that informed consent is not necessary.

Conclusion

Although emergency deliveries are rare events, they do occur. Emergency physicians must be aware of hospital policies regarding births in the emergency department as well as the resources that are available to support an emergency delivery. A woman who comes to the emergency department in labor should be assessed with a focused history and physical examination. If time permits, ultrasonography should be used to assess the fetal position in order to prepare for a normal vaginal or breech delivery. Complications should be anticipated: shoulder dystocia, umbilical cord prolapse, nuchal cord, and postpartum hemorrhage. If a pregnant woman goes into cardiac arrest, the physician should remember the ABCs, assess fundal height, and prepare for a cesarean section.

References

1. Brunette DD, Sterner SP. Prehospital and emergency department delivery: a review of eight years experience. *Ann Emerg Med*. 1989;18:1116-1118.
2. Elixhauser A, Machlin SR, Zodet MW, et al. Health care for children and youth in the United States: 2001 annual report on access, utilization, quality, and expenditures. *Ambul Pediatr*. 2002;2(6):419-437.
3. Stallard TC, Burns B. Emergency delivery and perimortem C-section. *Emerg Med Clin North Am*. 2003;21:679-693.
4. Burg MD, Beisbroeck D. Emergency delivery. In: Wolfson AB, ed. *Harwood-Nuss' Clinical Practice of Emergency Medicine*. 5th ed. Philadelphia, PA: Lippincott Williams & Wilkins; 2009:517-521.
5. VanRooyen MJ, Scott JA. Emergency delivery. In: Tintinalli JE, Stapczynski JS, Ma OJ, eds. *Emergency Medicine: A Comprehensive Guide*. 7th ed. New York, NY: McGraw-Hill; 2011:703-711.
6. Lydon-Rochelle M, Albers L, Gorwoda J, et al. Accuracy of Leopold maneuvers in screening for malpresentation: a prospective study. *Birth*. 1993;20:132-135.
7. Rouse DJ, St John E. Normal labor, delivery, and puerperium. In: Scott JR, Haney A, Karlan B, et al, eds. *Danforth's Obstetrics and Gynecology*. 9th ed. Philadelphia, PA: Lippincott Williams & Wilkins; 2003:35-56.
8. Gianopoulos JG. Emergency complications of labor and delivery. *Emerg Med Clin North Am*. 1994;12:201-217.
9. Archie CL. The course & conduct of normal labor & delivery. In: DeCherney AH, Nathan L, Goodwin TM, Laufer N, eds. *Current Diagnosis and Treatment Obstetrics & Gynecology*. 10th ed. New York, NY: Lange Medical Books/McGraw-Hill; 2007:203-211.
10. Mendelson MH, Lang JP. Postpartum emergencies. In: Wolfson AB, ed. *Harwood-Nuss' Clinical Practice of Emergency Medicine*. 5th ed. Philadelphia, PA: Lippincott Williams & Wilkins; 2009:522-527.
11. Brost BC, VanDorsten JP. Emergency vaginal delivery. In: Pearlman MD, Tintinalli JE, eds. *Emergency Care of the Woman*. New York, NY: McGraw-Hill; 1998:119-136.
12. Rahman J, Bhattee G, Rahman MS. Shoulder dystocia in a 16-year experience in a teaching hospital. *J Reprod Med*. 2009;54:378-384.

13. Kish K, Collea JV. Malpresentation and cord prolapse. In: DeCherney AH, Nathan L, Goodwin TM, Laufer N, eds. *Current Diagnosis and Treatment Obstetrics & Gynecology.* 10th ed. New York, NY: Lange Medical Books/McGraw-Hill; 2007:342-358.

14. Lin MG. Umbilical cord prolapse. *Obstet Gynecol Surv.* 2006;61:269-277.

15. Kung HC, Hoyert DL, Xu J, et al. Deaths: final data for 2005. *Natl Vital Stat Rep.* 2008;56(10):1-120.

16. Postpartum hemorrhage—acute. In: DISEASEDEX™ Emergency Medicine Summary in Micromedex 1.0. Greenwood Village, CO: Thomson Reuters (Healthcare) Inc; 2009.

17. Mirza FG, Gaddipati S. Obstetric emergencies. *Semin Perinatol.* 2009;33:97-103.

18. Katz VL, Dotters DJ, Droegemueller W. Perimortem cesarean delivery. *Obstet Gynecol.* 1986;68:571-576.

19. Katz V, Balderston K, DeFreest M. Perimortem cesarean delivery: were our assumptions correct? *Am J Obstet Gynecol.* 2005;192:1916-1921.

20. Capobianco G, Balata A, Mannazzu MC, et al. Perimortem cesarean delivery 30 minutes after a laboring patient jumped from a fourth-floor window: baby survives and is normal at age 4 years. *Am J Obstet Gynecol.* 2008;198:e15-e16.

CHAPTER 22

Resuscitation of the Critically Ill Neonate

Aaron Leetch and Alan Bedrick

IN THIS CHAPTER

Specialized equipment for neonatal resuscitation

Identification of the critically ill neonate
Airway/temperature
Breathing
Circulation

Drugs, dextrose, and diagnostics: postresuscitation care

Congenital heart disease

Other specific congenital anomalies

Withholding/discontinuing resuscitation

Introduction

Few things are as terrifying to an emergency physician as a cyanotic neonate after a precipitous emergency department delivery. Although most infants need little more than supportive care, the emergency department often selects for those in need of more intervention. Several maternal and fetal conditions can alert emergency physicians to the potential need for resuscitation (Table 22-1).[1] Because neonatal resuscitation is not commonplace in emergency departments, this chapter covers the most important aspects of the American Heart Association (AHA) guidelines,[2] with added tips for a successful resuscitation (Figure 22-1).

Resuscitation of a neonate immediately following delivery differs from that of adults, children, and even slightly older infants for one main reason—a neonatal resuscitation is almost exclusively focused on *respiration* as the key component of transition from fetal circulation. Even in neonatal intensive care units (NICUs) and delivery rooms, chest compressions and drugs are used only very infrequently.[3]

As an infant transitions from intrauterine life to extrauterine life, the first breath is the catalyst. The first breath promotes amniotic fluid in the lungs to absorb, umbilical vessels to constrict, and pulmonary arterioles to dilate.[4] As pulmonary arterial pressure decreases, blood preferentially flows to the lungs, allowing oxygenation and normal systemic circulation (Figure 22-2). For this reason, clearing the infant's airway and lungs, and thus stimulating that first breath, is crucial to survival.

KEY POINT
Neonatal resuscitation is almost exclusively a *respiratory* issue.

Also for this reason, most of the mainstays of adult resuscitation are not recommended for neonates by the AHA or the American Academy of Pediatrics. For example, the *only* drug used, according to AHA guidelines, is epinephrine.[2] There is no place for atropine, lidocaine, or cardioversion for a neonate with respiratory depression who requires resuscitation. If a neonate cannot be resuscitated with epinephrine, after all other measures have been used, the neonate cannot be resuscitated. Likewise, rapid-sequence intubation is not appropriate for a newly delivered critically ill infant; nearly all will tolerate endotracheal intubation without sedation. Once a neonate has established stable cardiorespiratory physiology (often in several days), he or she can then be treated according to the pediatric advanced life support (PALS) algorithm.

FIGURE 22-1.

Neonatal resuscitation algorithm. Intubation may be considered at any point in the algorithm. Adhere as closely as possible to the "golden minute" to address airway/warmth, breathing, and circulation.[2] (Source: American Heart Association, Inc.)

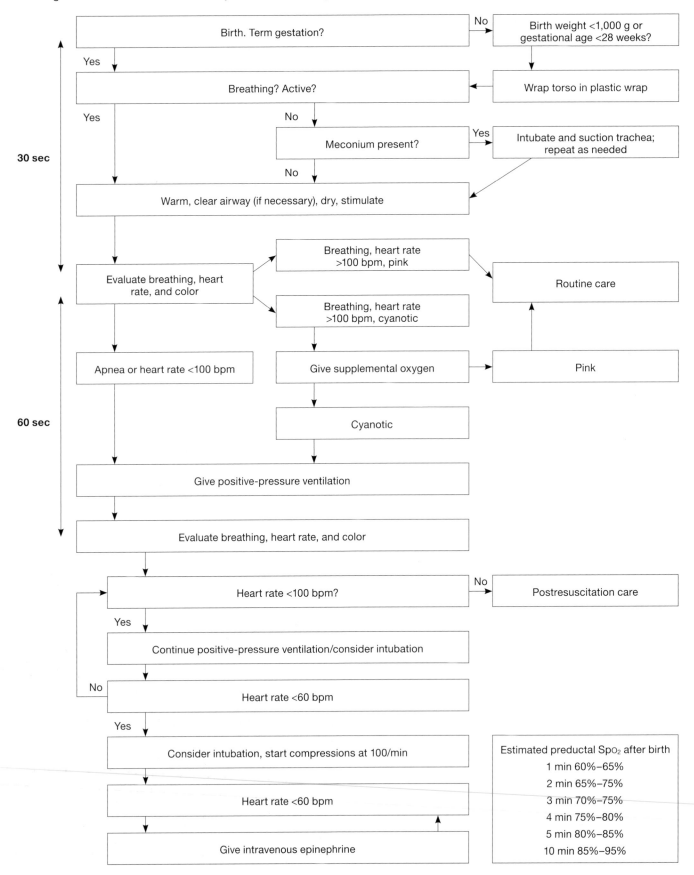

The *only* drug used in neonatal resuscitation after delivery is epinephrine.

Specialized Equipment for Neonatal Resuscitation

Aside from the typical advanced airway equipment, suction, intravenous lines, and monitors that are normally used for resuscitation, neonatal resuscitation requires preparation of a few specialized pieces of equipment (Table 22-2).[3] If a delivery can be anticipated, an overhead warmer should be prepared for the infant. Turn the warmer on and take everything off of it except for blankets and bulb suction; metallic equipment (eg, laryngoscopes) can become hot and burn infants or lose function (eg, endotracheal [ET] tubes). Deep-suction catheters (sizes 5F–14F), a meconium aspirator, and size 0 and 1 Miller laryngoscope blades are frequently necessary. Ideally, a flow-inflating bag (ie, bag-valve mask) attached to a pressure gauge should be used to monitor ventilatory pressures. A range of premature and full-term infant face masks and uncuffed ET tubes should be available because "appropriate size" is widely variable over even a few weeks of gestational age. Vascular access supplies should include 25-gauge catheters for peripheral access and umbilical catheters for central access. Scalp veins are also an option for vascular access in infants.

Ultrasonography is becoming a more readily available and well-used imaging modality in the emergency department. Birth weight and gestational age can be estimated using crown-to-rump length and biparietal measurements. Many ultrasound machines are programmed to convert these measurements into age and weight and can be useful when anticipating a difficult or premature delivery.

Identification of the Critically Ill Neonate

Immediately after birth, most neonates have some degree of cyanosis, pallor, poor muscle tone, or poor respiratory effort. It is what they do in the first 60 seconds that differentiates a healthy infant from a critically ill one. Newborns can be categorized as stable, purely cyanotic, or critical (Table 22-3).[4] Constant reevaluation of respiratory effort, heart rate, and color will aid in resuscitation. AHA guidelines allot 60 seconds for initial interventions, reevaluation, and initiation of positive-pressure ventilation (PPV) if indicated (Figure 22-2).[2] If there is no change in color, tone, or respiratory effort or if a child is bradycardic after this "golden minute," he or she is more likely to be critically ill. Contrary to popular belief, the Apgar score (Table 22-4) is not used to determine whether resuscitation is needed, although it is a good determinant of how the infant is responding to resuscitation efforts.

KEY POINT

The Apgar score is not used to determine whether resuscitation is needed.

Airway/Temperature

After an infant is delivered, start a timer to keep the resuscitation on pace (Figure 22-1). Providing warmth to a newborn is as important as clearing the airway, and the two can be done simultaneously. Newborns are highly susceptible to evaporative heat losses and will quickly decompensate if allowed to become hypothermic. Place the child under a radiant warmer and/or dry vigorously with warm blankets. Extremely premature infants (<28 weeks' gestation or weighing 1,000 g or less) should be wrapped in food-grade plastic wrap to prevent radiant heat losses.[5,6]

KEY POINT

Newborns are highly susceptible to evaporative heat losses and will quickly decompensate if allowed to become hypothermic.

PEARL

Providing warmth is as important as clearing the airway in neonates.

TABLE 22-1.

Maternal and fetal conditions predicting the need for resuscitation

Maternal
  Preeclampsia/eclampsia
  Diabetes mellitus
  Placental abruption
  Trauma
  Fever
  No prenatal care
  Illicit drug use

Fetal
  Meconium-stained amniotic fluid
  Early gestational age
  Known congenital anomalies
  Oligo/polyhydramnios
  Prolonged rupture of membranes

FIGURE 22-2.

Intrauterine and extrauterine cardiac flow. A. In utero, pulmonary arterial pressure is elevated and blood flows preferentially to the systemic circulation via right-to-left shunts. B. After the first breath, pulmonary arterial pressure decreases and the foramen ovale and ductus arteriosus close, allowing normal pulmonary and systemic flow.

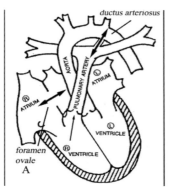
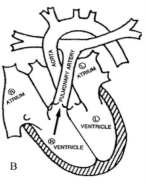

Place the infant in the sniffing position, being careful not to hyperextend the neck. If a neonate has obvious nasal or oral secretions, clear the mouth first and then the nose with bulb suction or a deep-suction catheter attached to wall suction. Infants are obligate nose breathers and must have a patent nasopharynx. However, if the neonate is breathing spontaneously and there is no obvious airway obstruction, suctioning should not be performed because it can cause a reflex bradycardia that further complicates resuscitation. If the neonate has not yet begun to cry or grimace, continue to vigorously dry the patient and stimulate by rubbing the back or flicking/slapping the feet.

KEY POINT

Infants are obligate nose breathers and must have a patent nasopharynx. However, if the neonate is breathing spontaneously and there is no obvious airway obstruction, suctioning should not be performed because it can cause a reflex bradycardia that further complicates resuscitation.

Infants with meconium-stained amniotic fluid at delivery are at risk for aspiration and the complications of aspiration pneumonia and respiratory compromise. Prevention of aspiration has been studied, resulting in new guidelines. Suctioning at the perineum is no longer recommended for infants who present with meconium, as it has not been shown to decrease the incidence of meconium aspiration.[6,7] Likewise, tracheal suctioning of vigorous infants with meconium staining does not appear to offer any benefit.[8] Although poorly studied, suctioning may offer a benefit to meconium-stained infants who are not vigorous and who are making no respiratory effort. These infants should not be stimulated prior to intubation, as they may aspirate meconium with their first breath. Instead, all infants with meconium staining who are not vigorous at birth should be intubated for tracheal suctioning to remove meconium from the proximal airway and minimize aspiration.

KEY POINT

All nonvigorous infants with meconium-stained fluid should be intubated for tracheal suctioning immediately after delivery.

Once tracheal intubation is achieved, attach a meconium aspirator to the ET tube (Figure 22-3).[3] This will serve as a conduit between the tube and wall suction. Once the aspirator is attached, occlude the thumb hole and gently remove the ET tube, thus suctioning the trachea. If meconium is thick or if there seems to be more in the trachea, repeat with a new tube. The AHA guidelines do not specify how many times tracheal suctioning should be repeated, but it is difficult to hold to the 60-second interval if suctioning is repeated more than two or three times. Infants who do not respond to repeated suction should proceed directly to positive-pressure ventilation, as discussed below. Still, most infants intubated for meconium will respond with a cry or respiratory effort, and prolonged intubation is usually not necessary. Because the ET tube in this scenario is used only for suction and not for ventilation, a smaller tube can be used to ensure quick access to very small airways. Other potential indications for immediate intubation include known or suspected congenital diaphragmatic hernia or extreme prematurity (<1,000 g or 28 weeks' gestation).

Neonatal Airways

Miller blades are recommended for neonates because their airways are more anterior and the epiglottis is more malleable and difficult to control. Size 0 blades are used for premature infants (<36 weeks) and size 1 for term infants (>36 weeks). Size 00 blades are available for extremely low-birth-weight infants (<28 weeks), but they can occlude the oropharynx and may be too short to reach the airway. All ET tubes used for neonatal resuscitation should be uncuffed, according to AHA guidelines. Because the size of neonatal airways varies so much depend-

TABLE 22-2.

Important neonatal resuscitation equipment

| Warm, clean blankets |
| Plastic wrap or bag |
| Bulb syringe |
| Suction catheters – 10F or 12F |
| Meconium aspirator |
| Bag-valve mask |
| Full-term and preterm face masks |
| Laryngeal mask airway – size 1 |
| Laryngoscope with Miller size 0 and 1 blades |
| Endotracheal tubes – sizes 2.5, 3.0, 3.5, 4.0 |
| End-tidal CO_2 detector |
| 25-gauge catheters |
| Umbilical line kit |
| Normal saline |
| Access to 1:10,000 epinephrine |

TABLE 22-3.

Clinical classification of neonates

Stable	Breathing
	Heart rate >100 beats/min
	No central cyanosis (pink oral mucous membranes)
Purely Cyanotic	Breathing
	Heart rate >100 beats/min
	Central cyanosis (blue mucous membranes)
Critical	Apnea
	or
	Heart rate <100 beats/min
	Central cyanosis

ing on gestational ages, the standard shorthand of (age+16)/4 for size and 3 × ET tube length for depth of insertion is not reliable. Correct sizing and depth of insertion can be estimated using weight or estimated gestational age (Table 22-5).[3]

FIGURE 22-3.

Tracheal aspiration for meconium. A. Perform endotracheal intubation with an ET tube of appropriate size. B. With the ET tube in the trachea, attach the meconium aspirator to the tube and then to wall suction. Occlude the thumb hole for suction. C. Maintain suction and gently withdraw the ET tube to aspirate. If meconium appears thick or infant does not respond with breaths or grimace, further attempts can be made with a new ET tube.

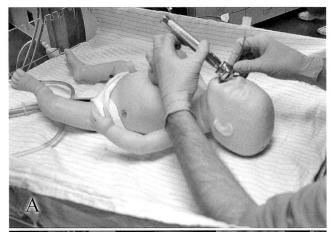

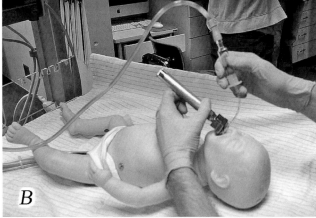

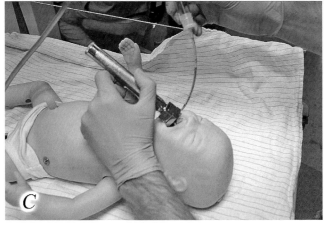

To reiterate, rapid-sequence intubation is never indicated in a neonatal resuscitation immediately postpartum. Placing a small towel under the neonate's shoulders may aid in aligning the airway. Their vocal cords lack the pearly appearance of an adult's or child's; the color is more nearly the color of the surrounding tissue. Weak respiratory effort can cause some movement of the cords, allowing distinction from the esophagus. Vocal cords can be identified by their physical proximity to the epiglottis. Once intubation is successful and confirmed (using examination and capnometry), the ET tube should be secured by bracing it against the gum and lip with one finger while an assistant tapes the tube in place. The airway is very short, so tracheal intubation can result in right mainstem bronchus placement or the tube can be dislodged with small flexion or extension of the neck. Towel rolls placed on either side of the head or a cervical collar can prevent movement. Confirm placement of all ET tubes with a chest radiograph. After the infant is intubated, be careful not to ventilate too vigorously, so as to avoid barotrauma or pneumothorax. All intubated infants should be reevaluated frequently for adverse sequelae of positive-pressure ventilation.

PEARL

Rapid-sequence intubation is never indicated immediately after delivery.

Breathing

After the initial steps, evaluation of the infant's respiratory effort, heart rate, and color should continue (Figure 22-2).[3] Stable infants may be observed. Infants with a heart rate faster than 100 beats/min and active respiratory effort but cyanosis (purely cyanotic infants) may simply need supplemental oxygen. Acrocyanosis (cyanosis limited to the hands and feet) can persist for hours and is not necessarily a sign of poor perfusion or oxygenation in newborns. Central cyanosis (cyanosis of the trunk, oral mucosa, or lips) always indicates poor perfusion or oxygenation and must be addressed immediately. Remember that a pulse oximeter placed on an acrocyanotic extremity can give falsely low oxygen levels. The AHA recommends placing a pulse oximeter on the right hand (preductal saturation) and aiming for normal oxygen saturation after 10 minutes.[2] The clinical picture is just as important as pulse oximetry for assessing respiratory status.[9]

PEARLS

A pulse oximeter placed on an acrocyanotic extremity can give falsely low oxygen levels.

Only central cyanosis (blue mucous membranes) requires intervention.

Oxygen can be delivered via any free-flowing mechanism (eg, face mask or tubing held in a cupped hand). Self-inflating devices such as a bag-valve mask must be squeezed to deliver oxygen and are not ideal for blow-by. After receiving blow-by oxygen, infants should show color change within several seconds. There is a concern among neonatologists that resuscitation on 100% oxygen can be detrimental to premature infants because of the high levels of free oxygen radicals. Prolonged oxygen use has been associated with complications such as retinopathy of prematurity and bronchopulmonary dysplasia, especially in infants born at less than 28 weeks' gestational age. Others suggest that decreased oxygen in resuscitation could lead to hypoxic-ischemic encephalopathy and intracranial hemorrhages. Current research is insufficient to make firm recommendations on resuscitation with room air.[6,10] Therefore, resuscitation with some concentration of oxygen above room air is recommended. Many neonatologists start resuscitation on 40% oxygen and titrate it as clinically indicated.

PEARL

Bag-valve-mask (BVM) ventilation of infants at 40 to 60 breaths/min

- With manometer: aim for peak airway pressures below 30–40 cm H_2O
- Without manometer: aim for gentle symmetric chest rise

Infants with a heart rate slower than 100 beats/min or apnea and those who do not improve after blow-by oxygen should receive positive-pressure ventilation via a BVM device, aiming for a respiratory rate of 40 to 60 breaths/min (Figure 22-2).[2] Infants are far more susceptible to barotrauma and pneumothorax than adults because of lower lung volumes. Therefore, a pressure gauge should be used with a flow-inflating bag to keep peak inspiratory pressures less than 30 to 40 cm H_2O in term infants and between 20 and 25 cm H_2O in preterm infants.[11] If a pressure gauge is unavailable, gently squeeze the bag only enough to provide symmetric chest rise. In cases in which BVM ventilation is ineffective and endotracheal intubation is unsuccessful, laryngeal mask airways can be used as rescue devices;

however, research into this method is limited to case studies.[12]

KEY POINT

Infants are far more susceptible to barotrauma and pneumothorax than are adults.

High airway pressures are easy to generate in newborns. Pneumothorax is not an uncommon event if peak inspiratory pressures are not monitored carefully on a manometer. However, dislodgement of the ET tube, obstruction with secretions, and mechanical failure of equipment are more common than pneumothorax. These should all be checked for before pneumothorax decompression. Congenital diaphragmatic hernia can cause unilateral absent breath sounds and tracheal deviation, and disastrous consequences can result from needle decompression or thoracostomy in these cases. Be aware of this condition and, if possible, obtain a chest film prior to decompression. If pneumothorax is suspected either clinically or on chest radiograph, needle decompression should be performed.[2] The AHA guidelines recommend placing an 18- or 20-gauge angiocatheter into the fourth intercostal space in the midaxillary line. A rush of air or fluid should occur, and the needle should be withdrawn, leaving the catheter in place. Attach the catheter to a three-way stopcock and aspirate the fluid or air with a 20-mL syringe. Secure the catheter in place prior to transport. A chest tube can be placed at the tertiary center.

Circulation

If infants do not respond to positive-pressure ventilation, their heart rate will eventually begin to drop. A neonatal heart rate is best measured by auscultation or by palpating the umbili-

---

TABLE 22-4.

Apgar mnemonic and scoring system

	0	1	2
Appearance (color)	Central cyanosis	Peripheral cyanosis	Pink
Pulse	Absent	<100 beats/min	>100 beats/min
Grimace (cry)	Absent	Grimace, no cry	Strong cry, cough
Activity (Tone)	Limp	Some flexion	Active motion
Respiratory effort	Apneic	Weak respirations	Strong respirations

---

TABLE 22-5.

Neonatal ET tube size and depth of insertion based on weight and gestational age[3]

Gestational age	Weight (g)	ET tube size	ET tube depth (at the lip)
<28 weeks	<1,000	2.5	6–7
28–34 weeks	1,000–2,000	3.0	7
34–38 weeks	2,000–3,000	3.5	8
>38 weeks	3,000–4,000	3.5	9
>38 weeks	>4,000	3.5–4.0 (rarely)	10

cus or the brachial artery. Any heart rate less than 60 beats/min requires chest compressions to ensure circulation and oxygen delivery to vital organs (Figure 22-2).[2] If a definitive airway has not yet been established, intubate and start chest compressions simultaneously. Perform chest compressions with two fingers over the middle of the chest or by encircling the chest with both hands and compressing with the thumbs. Evidence suggests that using the two-hand technique achieves greater systolic blood pressure and coronary perfusion and is recommended over the two-finger technique.[13] Perform chest compressions at a rate of 100 beats/min, alternating three compressions to one breath.[4] Heart rate and respiratory status should be reassessed frequently.

KEY POINT
Any heart rate less than 60 beats/min requires chest compressions to ensure circulation and oxygen delivery to vital organs.[2]

PEARL
The pulse in an infant is best palpated at the umbilical artery.

If vascular access has not yet been established, an umbilical central line should be placed (Figure 22-4).[3] Preparation should be similar to that for any other central line placement, using sterile technique and an antiseptic wash such as chlorhexidine or povidone-iodine. Place a sterile string or tie at the base of the umbilicus to aid in bleeding control. Using a scalpel, incise the umbilicus and identify two umbilical arteries (smaller) and one umbilical vein (larger). Use fine forceps to gently dilate the umbilical vein as needed and place an umbilical venous catheter into the vein. For emergency purposes, most catheters can be inserted to a depth of 5 cm and used immediately as a "low umbilical line." Suture the umbilical line into the skin, being careful to avoid the Wharton jelly (the gelatinous substance of which the umbilical cord is made), in a manner similar to that used for chest tubes. An abdominal radiograph should be ordered to confirm placement because umbilical lines that are placed too deeply can extend into the liver.

FIGURE 22-4.
Placement of an umbilical central line. A. Prep and drape the umbilicus in sterile fashion and place an umbilical tie at the base to control bleeding. B. Cut the umbilicus to expose the umbilical arteries and vein. The vein will be thin-walled compared with the thicker-walled arteries. C. Carefully dilate the umbilical vein with hooked forceps and cannulate the vein with an umbilical catheter. D. Attach a three-way stopcock and syringe and aspirate until blood flows easily. Pass the umbilical catheter to 5 cm for a low umbilical line.

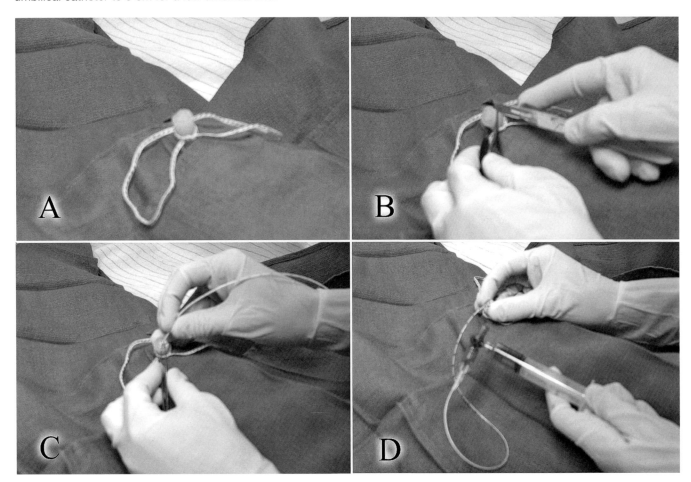

Drugs, Dextrose, and Diagnostics: Postresuscitation Care

If the heart rate continues to be less than 60 beats/min after an airway has been established, adequate ventilation has been given, and 30 seconds of chest compressions have been performed, epinephrine is the drug of choice, according to AHA guidelines (Figure 22-2).[2] Again, without adequate ventilation, cardiac resuscitation in newborns is futile. Once intravenous access has been established, use 1:10,000 strength epinephrine at 0.1 to 0.3 mL/kg rapid push (equal to 0.01–0.03 mg/kg).[14] This and other resuscitation drugs are listed with doses in Table 22-6. If the neonate's actual weight is unknown, use estimated weights from Table 22-5. Previous AHA guidelines recommended 0.3 to 1 mL/kg (0.03–0.1 mg/kg) of endotracheal epinephrine if intravenous access could not be obtained. However, recent research has shown endotracheal epinephrine to be unsatisfactory at previously recommended doses.[6,15] Therefore, intravenous administration of epinephrine is currently recommended. Continue chest compressions and reassess the heart rate after 30 seconds (Figure 22-2).[2]

Naloxone has traditionally been used at a dose of 0.1 mg/kg, but its role has never been studied. Use of naloxone in an infant with respiratory depression born to an opiate-addicted mother has been known to precipitate seizures.[16] In general, newborns thought to have respiratory depression from maternal opiate use should be given positive-pressure ventilation until opiates are metabolized rather than risk the potential adverse effect of naloxone-induced seizures.

PEARL

Use of naloxone in an infant with respiratory depression born to an opiate-addicted mother has been known to precipitate seizures.[16]

There is also a precedent and a theoretical basis for sodium bicarbonate use, but its effectiveness has not been well studied. During prolonged resuscitation, infants can develop severe acidosis. The administration of sodium bicarbonate is thought to improve the effectiveness of medications such as epinephrine and to prevent encephalopathy or death. Doses of 4 mL/kg of 5% sodium bicarbonate are given over several minutes in cases of confirmed acidosis on arterial or venous blood gas sampling. However, a few randomized controlled trials have shown no change in morbidity or mortality.[17]

Infants with evidence of blood loss (ie, known abruption, pallor, poor response to resuscitation) may need intravascular repletion. Isotonic crystalloids such as normal saline or Ringer lactate should be used cautiously at a dose of 10 to 20 mL/kg. Neonates are highly susceptible to fluid shifts and subsequent intraventricular hemorrhage and edema from rapid infusion of volume expanders, so crystalloids should be given slowly over 5 to 10 minutes.[3,18] Transfusion of blood products during the initial resuscitation is poorly studied and is neither recommended nor discouraged by AHA guidelines. In emergent cases, irradiated packed red blood cells free of cytomegalovirus can be transfused at 10 mL/kg; however, consultation with a neonatologist is recommended prior to initiating a transfusion.

Infants unresponsive to volume replacement may need inotropic or vasoactive pressor support. No one pressor has been shown to be superior in neonatal shock, but pressors should be selected based on the cause of the hypotension. Dopamine started at 2 mcg/kg/min is traditionally the pressor of choice in noncardiogenic shock, and milrinone started at 0.5 to 0.75 mcg/kg/min is the recommended pressor in cardiogenic shock.[12,14,19]

PEARL

If $D_{10}W$ is unavailable, dilute one ampule of $D_{50}W$ in 200 mL of sterile water to make $D_{10}W$.

Once an infant has been stabilized with a heart rate above 100 beats/min and stable respirations, the blood glucose concentration must be measured. A heelstick blood sugar concentration greater than 40 mg/dL is acceptable in a neonate[14]; anything less should be treated with a 2-mL/kg bolus of $D_{10}W$ infused over several minutes. $D_{50}W$ should not be used, as the osmotic load is too high. If $D_{10}W$ is unavailable, an ampule of $D_{50}W$ can be diluted in 200 mL of sterile water to yield $D_{10}W$. $D_{10}\frac{1}{4}NS$ should be used as maintenance fluid at a rate of 4 mL/kg/hr in term infants (based on 80–100 mL/kg/day) and 5 mL/kg/hr in preterm infants (based on 100–120 mL/kg/day). Smaller infants have a higher body surface-to-volume ratio and will lose fluids more quickly via insensible losses and thus require more fluids.

KEY POINT

A heelstick blood sugar concentration greater than 40 mg/dL is acceptable in a neonate[14]; anything less should be treated with a 2-mL/kg bolus of $D_{10}W$ infused over several minutes.

TABLE 22-6.

Common drugs used in neonatal resuscitation[14]

Resuscitation Medications
- Epinephrine (1:10,000)
  - 0.1–0.3 mL/kg IV
  - 0.3–1 mL/kg ET tube
- $D_{10}W$, 2 mL/kg
- Crystalloid/blood products, 10–20 mL/kg
- Naloxone, 0.01 mg/kg[a]
- Sodium bicarbonate, 4 mg/kg[a]

Postresuscitation
- Vitamin K, 0.5–1 mL IM

Cardiac
- Prostaglandin E_1, 0.05–0.1 mcg/kg/min
- Dopamine, 2 mcg/kg/min, starting dose
- Milrinone, 0.5–0.75 mcg/kg/min
- Furosemide, 1–2 mg/kg

Antibiotics/Antivirals
- Ampicillin, 50–100 mg/kg
- Gentamicin, 3 mg/kg
- Acyclovir, 20–30 mg/kg[a]

[a]Discuss with neonatologist prior to use.

PEARL

Start intravenous maintenance fluids and give intramuscular vitamin K prior to transfer.

- Term infants: $D_{10}\frac{1}{4}NS$ at 4 mL/kg/hr; vitamin K, 1 mg

- Preterm infants: $D_{10}\frac{1}{4}NS$ at 5 mL/kg/hr; vitamin K, 0.5 mg

All newborns require vitamin K to prevent hemorrhagic disease of the newborn. Vitamin K is given in a dose of 0.5 to 1 mg IM[14]; give 1 mg to larger infants and 0.5 mg to premature infants. Vitamin K should be given to all infants within an hour of birth regardless of their clinical condition. If the infant will be transferred to a tertiary NICU, give vitamin K prior to transfer. Erythromycin ophthalmic ointment should also be placed on both eyes to prevent gonococcal and chlamydial infections. This, however, is not emergent and can be delayed in a critically ill infant until a tertiary center is reached.

PEARL

Vitamin K should be given to all infants within an hour of birth regardless of their clinical condition.

Prostaglandin E_1 (PGE_1) is given as a drip at 0.05 to 0.1 mcg/kg/min to newborns with ductal-dependent congenital heart disease; the indications are discussed later in this chapter.[14] The well-known adverse effect of PGE_1 is apnea; however, the occurrence of apnea is rare except with high doses. Infants receiving PGE_1 do not necessarily need to be intubated empirically or for transport.[20] Instead, they should be monitored closely for signs of respiratory distress or cardiovascular compromise, and the drip should be decreased to the lowest effective dose possible to achieve good oxygenation.

Herpes simplex virus, although uncommon, can be deadly in infants. Signs and symptoms suggestive of herpetic infection include vesicular skin lesions and seizures; the neonate is at risk if the mother has active genital (not oral) lesions at the time of delivery. The virus should be treated initially with acyclovir: 20 mg/kg for newborns of less than 35 weeks' gestational age and 30 mg/kg for those born after 35 weeks' gestation.[14] Consultation with a neonatologist is recommended prior to initiation of acyclovir.

Important urgent laboratory studies to obtain on a neonate following resuscitation include a complete blood count with differential and platelets (CBC), electrolytes, blood cultures, and an arterial blood gas (ABG). The NICU will also want a blood type with Coombs test to check for ABO incompatibility as well as total and direct bilirubin levels to monitor for jaundice. A chest film should be obtained to evaluate for aspiration, pneumonia, and ET tube placement, if necessary.

PEARL

Postresuscitation laboratory tests

- CBC with differential and platelets

- Electrolytes, BUN, creatinine, and total and direct bilirubin

- ABG, blood cultures

- Type and screen with direct/indirect Coombs test

Respiratory status is still the utmost concern after resuscitation. Serious causes of respiratory compromise include sepsis, meconium aspiration, neonatal respiratory distress syndrome (due to lack of surfactant in premature infants), congenital diaphragmatic hernia, and a myriad of genetic disorders. However, sepsis is the most common serious cause. Intubated infants should be monitored for signs of pneumothorax, including hypoxia and high peak inspiratory pressures. Nonintubated infants should be monitored for work of breathing. Grunting, retractions, and sustained respiratory rates greater than 70 breaths/min can be indicators of impending respiratory compromise.

PEARL

Grunting, retractions, and sustained respiratory rates greater than 70 breaths/min can be indicators of impending respiratory compromise.

Any infant with a difficult resuscitation, a history of maternal fever, or evidence of respiratory distress after delivery should be assumed septic until proved otherwise. Ampicillin, 50 to 100 mg/kg per dose, and gentamicin, 3 mg/kg per dose, should be given empirically after blood cultures are drawn.[14]

KEY POINT

Any infant with a difficult resuscitation, a history of maternal fever, or evidence of respiratory distress after delivery should be assumed septic until proved otherwise.

Newborns should be kept warm using an overhead warmer, warm blankets, or maternal skin-to-skin contact. However, new studies are proposing a role for induced hypothermia in infants

TABLE 22-7.

Common congenital heart diseases

Persistently cyanotic	Low cardiac output	Congestive heart failure
Blue baby	*Gray baby*	*Wet, tired baby*
- Tetralogy of Fallot	*Think sepsis first*	- Ventricular septal defect
- Pulmonary stenosis/atresia	- Coarctation of the aorta	- Atrial septal defect
- Tricuspid atresia	- Interrupted aorta	- Patent ductus arteriosus
- Transposition of great arteries	- Hypoplastic left heart syndrome	
- Truncus arteriosus	- Aortic stenosis	
- Total anomalous pulmonary venous return	- Arrhythmias	

with suspected intra-uterine asphyxia and profound metabolic acidosis.[21,22] Infants with moderate encephalopathy had a survival benefit when cooled to 33.5°C. However, this strategy is not to be used routinely and should be discussed with a neonatologist prior to initiation. As a general rule, normothermia should be the goal for newborns.

Congenital Heart Disease

Undiagnosed congenital heart disease (CHD) is always a concern in precipitous deliveries. Identifying the exact structural defect in congenital heart disease is not nearly as important as identifying and treating the pathophysiology behind it. Critical cardiac lesions in neonates will present in three ways: 1) persistent cyanosis, 2) low cardiac output, and 3) congestive heart failure (Table 22-7).[23] Any neonate with these signs or symptoms should have a chest film and an ECG. Early consultation with a pediatric cardiologist should be obtained. An echocardiogram should be considered early.

Persistent cyanosis in an infant *without respiratory distress* can be a manifestation of cardiac lesions, persistent pulmonary hypertension, or lung disease.[23] These infants often appear "comfortably blue" and usually will have a loud murmur on examination. Parenchymal lung disease is normally easily identified on a chest film; however, a hyperoxia test should be used for better diagnosis. The hyperoxia test involves comparing arterial oxygen saturation on room air with saturation on 100% oxygen. Measure Po_2 using a pre- and post-oxygenation ABG measurement. A Po_2 of less than 100 mm Hg is suggestive of CHD with significant right-to-left shunting. Importantly, an infant with persistent pulmonary hypertension can have a negative

hyperoxia test. Any neonate with a failed hyperoxia test should receive PGE_1 for both a therapeutic and a diagnostic trial. Total anomalous pulmonary venous return (TAPVR) is the one cardiac abnormality that will produce a normal hyperoxia test and will not respond to PGE_1. The quickest way to diagnose this condition is with an echocardiogram. Emergent surgical intervention is the only treatment. Classic chest radiographic findings in persistently cyanotic infants include a boot-shaped heart in those with tetralogy of Fallot, a "snowman" appearance in those with TAPVR, and an "egg-on-a-string" appearance in those with transposition of the great arteries.

PEARL

The hyperoxia test

- Obtain ABG measurements on room air and 100% O_2
- Po_2 >100 mm Hg = Primary pulmonary disease = No PGE_1
- Po_2 <100 mm Hg = CHD with right-to-left shunting or persistent pulmonary hypertension = Trial of PGE_1

Pitfalls

- Pulse oximetry is *not* an acceptable substitute for Po_2
- Neonates with TAPVR can have a Po_2 >100 mm Hg and no response to PGE_1

Poor cardiac output manifests as pale-gray infants with poor peripheral pulses and often no murmur.[23] These neonates appear septic and should be treated with intravenous fluid resuscitation and antibiotics initially because sepsis is far more common than CHD. In patients who do not respond to initial sepsis treatment, CHD should be considered. Comparing pulse ox-

TABLE 22-8.

Common congenital anomalies requiring immediate intervention

Disorder	Examination findings	Interventions
Congenital diaphragmatic hernia	Respiratory distress	Immediate intubation
	Scaphoid abdomen	Nasogastric tube placement for decompression
	Bowel above the diaphragm on chest film	
Gastroschisis	Evisceration of bowel through abdominal wall defect without a protective sac	Cover bowel in wet, sterile saline gauze, then in a plastic cellophane bag
		Avoid touching or twisting bowel as much as possible
		Nasogastric tube placement for decompression
		Ampicillin/gentamicin
Omphalocele	Evisceration of bowel through abdominal wall defect with a protective sac	Cover bowel in wet, sterile saline gauze, then in plastic cellophane
		Avoid touching or twisting bowel as much as possible
		Nasogastric tube placement for decompression
Choanal atresia	Respiratory distress	Immediate endotracheal intubation
	Inability to pass nasogastric tube	

imetry on a preductal extremity (right arm) and postductal extremity (left leg) can identify aortic lesions such as coarctation or interrupted aortic arch. Blood pressures in the four extremities may show higher preductal blood pressures compared with postductal pressures. An early echocardiogram in these patients will reveal lesions such as hypoplastic left heart disease or aortic stenosis that are ductal-dependent but not readily identifiable by examination. If an echocardiogram cannot be obtained, a trial of PGE_1 is warranted. Again, early consultation with a pediatric cardiologist is essential. Tachyarrhythmias or congenital heart block are exceedingly rare but can be identified quickly from the heart rate and cardiac monitor reading and confirmed on ECG. In supraventricular tachycardia, adenosine is dosed at 0.05 to 0.1 mg/kg in stable patients, and synchronized cardioversion is used at 0.5 J/kg in unstable patients. Congenital complete heart block needs emergent pacemaker placement.

Congestive heart failure does not immediately manifest at birth but rather takes several weeks to months for the right ventricle to start to fail as the left-to-right shunts become right-to-left shunts.[23] Infants will have symptoms of lethargy, poor feeding, or sweating or cyanosis with feeds. Tachypnea, hepatomegaly, failure to thrive, and murmurs are common findings. These infants will also appear septic but will actually worsen with administration of intravenous fluids. A chest film will likely show cardiomegaly with pulmonary congestion, and an echocardiogram will confirm the diagnosis. Use of diuretics such as furosemide, 0.5 to 1 mg/kg, can help improve oxygenation, and inotropes such as milrinone, 0.5 to 0.75 mcg/kg/min, can improve cardiac output.[14]

Other Specific Congenital Anomalies

Several congenital anomalies are common to NICU settings but are rarely encountered in emergency departments. After stabilization, neonates with these anomalies should be transferred to a tertiary care NICU for further management. Specific emergent interventions are presented in Table 22-8.[24]

Withholding or Discontinuing Resuscitation

A neonatal resuscitation is difficult enough without the consideration of withdrawal of care. However, there are appropriate times to withdraw resuscitative efforts if the parents are in agreement.[25–27] Infants born at less than 23 weeks' gestational age or with a birth weight less than 500 g have a high mortality rate and even higher morbidity rate. Similarly, infants without respiratory effort or pulse after 10 minutes of resuscitation have high mortality rates and severe neurologic deficits. In these circumstances, cessation or withholding of resuscitative measures should be discussed with the parents. Severe congenital abnormalities such as anencephaly and trisomy 13 are also considered to be incompatible with life, and resuscitation may be withheld. However, emergency physicians are not expected to be experts on congenital anomalies and should always err on the side of resuscitation if they are unsure of the infant's prognosis.

Conclusion

Few things are as stressful for the emergency physician as resuscitating a critically ill neonate following a precipitous emergency department delivery. Most critically ill neonates have a respiratory cause of their distress; therefore, the airway should be assessed and ventilation should be supplied within the first 60 seconds after evaluation. Equally important as assessing respiratory status is keeping the neonate warm and dry. Neonates who remain bradycardic despite supplemental oxygen and positive-pressure ventilation require compressions and possibly epinephrine. Once resuscitated, critically ill neonates should receive intravenous fluids containing dextrose, vitamin K, and broad-spectrum antibiotics. Congenital heart disease should be suspected in neonates not responding to these therapies. With a systematic approach to the critically ill neonate, the emergency physician can ultimately reduce morbidity and mortality.

References

1. Sutton L, Sayer GP, Bajuk B, et al. Do very sick neonates born at term have antenatal risks? 2. Infants ventilated primarily for problems of adaptation to extra-uterine life. *Acta Obstet Gynecol Scand.* 2001;80:905-916.
2. Kattwinkel J, Perlman JM, Aziz K, et al. Special Report—Neonatal Resuscitation: 2010 American Heart Association Guidelines for Cardiopulmonary Resuscitation and Emergency Cardiovascular Care. *Pediatrics.* 2010;126:e1400-e1413.
3. Katwinkel J, ed. *Textbook of Neonatal Resuscitation.* 6th ed. Oak Grove Village, IL: American Academy of Pediatrics and American Heart Association; 2011.
3. Clyman R. Mechanisms regulating closure of ductus arteriosus. In: Polin RA, Fox WW, Abman S, eds. *Fetal and Neonatal Physiology.* 3rd ed. Philadelphia, PA: WB Saunders; 2003:743-748.
4. Vohra S, Frent G, Campbell V, Abbott M, Whyte R. Effect of polyethylene occlusive skin wrapping on heat loss in very low birth weight infants at delivery: a randomized trial. *J Pediatr.* 1999;134:547-551.
5. Saugstad OD. New guidelines for newborn resuscitation. *Acta Paediatr.* 2007;96(3):333-337.
6. Vain NE, Szyld EG, Prudent LM, Wiswell TE, Aguilar AM, Vivas NI. Oropharyngeal and nasopharyngeal suctioning of meconium-stained neonates before delivery of their shoulders: multicentre, randomised controlled trial. *Lancet.* 2004;364:597-602.
7. Wiswell TE, Gannon CM, Jacob J, et al. Delivery room management of the apparently vigorous meconium-stained neonate: results of the multicenter, international collaborative trial. *Pediatrics.* 2000;105:1-7.
8. Toth B, Becker A, Seelbach-Gobel B. Oxygen saturation in healthy newborn infants immediately after birth measured by pulse oximetry. *Arch Gynecol Obstet.* 2002;266:105-107.
9. Davis PG, Tan A, O'Donnell CP, Schulze A. Resuscitation of newborn infants with 100% oxygen or air: a systematic review and meta-analysis. *Lancet.* 2004;364:1329-1333.
10. Vyas H, Milner AD, Hopkin IE, Boon AW. Physiologic responses to prolonged and slow-rise inflation in the resuscitation of the asphyxiated newborn infant. *J Pediatr.* 1981;99:635-639.
11. Paterson SJ, Byrne PJ, Molesky MG, Seal RF, Finucane BT. Neonatal resuscitation using the laryngeal mask airway. *Anesthesiology.* 1994;80:1248-1253.
12. Houri PK, Frank LR, Menegazzi JJ, Taylor R. A randomized, controlled trial of two-thumb vs two-finger chest compression in a swine infant model of cardiac arrest. *Prehosp Emerg Care.* 1997;1:65-67.
13. Lee C, Custer J, Rau R. Drug doses. In: Custer J, Rau R, eds. *The Harriet Lane Handbook: A Manual for Pediatric House Officer.* 18th ed. Philadelphia, PA: Mosby; 2009.
14. Barber CA, Wyckoff MH. Use and efficacy of endotracheal versus intravenous epinephrine during neonatal cardiopulmonary resuscitation in the delivery room. *Pediatrics.* 2006;118:1028-1034.
15. Gibbs J, Newson T, Williams J, Davidson DC. Naloxone hazard in infant of opioid abuser. *Lancet.* 1989;2(8655):159-160.
16. Lokesh L, Kumar P, Murki S, Narang A. A randomized controlled trial of sodium bicarbonate in neonatal resuscitation—effect on immediate outcome. *Resuscitation.* 2004;60:219-223.
17. So KW, Fok TF, Ng PC, Wong WW, Cheung KL. Randomised controlled trial of colloid or crystalloid in hypotensive preterm infants. *Arch Dis Child Fetal Neonatal Ed.* 1997;76:F43-F46.
18. Noori S, Friedlich P, Seri I. Pathophysiology of neonatal shock. In: Polin RA, Fox WW, Abman S, eds. *Fetal and Neonatal Physiology.* 3rd ed. Philadelphia, PA: WB Saunders; 2003:772–782.
19. Meckler GD, Lowe C. To intubate or not to intubate? Transporting infants on prostaglandin E1. *Pediatrics.* 2009;123:e25-e30.

20. Gluckman PD, Wyatt JS, Azzopardi D, et al. Selective head cooling with mild systemic hypothermia after neonatal encephalopathy: multicentre randomised trial. *Lancet.* 2005;365:663-670.

21. Donovan EF, Fanaroff AA, Poole WK, et al. Whole-body hypothermia for neonates with hypoxic-ischemic encephalopathy. *N Engl J Med.* 2005;353:1574-1584.

22. Brooks PA, Penny DJ. Management of the sick neonate with suspected heart disease. *Early Hum Dev.* 2008;84:155-159.

23. Stoll B, Adams-Chapman I. Delivery room emergencies. In: Behrman R, Kliegman R, Jenson HB, Stanton BF, eds. *Nelson Textbook of Pediatrics.* 18th ed. Philadelphia, PA: Saunders Elsevier; 2007:1532.

24. Draper ES, Manktelow B, Field DJ, James D. Tables for predicting survival for preterm births are updated. *BMJ.* 2003;327:872.

25. Jain L, Ferre C, Vidyasagar D, Nath S, Sheftel D. Cardiopulmonary resuscitation of apparently stillborn infants: survival and long-term outcome. *J Pediatr.* 1991;118:778-782.

26. Haddad B, Mercer BM, Livingston JC, Talati A, Sibai BM. Outcome after successful resuscitation of babies born with Apgar scores of 0 at both 1 and 5 minutes. *Am J Obstet Gynecol.* 2000;182:1210-1214.

CHAPTER 23

Pediatric Resuscitation

Jenny S. Mendelson and Chad D. Viscusi

Introduction

Children account for more than 30 million annual visits to emergency departments in the United States, or 25% to 35% of the total number of visits.[1] Despite the enormity of this number, many emergency physicians confess to feeling less prepared to handle pediatric than adult patients. This discomfort is magnified when it comes to caring for a critically ill or crashing child.[2] Most emergency physicians see relatively few critically ill pediatric patients and thus have few opportunities to refine their skills in advanced pediatric life-saving techniques. Therefore, familiarity and practice with pediatric resuscitation algorithms are paramount.

Initial Assessment

When facing a critically ill pediatric patient, an adept emergency physician must be able to make a rapid global clinical assessment. One approach to this initial assessment is the pediatric assessment triangle (PAT). This is a widely published and recognized tool used to assess children of all ages with all levels of illness and injury. The PAT focuses attention on three components—appearance, work of breathing, and circulation—facilitating a rapid assessment and triage of patients into categories of "sick" or "not sick." The PAT does not require a stethoscope or monitoring equipment and can be completed in less than 30 seconds.[3]

To assess the general appearance of the child, the "tickles" (TICLS) mnemonic can be used. The following features should be assessed: **t**one (moving and resisting examination versus being limp and listless), **i**nteractiveness (alert and attentive versus uninterested or unresponsive), **c**onsolability (comforted by caregiver versus agitated and crying), **l**ook/gaze (fixing on faces or toys versus staring aimlessly and unfocused), and **s**peech/cry (cry is loud and strong versus weak and hoarse). The TICLS assessment can identify more subtle abnormalities than the traditional "AVPU" (alert, voice, pain, unresponsive) scale. For instance, a child can be on the verge of respiratory failure and still remain "alert."

After the general appearance is assessed, the child's work of breathing should be evaluated. Unlike in adults, work of breathing in a child is often a better assessment of oxygenation and ventilation status than breath sounds and respiratory rate. The child should be evaluated for abnormal audible airway sounds, abnormal positioning, retractions, and flaring. The predominant signs of respiratory distress in children are outlined in Table 23-1. Once a child in respiratory distress tires, these signs may become less apparent. Slowing of the respiratory rate and shallow breathing can signal impending respiratory failure.

FIGURE 23-1.

Algorithm for tachycardia in pediatric patients.[20] (Source: American Heart Association, Inc.)

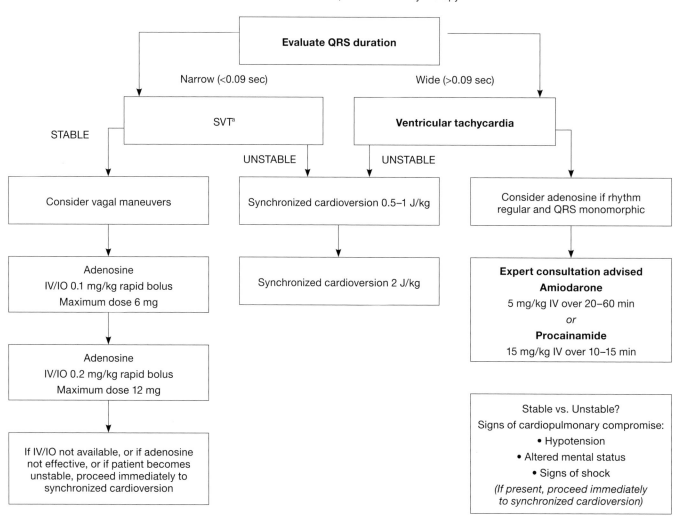

FIGURE 23-2.

Algorithm for cardiac arrest in pediatric patients.[20] (Source: American Heart Association, Inc.)

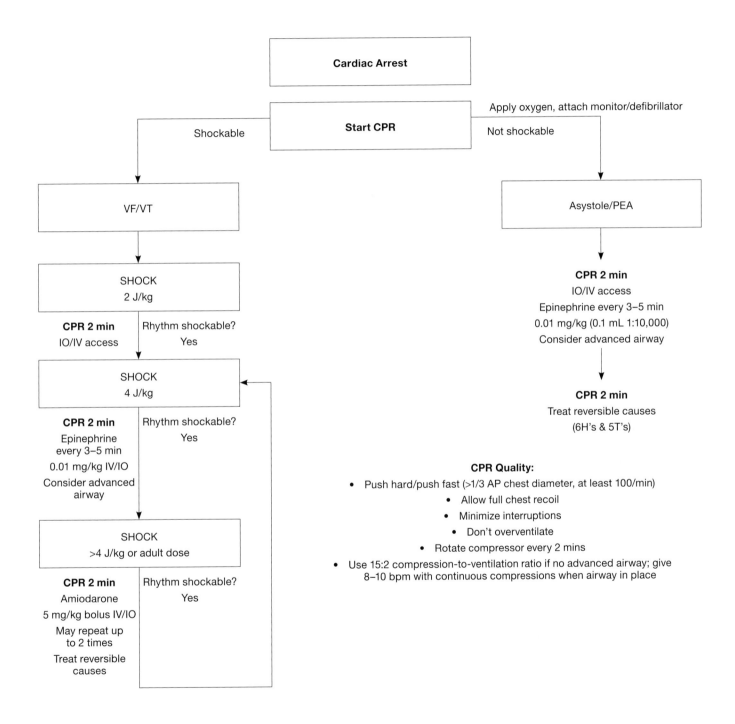

FIGURE 23-3.

Algorithm for bradycardia in pediatric patients.[20] (Source: American Heart Association, Inc.)

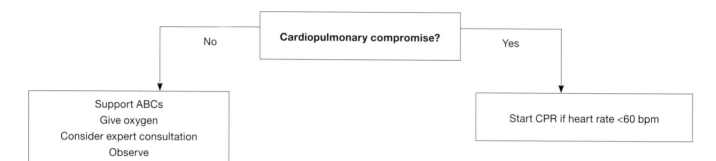

**Bradycardia
w/ pulse and poor perfusion**

Identify and treat underlying cause
• Maintain patent airway, assist breathing if necessary
• Apply oxygen, cardiac monitors, oximetry; obtain IV/IO access
• 12-lead ECG if available, but do not delay therapy

Cardiopulmonary compromise?

No

Yes

Support ABCs
Give oxygen
Consider expert consultation
Observe

Start CPR if heart rate <60 bpm

Epinephrine
0.01 mg/kg IV/IO (0.1 mL 1:10,000)
Repeat every 3–5 min
Atropine
0.02 mg/kg IV/IO
Use for increased vagal tone
or primary AV block
Consider transthoracic or transvenous
pacing
Treat underlying causes

**If pulseless arrest develops, proceed to
cardiac arrest algorithm (Figure 23-2).**

PEARL

Slowing of the respiratory rate and shallow breathing can signal impending respiratory failure.

The final component of the PAT is an assessment of the circulation to the skin, looking for pallor, mottling, and cyanosis. Cyanosis, while certainly a clear and dramatic sign, has significant limitations as a diagnostic tool. It depends on the amount of hemoglobin in the blood and the status of the peripheral circulation. A child with severe anemia, for example, may have significant hypoxia without any visible cyanosis. Conversely, a very young infant whose hemoglobin has not yet fallen from the high levels found at birth may have peripheral cyanosis despite a normal central blood oxygen concentration.

The PAT gives a quick reflection of the adequacy of ventilation, oxygenation, and central nervous system function and subsequently assists with early recognition and prioritization of problems. Combining the three elements of the PAT can establish severity. A child with a normal appearance and increased work of breathing is in respiratory distress. Abnormal appearance and increased work of breathing can be signs of early respiratory failure. Abnormal appearance and abnormally decreased work of breathing are seen in late respiratory failure. Abnormal appearance and decreased circulation indicate shock and should prompt rapid progression through the pediatric primary survey to initiate resuscitation.

Along with the primary assessment, one of the first steps in the evaluation of a critically ill child should be a measurement of weight. If the weight is unknown or cannot be determined immediately, it can be estimated by the following formula:

$$\text{Weight (kg)} = 2 \times \text{age (years)} + 10$$

However, it is preferable to use a resuscitation tool such as a Broselow tape, which provides recommended equipment sizes and drug doses based on the patient's length. This eliminates the need to estimate the patient's age and weight and reduces the risk of error based on miscalculation during times of high stress.[4]

KEY POINTS

Briefly assess the patient's appearance, work of breathing, and circulation. This will allow you to determine the severity of the patient's condition and direct further management.

Use a length-based resuscitation tape (eg, Broselow tape) to determine equipment sizes and drug doses.

Pediatric Primary Survey: The ABCs

In contrast to the PAT, which can be performed in any order, the pediatric primary survey is an ordered, comprehensive, hands-on evaluation of cardiopulmonary status. The sequence of interventions is crucial. First and foremost, the airway must be evaluated and secured. Breathing must be supported or controlled. Circulation and perfusion must be reestablished or enhanced. As in adults, the primary survey provides a specific, regimented approach for identifying and treating life threats before moving to the next step. Although the steps in the survey are the same as for adults, the differences in the anatomy and physiology of children can make diagnosis and management challenging.

Airway

As with adults, the primary reasons for pediatric airway management include inadequate oxygenation, inadequate ventilation, or inadequate airway protection. However, not every critically ill child needs to be intubated. Well-performed noninvasive ventilation is usually sufficient, and several studies have shown that it is safer and as effective as endotracheal (ET) intubation, especially in the prehospital setting.[5-7] Effective bag-valve-mask (BVM) ventilation is one of the most critical resuscitation skills to master. Consideration should be given to several anatomic and physiologic differences between pediatric and adult airways when managing a child with respiratory distress or respiratory failure. As children grow, their anatomy and physiology become more similar to those of adults, and by age 8, the airway is thought to approximate the adult form.

Anatomic features of the pediatric patient that affect airway management include a more prominent occiput, a relatively large tongue, small nasal passages, hypertrophied lymphoid tissue, a short trachea, a long epiglottis, and a larynx that is more anterior and more cephalad than in adults.[8] When the child is lying on a flat surface, the size of the occiput causes neck flexion and potential airway compromise. This can be overcome

TABLE 23-1.

Signs of respiratory distress in children

Abdominal breathing
Accessory muscle use
Diaphoresis
Grunting
Nasal flaring
Retractions
Tachypnea
Tripod positioning

TABLE 23-2.

Endotracheal tube and laryngoscope blade sizes

Size of uncuffed ET tube = (age in years / 4) + 4
Size of cuffed ET tube (after age 2) = (age in years / 4) + 3.5
Suggested laryngoscope blades • Premature infant: #0 Miller blade (straight) • Term infant, small child: #1 Miller blade (straight) • Child <8 years old: #2 Macintosh blade (curved) • Adolescent/adult: #3 Macintosh blade (curved)

by placing a towel roll behind the infant's shoulders. However, overextension of the neck can also result in airway obstruction. Infants are obligate nose breathers until age 3 to 6 months, and during this time even minor congestion can lead to obstruction. The infant's tongue is larger in proportion to the oral cavity and can easily obstruct the airway. The epiglottis is longer and omega shaped and is positioned in a short neck close to prominent adenoid and tonsillar tissue. The long epiglottis can obscure the laryngoscopic view of the cords, and this can be overcome by direct elevation using a straight blade (Miller) rather than indirect elevation using a curved blade (Macintosh) placed in the vallecula. The glottic opening lies at approximately the level of C2 or C3 in an infant or child, as opposed to C3 or C4 in the adolescent or adult. This superior (cephalad) and anterior placement can make the airway difficult to see behind the tongue on laryngoscopy. Because the cricoid ring is the narrowest portion of the pediatric airway, as opposed to the vocal cords in adults, it is possible that the tube will pass through the cords but not any further.[9] Finally, the diameter of the pediatric airway is much smaller than the adult airway, making it far more vulnerable to obstruction by foreign objects and edema. Minor narrowing from respiratory infection or bronchospasm can result in profound airway compromise.

Physiologic differences between children and adults that complicate airway management include increased oxygen consumption and metabolic rate and decreased pulmonary reserve. Infants have 40% the functional residual capacity (FRC) of adults while awake and only 10% the FRC of adults while asleep. This decreased FRC means infants have less oxygen available for gas exchange during exhalation or apnea. Additionally, infants have a higher metabolic rate than adults, consuming at least 6 mL of oxygen per minute, compared with only 3 mL/min in an adult. All these factors cause infants and children to desaturate much more rapidly than adults during periods of apnea,

despite adequate preoxygenation.[9] These factors also conspire to give the intubator less time for direct laryngoscopy in a sick child. The infant and small child are at further risk of respiratory problems because of their immature physiologic responses. The infant may become apneic and bradycardic in response to a hypoxic challenge instead of increasing the respiratory effort and heart rate.[10]

KEY POINT

Physiologic differences between children and adults that complicate airway management include increased oxygen consumption and metabolic rate and decreased pulmonary reserve.

Adequate positioning and airway clearance can be all that is needed to relieve obstruction. The first step should be to place the child in the "sniffing position," with neck extended and chin lifted. If there is concern about cervical spinal injury, a jaw thrust should be used instead. If the jaw thrust is ineffective, it is necessary to use the head-tilt/chin-lift technique to establish a patent airway. Supplemental oxygen should be supplied and secretions cleared by suctioning. Placement of a nasal or oral airway can relieve obstruction caused by a large tongue. Oral airways should be used only in patients without a gag reflex. The appropriate size can be determined by holding the oral airway next to the child's face; with the flange held at the corner of the mouth, the tip of the airway will reach the angle of the mandible. Using the correct size is crucial, as an airway that is too small can push the tongue down and worsen obstruction, whereas an airway that is too large can cause pharyngeal trauma. Nasal airways can be used in awake patients but cannot be used if there is possible basilar skull fracture or coagulopathy. They should be used cautiously in infants because an infant's hypertrophied adenoids and tonsils can be traumatized by airway insertion, resulting in bleeding. The risk of bleeding can be minimized by inserting the bevel away from the nasal septum. The appropriately sized nasal airway should reach from the nostril to the tragus of the ear when held against the face, and its width should be less than that of the nostril.

Although BVM ventilation should be considered the "gold standard" for initial airway management, tracheal intubation offers the advantage of long-term airway maintenance and some

TABLE 23-3.

Evaluating the difficult airway using the LEMON mnemonic. Adapted with permission from "The Difficult Airway Course: Emergency," Airway Management Education Center, www.theairwaysite.com, and from Murphy MF, Walls RM. Identification of the difficult and failed airway. In: Walls RM, Murphy MF, eds. *Manual of Emergency Airway Management.* 3rd ed. Philadelphia, PA: Lippincott Williams & Wilkins; 2008:81-93.

L: Look externally (short neck, large tongue, micrognathia)
E: Evaluate the 3-3-2 rule (incisor distance <3 fingerbreadths, hyoid/mentum distance <3 fingerbreadths, thyroid-to-mouth distance <2 fingerbreadths)
M: Mallampati (Mallampati score ≥ 3)
O: Obstruction and obesity (presence of any condition that could cause an obstructed airway)
N: Neck mobility (limited neck mobility)

TABLE 23-4.

Equipment needed for intubation (the SOAP ME mnemonic)

S: Suction (catheters and Yankauer tips)
O: Oxygen (nasal cannula, oxygen flow, masks, and appropriate bag)
A: Airway (appropriate ET tube, oral/nasal airway, stylets, laryngoscope with functioning light and appropriate blades)
P: Pharmacology (RSI medications)
ME: Monitoring equipment (end-tidal CO_2 detector, stethoscope, monitors)

protection from aspiration of gastric contents.[11] Determining the appropriate size of airway equipment can be challenging in children. If a length-based resuscitation tape is not available, an age-based formula can be used to estimate ET tube size (Table 23-2). This has been found to be more accurate than estimating ET tube size based on the width of the patient's fifth finger.[12] When preparing for intubation, tubes half a size smaller and half a size larger should be available. The depth of ET tube insertion in centimeters is approximately three times the uncuffed ET tube size. In the past, the use of cuffed tubes in children younger than 8 years was discouraged. However, this practice is becoming increasingly common. The use of either a cuffed or an uncuffed ET tube is acceptable, and a cuffed tube is now considered preferable in many cases. The conventional thought was that cuffed tubes increased the risk of ischemic damage to the tracheal mucosa, thus risking the complication of subglottic stenosis. Newer ET tubes are designed to be high volume and low pressure, resulting in a seal at lower pressure. When used in

controlled settings with frequent cuff pressure monitoring (typically in a pediatric ICU), cuffed tubes have not been shown to increase the risk of postextubation stridor or reintubation rates.[13–15] Additionally, cuffed ET tube use minimizes the risk of air leak, thus optimizing ventilation with higher pressures and resulting in more consistent ventilation. The use of cuffed tubes can also decrease the need to exchange inappropriately sized ET tubes.[9]

KEY POINT

Use a cuffed ET tube for children 2 years and older.

PEARL

When used in controlled settings with frequent cuff pressure monitoring (typically in a pediatric ICU), cuffed tubes have not been shown to increase the risk of postextubation stridor or reintubation rates.[13–15]

The key to successful intubation is using a standard procedure every time. Every patient in the emergency department is generally presumed to have a full stomach; therefore, rapid-sequence intubation (RSI) should be the norm. The risks of intubation should be considered. As with adults, the LEMON mnemonic may be used to predict difficult airways, although this technique has not been validated for use in children (Table 23-3). Gather appropriately sized equipment, including alternative airway management devices, and medications that will be used. Another mnemonic that may be helpful is "SOAP ME" (Table 23-4). Preoxygenate the patient, keeping in mind that even when appropriately oxygenated, the child will desaturate much more rapidly than an adult. Deliver RSI medications (Table 23-5) only when you are confident that BVM ventilation will be successful. The Sellick maneuver (cricoid pressure) may be used to decrease the chance of regurgitation by pressing the cricoid cartilage firmly against the esophagus. Studies have shown the positive effects of the Sellick maneuver in infants as young as 2 weeks.[16] However, this must be done cautiously in infants because too much pressure can collapse their pliable airways. One technique that may be used to improve visualization is to have the intubator use his or her own left fifth finger (while holding the laryngoscope) to provide gentle cricoid pressure. This allows the physician to manipulate the cricoid ring, helping to bring the glottis into view.

TABLE 23-5.

Pediatric RSI drugs. From: *EMRA Pediatric Qwic Card.* Dallas, TX: Emergency Medicine Residents Association; 2008. Used with permission of Dale Woolridge, MD, PhD.

Pretreatment

- Atropine (0.02 mg/kg IV/ET tube)—Minimum, 0.1 mg; use to decrease bradycardia from vagal stimulation; always use in patients <5 years old and before second dose of succinylcholine
- Lidocaine (1 mg/kg IV/ET tube)—To blunt theoretical increase in intracranial pressure (ICP)

Induction

- Etomidate (0.2–0.6 mg/kg IV)—Less hypotension than some sedatives
- Fentanyl (2–5 mcg/kg IV)—Can cause chest wall rigidity if given rapidly
- Ketamine (1–2 mg/kg IV)—Preferred in presence of bronchospasm; avoid if increased ICP is suspected
- Thiopental (3–5 mg/kg IV)—Preferred if increased ICP is suspected; use ½ dose in the presence of hypotension
- Midazolam (0.2–0.3 mg/kg IV)—Causes low blood pressure, heart rate, and respiratory rate

Paralysis

- Succinylcholine (1–2 mg/kg IV)—Pretreat with atropine in patients younger than 5 years and before all subsequent doses; avoid if hyperkalemia or renal failure is suspected or if the patient has a history of malignant hyperthermia or neuromuscular disease
- Rocuronium (0.6–1.2 mg/kg IV)—Onset in 1 min; lasts 30 min

Delayed onset paralytics, *not suited for RSI:*

- Pancuronium (0.04–0.1 mg/kg IV)—Avoid in asthmatic patients (histamine release) and patients with renal failure
- Vecuronium (0.08–0.1 mg/kg IV)—Onset in 1–3 min; lasts 90 min
- Cisatracurium (0.1–0.3 mg/kg IV)—Onset in 13 min; lasts 30–60 min

---

TABLE 23-6.

Comparison of LMA and ET tube size

Weight (kg)	Laryngeal mask airway	ET tube
<5	1	3.5
5–10	1.5	4
10–20	2	4.5
20–30	2.5	5
>30	3	6

Once the ET tube has been passed, confirm placement using clinical evaluation (gentle symmetric chest rise, equal bilateral breath sounds, condensation in the tube) as well as an end-tidal CO_2 detector. If breath sounds are heard over the stomach, do not remove the tube immediately—breath sounds are easily transmitted in infants and small children. Gurgling sounds suggest esophageal intubation, necessitating tube removal. Pediatric end-tidal CO_2 detectors should be used in patients weighing less than 15 kg and adult end-tidal CO_2 detectors in patients weighing more than 15 kg. End-tidal CO_2 detectors may not reliably confirm placement in instances of low pulmonary blood flow (eg, cardiac arrest or massive pulmonary embolism).[17] If any uncertainty remains, perform careful direct laryngoscopy to verify that the ET tube passes through the vocal cords. Finally, obtain a chest film to confirm proper tube position in the midtrachea.

As in adults, if a child develops problems with oxygenation or ventilation after intubation, use the "DOPE" mnemonic to consider potential reasons for this decompensation: **d**islodgement, **o**bstruction, **p**neumothorax, or **e**quipment malfunction/failure. Dislodgement is a frequent problem in small children because of their short trachea length. Small pediatric ET tubes are also more easily obstructed than larger, adult-sized tubes. When a problem arises, take the child off the ventilator and bag to ventilate manually. This will eliminate ventilator malfunction as a source of the problem and allow the clinician to use the ease of bagging to assess lung compliance as well as possible tube obstruction. Auscultate to check for tube position or dislodgement, and use a suction catheter to attempt to clear secretions from the tube. If equipment malfunction, obstruction, and displacement have been eliminated as causes, consider an underlying pneumothorax. If the patient is in extremis, needle decompression can be performed. In the stable patient, check a chest radiograph to evaluate tube placement and assess for pneumothorax.[9]

Difficult Airway

When traditional intubation techniques fail, alternative methods must be employed. It is critical to recognize the difficult airway before giving induction agents and paralytics. Findings that predict a difficult airway include limited mouth opening, cervical spine immobility, small mouth, prominent central incisors, short neck, large tongue, obesity, laryngeal edema, and mandibular or midface dysmorphology or trauma.[8] Consider using the "LEMON" mnemonic (Table 23-3), as discussed previously. In the absence of these findings, an unanticipated difficult pediatric airway is uncommon. If a difficult airway is predicted, video laryngoscopy is an increasingly common alternative airway method. Numerous video laryngoscope devices, available in pediatric sizes and even neonatal sizes, can offer improved success rates as well as facilitate teaching to novice intubators.[18,19]

If the child cannot be intubated using standard techniques, effective BVM ventilation should be provided. If this is successful, the clinician has time to optimize further attempts by repositioning the child and having the most skilled individual available repeat the laryngoscopy. If ventilation is still not achieved, the laryngeal mask airway (LMA) may be employed as a rescue device (Table 23-6). The most recent American Heart Association (AHA) recommendations for pediatric advanced life support state that "when BVM ventilation is unsuccessful and when endotracheal intubation is not possible, the LMA is an acceptable adjunct when used by experienced providers."[20] However, the guidelines advise caution, stating that complications associated with LMA insertion occur more frequently in young children than in adults. The esophageal-tracheal combination tube, or Combitube, is another alternative device for the "can't intubate/can't ventilate" situation. Unfortunately, it is not available in sizes appropriate for most children. The smallest version is recommended for use in "small adults" (4 to 6 feet tall).

If endotracheal intubation fails and ventilation is unsuc-

TABLE 23-7.

Initial pediatric ventilator settings

Pressure control (weight <10 kg)
- Peak inspiratory pressure = 20–30 cm H_2O
- PEEP = 3–5 cm H_2O
- F_{IO_2} = 100%
- RR = Age appropriate

Volume control (weight >10 kg)
- Tidal volume = 8–10 mL/kg
- PEEP = 5 cm H_2O
- F_{IO_2} = 100%
- RR = Age appropriate

TABLE 23-8.

Average vital signs by age. From: *EMRA Pediatric Qwic Card.* Dallas, TX: Emergency Medicine Residents Association; 2008. Used with permission of Dale Woolridge, MD, PhD.

Age	Weight (kg)	Heart Rate (bpm)	Respiratory Rate (breaths per minute)	Systolic Blood Pressure (mm Hg)
Newborn	3.5	130–150	40	70
3 mo	6	140	30	90
6 mo	8	130	30	90
1 yr	10	120	26	90
2 yr	12	115	26	90
3 yr	15	110	24	90
4 yr	17	100	24	90
6 yr	20	100	20	95
8 yr	25	90	20	95
10–12 yr	30–40	85	20	100

cessful with alternative airway devices, an invasive airway technique should be used. Options include needle cricothyrotomy and surgical cricothyrotomy. Needle cricothyrotomy is the easier and safer method of the two for temporary ventilatory support in the emergency department. This is a temporary measure because, although oxygenation can be preserved, ventilation is often marginal. Insert a 14-gauge catheter over a needle into the cricothyroid membrane while aspirating back. When free flow of air into the syringe is obtained, the position is correct. Consider placing a small amount of sterile saline in the syringe to assist in the detection of aspirated air. Once cannulated, the catheter can be connected directly to an adapter device, or it may be attached to the barrel of a 3-mL syringe and then to a resuscitation bag via the hub of a 7.0 ET tube. For children younger than 5 years, needle cricothyrotomy with bag ventilation is preferred. For children aged 5 to 10 years, bag ventilation or transtracheal jet ventilation may be used. Children older than 10 years should be of adequate size to allow placement of a larger-bore cricothyroid tube using Seldinger technique.

KEY POINT

When managing a difficult airway, do not continue to do the same thing and expect a different result. Move on to adjunctive airway devices.

PEARL

For children younger than 5 years, needle cricothyrotomy with bag ventilation is preferred. For children aged 5 to 10 years, bag ventilation or transtracheal jet ventilation may be used. Children older than 10 years should be of adequate size to allow placement of a larger-bore cricothyroid tube using Seldinger technique.

Breathing

When a child shows evidence of respiratory distress, the first step after airway positioning and clearance is simply to provide supplemental oxygen. Although oxygen delivered by nasal cannula or face mask is preferred and provides a higher inspired

TABLE 23-9.

Reversible causes of dysrhythmia, shock, and cardiorespiratory arrest

Six H's
- Hydrogen ion (acidosis)
- Hypoglycemia
- Hypothermia
- Hypo/Hyperkalemia
- Hypoxia
- Hypovolemia

Five T's
- Tamponade
- Tension pneumothorax
- Thrombosis (coronary or pulmonary)
- Toxins
- Trauma

FIO_2, blow-by oxygen is an effective alternative for an agitated child who does not tolerate having something on his or her face.

If inadequate oxygenation and ventilation persist, assisted ventilation may be necessary. As mentioned above, BVM ventilation is the technique of choice for airway management during the initial phase of resuscitation. BVM ventilation is usually simple and effective, yet, like everything in pediatrics, requires appropriately sized equipment. A mask that fits properly covers the child's chin, mouth, and nose. A mask that is too large covers the eyes and extends over the tip of the chin, and one that is too small does not cover the nose and mouth effectively and cannot make a seal. In the emergency department, a self-inflating resuscitation bag is most commonly used. This device does not require attachment to high-flow oxygen to function, although this is a common practice. When using BVM ventilation, take care not to compress the soft tissues of the neck in a young child. Hold the mask using the E-C clamp—using the thumb and index finger on the left hand to form a C that holds the mask onto the child's face and using the other three fingers to form an E along the angle of the jaw. Pull the child's jaw up to the mask rather than pushing the mask down on the face. Squeeze the bag only until chest rise is seen. Normal tidal volume is 6 to 8 mL/kg, but with the dead space of the device, one can estimate the volume needed as 10 mL/kg.[9] Avoid overventilation, as this can lead to gastric distention and difficulty ventilating because of an elevated hemidiaphragm.[21]

Hyperventilation is not recommended and can actually be harmful. Increased respiratory rates cause increased intrathoracic pressure, thereby decreasing venous return and coronary perfusion pressure. This has been shown to decrease survival.[22] Hyperventilation also drives down the PCO_2, resulting in cerebral vasoconstriction and hypoperfusion. Mild hyperventilation to a goal PCO_2 of 30 to 35 mm Hg should be reserved for patients with signs of impending cerebral herniation and those with suspected pulmonary hypertension. Once an advanced airway is in place, respirations should be administered simultaneously with chest compressions, at a rate of 8 to 10 breaths/min.[23]

KEY POINTS

Effective bag-mask ventilation may obviate the need for intubation. Prolonged delivery of unnecessarily high oxygen concentrations should be avoided. Do not hyperventilate the patient.

Do not overventilate. Use an age-appropriate rate and a tidal volume of 8–10 mL/kg.

Initial ventilator settings in the critically ill child are based on normal physiologic parameters for a healthy child of similar weight and age. A positive end-expiratory pressure (PEEP) of 5 cm H_2O is a good starting point. Many ventilators are designed to deliver both pressure and volume control modes of ventilation. Either may be used, but consider pressure mode in infants and smaller children weighing less than 10 kg (Table 23-7). Use either, with the goals of gentle chest rise, good air exchange, and delivery of a tidal volume of about 8 to 10 mL/kg. The target respiratory rate varies with the patient's age. Good starting points are rates of 30 breaths/min for infants, 20 for children, and 16 for older children and teenagers. Inspiratory time should be set between 0.5 and 1 second to target an inspiratory-to-expiratory ratio of 1:3 and allow adequate time in the exhalation phase of the respiratory cycle for carbon dioxide elimination. In patients demonstrating obstruction such as asthmatics, a larger ratio of 1:5 may be required. Avoid plateau pressures greater than 30 cm H_2O to minimize barotrauma. Obtain a blood gas measurement shortly after placing the patient on the ventilator to assess the effectiveness of ventilation.

PEARL

Avoid plateau pressures greater than 30 cm H_2O to minimize barotrauma.

Circulation

Rapidly assess the circulation to determine the adequacy of cardiac output and perfusion. Add to the PAT assessment of skin perfusion with a hands-on assessment of heart rate, pulse quality, level of consciousness, capillary refill, extremity temperature, skin color, urine output, and blood pressure.[3]

Cardiac Arrest

Approximately 16,000 American children (8–20 per 100,000 children) suffer a cardiac arrest each year.[24] If a child is unresponsive and not breathing, take up to 10 seconds to check for a carotid, femoral, or brachial pulse. If no pulse is present, begin cardiopulmonary resuscitation (CPR) along with assisted ventilation. The new AHA guidelines focus on performing high-quality CPR with minimal interruptions. In fact, the recommended universal sequence has been changed from ABC to CAB to emphasize the importance of initiating chest compressions immediately after cardiopulmonary arrest.[25] To

perform chest compressions for children (approximately 1 year of age to puberty), use the heel of one or two hands to depress the lower half of the sternum to a depth of at least one third of the anteroposterior (AP) chest diameter or about 5 cm.[26] For children, the compression-to-ventilation ratio is 30:2 for lone rescuers and 15:2 for two rescuers. For infants younger than 1 year, the AHA recommends that lone rescuers use two fingers to depress the sternum at least one third the depth of the chest or about 4 cm. The "two-thumb/encircling hands" technique is recommended when two or more health care providers are present. One rescuer's thumbs should forcefully compress the lower third of the sternum, but there are no data to support circumferential squeezing of the thorax.[25] The two-thumbs technique is preferred because it improves coronary artery perfusion pressure and may generate higher systolic and diastolic blood pressures. When performing chest compressions, rescuers should aim for a rate of at least 100 compressions/min, allow full chest recoil at the end of each compression, and be relieved by a different rescuer after 2 minutes to decrease rescuer fatigue. This switch should be performed in less than 5 seconds to minimize interruptions in CPR. In neonates, compressions and ventilations should be given in a 3:1 ratio of compressions to ventilations, with 90 compressions and 30 breaths in 1 minute, for a total of 120 events per minute. When compressions are given continuously, the rate should be 120 compressions per minute.[27]

Because pediatric cardiac arrest is most commonly caused by respiratory failure or shock, in up to 50% of cases, return of spontaneous circulation can be established with chest compressions and ventilation alone.[28,29] Even though early, high-quality CPR is key, studies have shown that when CPR is performed, it is often suboptimal, with compressions that are too few, too

TABLE 23-10.

Signs and symptoms of shock states in children

Hypovolemic	Cardiogenic	Distributive
Weak, pale, lethargic	Weak, pale, lethargic	Weak, pale lethargic
Tachypnea (to compensate for metabolic acidosis)	Tachypnea, retractions	Apnea, respiratory distress
Pale, mottled skin	Pale, mottled skin	Pale, mottled skin
Sunken eyes	Cool extremities	Cool or warm extremities
Dry mucous membranes	Hepatomegaly	Tachycardia
Poor skin turgor	Pulmonary edema	Hypotension
Delayed capillary refill	Tachycardia	History of source—allergen trigger, spinal cord injury, infection, etc.
Cool extremities	Arrhythmia	
Tachycardia	Heart murmur	
Hypotension (late finding)	Hypotension	
History of source—vomiting, diarrhea, hemorrhage, etc.	History of source—congenital heart disease, etc.	

shallow, and too weak. Ventilations are often excessive, with too many interruptions in chest compressions.[30,31] To maximize the effectiveness of compressions, the AHA stresses the need to "push hard and push fast." Interruptions in compressions should be minimized because they decrease the rate of return to spontaneous circulation. Rhythm checks should be performed every 2 minutes and result in only brief interruptions in chest compressions. Once an advanced airway is in place, compressions and breaths should be performed continuously without interruption.[20] These recommendations are all focused on improving myocardial, cerebral, and systemic perfusion to maximize the likelihood of recovery.

KEY POINTS

When CPR is necessary, push hard and push fast, minimize interruptions, allow time for chest recoil, and check rhythm quickly every 2 minutes of CPR.

Universal compression:ventilation ratio of 30:2 (lone rescuer) or 15:2 (two rescuers). Once an advanced airway is in place, deliver simultaneous ventilations and compressions, with a ventilation rate of 8 to 10 breaths/min.

Arrhythmias

Rhythm disturbances in children can be organized into three general categories: fast, slow, and pulseless (Figures 23-1, 23-2, 23-3). The clinical presentation of arrhythmia can range tremendously from nonspecific signs and symptoms in a stable child to profound respiratory distress, shock, or arrest. Remember—vital signs are vital (Table 23-8).

The most likely cause of bradyarrhythmia in children is hypoxia. When faced with a bradycardic child, first and foremost supply oxygen and support respirations. Chest compressions should be started when the heart rate is less than 60 beats/min and the child shows signs of poor perfusion, such as hypotension, altered mental state, or signs of shock. If bradycardia persists despite good CPR, give epinephrine, 0.01 mg/kg (0.1 mL/kg of 1:10,000), IV/IO. This dose may be repeated every 3 to 5 minutes. If vagal stimulation or cholinergic drug toxicity is suspected, consider atropine, 0.02 mg/kg IV/IO (minimum dose 0.1 mg; maximum single dose 0.5 mg in a child and 1 mg in an adolescent). This dose can be repeated to a maximum total dose of 1 mg in a child and 2 mg in an adolescent. Consider cardiac pacing if the bradycardia is caused by complete heart block or sinus node dysfunction, especially if it is associated

TABLE 23-11.

Infusion rates for vasoactive medications

Dobutamine, 2–20 mcg/kg/min
Dopamine, 2–20 mcg/kg/min
Epinephrine, 0.1–1 mcg/kg/min
Norepinephrine, 0.1–2 mcg/kg/min
Vasopressin, 0.5 mU/kg/hr

with congenital or acquired heart disease. If, at any point, the child progresses to pulseless electrical activity (PEA), switch to the PEA algorithm.[20,32]

When tachycardia is present and the patient is stable with a palpable pulse and adequate perfusion, administer oxygen, support ventilation, establish intravenous access, and obtain an electrocardiogram to evaluate the QRS duration. Narrow complex (<0.09 sec) tachycardia is most likely sinus tachycardia or supraventricular tachycardia (SVT). Rapid heart rates in children are most commonly due to sinus tachycardia. Although sinus tachycardia is not usually in itself harmful, the underlying cause should be identified and corrected. Common causes include hypoxemia, hypovolemia, hyperthermia, fever, toxins, pain, and anxiety. SVT is the most common tachyarrhythmia in children and typically presents with a heart rate faster than 180 beats/min in children and faster than 220 beats/min in infants (but the rate can reach as high as 300 beats/min). If the child is stable, the treatment of choice is vagal stimulation if it will not significantly delay chemical or electrical cardioversion. In infants and young children, apply a bag of ice/water slurry to the face firmly (but do not occlude the airway). In older children, have the child try Valsalva maneuvers such as blowing through a straw and bearing down or use carotid massage. Do not apply ocular pressure, as this can damage the retina. If vagal maneuvers fail to break the rhythm, adenosine should be given as a rapid intravenous bolus of 0.1 mg/kg (maximum initial dose 6 mg). This dose can be doubled on the second attempt to 0.2 mg/kg with a maximum dose of 12 mg. Remember to administer adenosine fast, followed by an immediate flush of 5 to 10 mL of normal saline. Rapid infusion is necessary because of the very short half-life of the medication. It is best achieved by using two syringes attached to a stopcock to allow the flush to go in as fast as possible. If adenosine fails, consider electrical cardioversion with sedation, amiodarone, or procainamide. These antiarrhythmic agents prolong the QT interval, must be infused slowly, and should not be used concurrently without expert consultation because they can precipitate torsade de pointes. Verapamil should not be used in infants because it has caused shock and cardiac arrest in this population.[33] If the patient becomes unstable or if perfusion is poor, proceed immediately to synchronized cardioversion with 0.5 to 1 J/kg. This can be repeated at 2 J/kg if the initial attempt is unsuccessful. Record a rhythm strip continuously during all chemical and electrical rhythm conversion attempts.[20,32]

PEARL

SVT is the most common tachyarrhythmia in children and typically presents with a heart rate faster than 180 beats/min in children and faster than 220 beats/min in infants (but the rate can reach as high as 300 beats/min).

Wide complex (>0.09 sec) tachycardia is usually ventricular, but it can be supraventricular with aberrant conduction. If perfusion is poor or if the child is unstable, proceed directly to synchronized cardioversion, as discussed above (0.5–1 J/kg, then 2 J/kg if unsuccessful). If perfusion is adequate, consider giving a dose of adenosine to determine if the rhythm is SVT with aberrant conduction. If the patient is in stable ventricular tachycardia, consider expert consultation for guidance regarding pharmacologic conversion with amiodarone or procainamide. These drugs must be given slowly while carefully monitoring the patient for electrocardiographic and blood pressure changes. Slow or stop drug infusion if the QRS interval widens or the blood pressure falls during drug administration.[20]

The electrocardiographic rhythm of a patient in pulseless cardiopulmonary arrest can fall into one of two categories: 1) ventricular tachycardia (VT)/ventricular fibrillation (VF) or 2) PEA/asystole. This distinction is critical, as survival is much more likely after arrests presenting with VT/VF than with PEA/asystole.[24,34,35] If VF or VT is present, or in the case of sudden witnessed collapse (which is presumed to be VF), proceed immediately to defibrillation. The defibrillation success rate decreases by approximately 5% to 10% with every minute of delay.[36] After one shock (not three as previously recommended) of 2 J/kg unsynchronized, resume CPR. After 2 minutes of CPR, check the rhythm and defibrillate again using 4 J/kg. Make every attempt to minimize interruption of chest compressions. Give epinephrine, 0.01 mg/kg (0.1 mL/kg of 1:10,000) IV/IO and repeat every 3 to 5 minutes. Perform another 2 minutes of CPR. If a shockable rhythm persists, deliver a third shock of more than 4 J/kg (maximum dose not to exceed 10 J/kg or the adult dose). If cardioversion is still unsuccessful after the third defibrillation attempt, continue CPR and consider the administration of an antiarrhythmic drug: amiodarone (5 mg/kg IV/IO), or lidocaine (1 mg/kg IV/IO) if amiodarone is not available. Magnesium sulfate (25–50 mg/kg IV/IO, maximum 2 g) should be given by rapid infusion for polymorphic VT or torsade de pointes. If the rhythm is PEA or asystole, it is not amenable to electrical cardioversion or defibrillation. Give epinephrine as above, repeating every 3 to 5 minutes, followed each time by 2 minutes of high-quality CPR. Search for possible contributing and potentially reversible factors—think of "the 6 H's and 5 T's" (Table 23-9)—and rapidly correct any identified irregularities.[20] If spontaneous circulation returns, proceed to meticulous post-cardiac arrest care.

KEY POINT

Defibrillate using a single shock of 2 J/kg followed by immediate resumption of 2 minutes of CPR. If a shockable rhythm persists, deliver 4 J/kg, epinephrine, and another 2 minutes of high-quality CPR. A third shock with more than 4 J/kg, with a maximum of 10 J/kg or the adult dose, and administration of amiodarone are recommended if attempts at defibrillation fail to restore a perfusing rhythm.

Shock

Shock is a state of inadequate perfusion resulting in inadequate substrate (oxygen, glucose) delivery to the vital organs. The management goal is early recognition to prevent tissue damage and progression to cardiopulmonary arrest. The underlying causes of shock can be divided into three main categories: hypovolemic, cardiogenic, and distributive (Table 23-10). Hypovolemic shock, the most common cause of shock in pediatric patients, is characterized by an inadequate circulating intravascular volume. It often results from dehydration or hemorrhage.

Distributive shock is characterized by inadequate distribution of fluid volume. This is usually caused by systemic vasodilation that leads to functional hypovolemia. Septic shock and anaphylactic shock are types of distributive shock that lead to this fluid shifting. Cardiogenic shock is characterized by myocardial dysfunction. Fluid volume can be normal or even slightly increased, but the diminished pump function of the myocardium impairs cardiac output.

Although shock is associated with hypotension, do not over-rely on blood pressure measurements. Because of strong compensatory responses, children are able to maintain cardiac output and blood pressure by significant increases in heart rate and systemic vascular resistance. Many children have normal or even slightly elevated blood pressures during the early stages of shock. With acute hemorrhage, blood pressure can be maintained in a normal range until approximately 30% of the circulating blood volume has been lost. Once uncompensated shock ensues, it can progress rapidly to terminal shock unresponsive to therapy. Hypotension is a late and ominous sign of shock in pediatric patients. Every effort should be made to recognize and treat shock states before decompensation occurs.[37]

KEY POINT

It is necessary to recognize and treat shock *before* hypotension occurs in children.

PEARL

Many children have normal or even slightly elevated blood pressures during the early stages of shock. With acute hemorrhage, blood pressure can be maintained in a normal range until approximately 30% of the circulating blood volume has been lost.

Resuscitation options for the treatment of shock vary widely depending on the etiology. Regardless of the cause, the goal is to rapidly restore tissue perfusion. Initially, administer supplemental oxygen, place monitors, and expediently obtain intravenous or intraosseous access. Give volume-expanding isotonic crystalloids (normal saline or lactated Ringer solution) in a bolus of 20 mL/kg *as fast as possible*. Reassess the child after each bolus and repeat if there is still evidence of poor perfusion.

KEY POINT

In shock, rapid fluid resuscitation is crucial. Give 20 mL/kg × 3 boluses within the first 15 to 20 minutes. If shock persists, consider packed red blood cells and pressors.

To deliver boluses this rapidly, consider a manual push-pull technique or delivery via pressure bag. Infusion by gravity is not rapid enough.[39] Packed red blood cells (given in 10-mL/kg aliquots) is the resuscitation fluid of choice for volume expansion, especially when signs of shock persist after 40 to 60 mL/kg crystalloid has been administered. Although the evidence for this in children is not as clear as in adults, the Society of Critical Care Medicine recommends maintaining a hemoglobin concentration of 8 to 10 g/dL to improve oxygen-carrying capacity and tissue perfusion.[40] If there is a concern about cardiogenic shock, give smaller volumes more slowly while watching carefully for signs of worsening cardiac function or volume overload.[32]

If fluid resuscitation is insufficient to restore perfusion, add vasopressor support (Table 23-11). In children, the choice of vasoactive agent should be tailored to the patient and the clinical situation. The initial pressor of choice is often dopamine. Start at 5 mcg/kg/min and titrate up by 2.5 mcg/kg/min every few minutes until perfusion improves and/or the target blood pressure is achieved (usually a mean arterial blood pressure of 65 mm Hg). Dopamine-resistant shock is diagnosed if inadequate perfusion persists after titration to 20 mcg/kg/min. In dopamine-resistant shock, consider the administration of norepinephrine (start at 0.05 mcg/kg/min and then titrate by 0.05–0.1 mcg/kg/min every 3–5 min to a maximum dose of 2 mcg/kg/min) or epinephrine (start at 0.05 mcg/kg/min and then titrate by 0.05–0.1 mcg/kg/min every 3–5 min to a maximum dose of 1 mcg/kg/min). In cases of myocardial dysfunction, dobutamine may improve cardiac output by improving contractility, rate, and myocardial relaxation (start at 2.5 mcg/kg/min and then titrate by 2.5 mcg/kg/min every 3–5 min).[40]

PEARL

The Society of Critical Care Medicine recommends maintaining a hemoglobin concentration of 8 to 10 g/dL to improve oxygen-carrying capacity and tissue perfusion.[40]

In children, the choice of vasoactive agent should be tailored to the patient and the clinical situation. The initial pressor of choice is often dopamine.

Hypoglycemia can develop rapidly in shock states in response to high glucose utilization and low glycogen stores. Monitor for this and other electrolyte abnormalities and correct them if necessary. In sepsis, promptly administer broad-spectrum antibiotics after appropriate cultures have been obtained.

Vascular Access

Even with adequate CPR, resuscitation drugs may be needed to restore a perfusing rhythm. Additionally, rapid fluid resuscitation may prevent a shocky patient from progressing to cardiorespiratory failure. Pediatric intravenous placement can be difficult in the hands of an inexperienced clinician, and this is only made harder by the stress of a code situation. In a crashing or coding patient, do not waste time attempting to place a central line; if peripheral intravenous access cannot be secured rapidly (ie, after three attempts), move immediately to intraosseous placement.

Intraosseous lines are now being recommended for resuscitation in all age groups, from premature infants to adults, as a rapid, safe, effective option for vascular access.[41] New devices, including spring-loaded needles and powered drills, can facilitate proper placement. Complications are similar to those associated with traditional intraosseous needles, including needle displacement, fracture, infection, and compartment syndrome. Nevertheless, the ease and rapidity of placement, as well as the effectiveness of drug delivery, make this an ideal technique for use during a pediatric resuscitation. The AHA recommends intraosseous access over endotracheal drug delivery and notes that it can be used for administration of fluids (including blood products) and medications (including pressors) and for initial blood sampling.[20] Equipment for intraosseous access should be readily available, and caregivers should be familiar with its use.

If attempts at intravenous and intraosseous line placement fail, some medications may be given via the endotracheal route. Certain lipid-soluble drugs such as lidocaine, epinephrine, atropine, and naloxone ("LEAN") can be delivered endotracheally. Although optimal endotracheal doses are not known, most experts recommend double or triple the typical intravenous dose for lidocaine, atropine, and naloxone and 10 times the typical dose for epinephrine (0.1 mg/kg or 0.1 mL/kg of a 1:1,000 concentration) when given endotracheally. If this route is used, follow the drug dose with a 5-mL normal saline flush. In neonates, this may be too large a volume, so instead dilute the drug to 1 to 2 mL with normal saline and give directly or use a 5F feeding catheter inserted down the ET tube, followed by 0.5 mL saline. In both cases, give several assisted bag ventilations immediately to help distribute the drug deep into the bronchial tree. Overall, the endotracheal route is discouraged because of "erratic and inconsistent" drug absorption and potential toxicity.[41]

Postresuscitation Care

Despite our best efforts, most victims of pediatric cardiopulmonary arrest will not be resuscitated successfully. When reperfusion is achieved, the immediate postresuscitation phase is critical. During this period, patients are at high risk for brain injury, ventricular arrhythmias, and extension of reperfusion injuries. Interventions during this period are aimed at minimizing reperfusion injury and supporting cellular recovery. Hyperthermia following cardiac arrest and anoxic brain injury in children are common and should be avoided. Mild induced hypothermia can be employed in children as in adults and may improve outcomes.[24,42]

KEY POINT

During resuscitation, give medications intravenously or intraosseously; use endotracheal delivery as a last resort (the absorption is inconsistent).

Conclusion

Unstable pediatric patients present unique challenges in the emergency department. By being aware of the different anatomy and physiologic responses in children and being familiar with and prepared for pediatric procedures, the emergency physician will be able to deliver focused, effective emergency care to critically ill children.

References

1. Weiss HB, Mathers LJ, Forjuoh SN, Kinnane JM. *Child and Adolescent Emergency Department Visit Data Book*. Pittsburgh, PA: Center for Violence and Injury Control, Allegheny University of the Health Sciences; 1997.
2. Langham M, Keshavarz R, Richardson L. How comfortable are emergency physicians with pediatric patients? *J Emerg Med*. 2004;26:465-469.
3. Dieckmann RA. Pediatric assessment. In: Gausche-Hill M, Fuchs S, Yamamoto L, eds. *APLS: The Pediatric Emergency Medicine Resource*. 4th ed. Sudbury, MA: American Academy of Pediatrics and American College of Emergency Physicians; 2007:20-51.
4. Luten R, Wears RF, Broselow J, et al. Managing the unique size-related issues of pediatric resuscitation: reducing cognitive load with resuscitation aids. *Acad Emerg Med*. 2002;9:840-847.
5. Gausche M, Lewis RJ, Stratton SJ, et al. Effect of out-of-hospital pediatric endotracheal intubation on survival and neurological outcome: a controlled clinical trial. *JAMA*. 2000;283:783-790.

6. Stockinger ZT, McSwain NE Jr. Prehospital endotracheal intubation for trauma does not improve survival over bag-valve-mask ventilation. *J Trauma.* 2004;56:531-536.

7. Pitetti R, Glustein JZ, Bhende MS. Prehospital care and outcome of pediatric out-of-hospital cardiac arrest. *Prehosp Emerg Care.* 2002;6:283-290.

8. Sullivan KJ, Kissoon N. Securing the child's airway in the emergency department. *Pediatr Emerg Care.* 2002;18:108-124.

9. Santillanes G, Gausche-Hill M. Pediatric airway management. *Emerg Med Clin North Am.* 2008;26:961-975.

10. Stewart C. Managing the pediatric airway in the ED. *Pediatr Emerg Med Pract.* 2006;3:1-24.

11. Bingham RM, Proctor LT. Airway management. *Pediatr Clin North Am.* 2008;55:873-886.

12. King BB, Baker MD, Braitman LE, et al. Endotracheal tube selection in children: a comparison of four methods. *Ann Emerg Med.* 1993;22:530-534.

13. Khine HH, Corddry DH, Kettrick RG, et al. Comparison of cuffed and uncuffed endotracheal tubes in young children in general anesthesia. *Anesthesiology.* 1997;86:627-631.

14. Newth CJ, Rachman B, Patel N, et al. The use of cuffed versus uncuffed endotracheal tubes in pediatric intensive care. *J Pediatr.* 2004;144:333-337.

15. Deakers TW, Reynolds G, Stretton M, et al. Cuffed endotracheal tubes in pediatric intensive care. *J Pediatr.* 1994;125:57-62.

16. Moynihan RJ, Brock-Utne JG, Archer JH, et al. The effect of cricoid pressure on preventing gastric insufflation in infants and children. *Anesthesiology.* 1993;78:652-656.

17. Li J. Capnography alone is imperfect for endotracheal tube placement confirmation during emergency intubation. *J Emerg Med.* 2001;20:223-229.

18. Kim JT, Na HS, Bae JY, et al. GlideScope video laryngoscope: a randomized clinical trial in 203 paediatric patients. *Br J Anaesth.* 2008;101:531-534.

19. Nouruzi-Sedeh P, Schurmann M, Groeben H. Laryngoscopy via Macintosh blade versus GlideScope success rate and time for endotracheal intubation in untrained medical personnel. *Anesthesiology.* 2009;110:32-37.

20. Kleinman ME, Chameides L, Schexnayder SM, et al. Part 14: Pediatric Advanced Life Support: 2010 American Heart Association Guidelines for Cardiopulmonary Resuscitation and Emergency Cardiovascular Care. *Circulation.* 2010;122 suppl 3:S876-S908.

21. Berg MD, Ahamed IH, Berg RA. Severe ventilatory compromise due to gastric distension during pediatric cardiopulmonary resuscitation. *Resuscitation.* 1998;36:71-73.

22. Aufderheide T, Lurie K. Death by hyperventilation: a common and life-threatening problem during cardiopulmonary resuscitation. *Crit Care Med.* 2004;32(9 suppl):S345-S351.

23. Doniger SJ, Sharieff GQ. Pediatric resuscitation update. *Emerg Med Clin North Am.* 2000;25:947-960.

24. Topjian AA, Nadkarni VM, Berg RA. Cardiopulmonary resuscitation in children: advances in science, techniques, and outcomes. *Curr Opin Crit Care.* 2009;15:203-208.

25. Berg MD, Schexnayder SM, Chameides L, et al. Part 13: Pediatric Basic Life Support: 2010 American Heart Association Guidelines for Cardiopulmonary Resuscitation and Emergency Cardiovascular Care. *Circulation.* 2010;122[suppl 3]:S862-S875.

26. Stevenson A, McGowan J, Evans A, et al. CPR for children: one hand or two? *Resuscitation.* 2005;64:205-208.

27. Kattwinkel J, Perlman JM, Aziz K, et al. Part 15: Neonatal Resuscitation: 2010 American Heart Association Guidelines for Cardiopulmonary Resuscitation and Emergency Cardiovascular Care. *Circulation.* 2010;122[suppl 3]:S909-S919.

28. Young KD, Gausche-Hill M, McClung CD, et al. A prospective, population-based study of the epidemiology and outcome of out-of-hospital pediatric cardiopulmonary arrest. *Pediatrics.* 2004;114:157-164.

29. Berg MD, Nadkarni VM, Berg RA. Cardiopulmonary resuscitation in children. *Curr Opin Crit Care.* 2008;14:254-260.

30. Donoghue AJ, Nadkarni VM, Berg RA, et al. Out-of-hospital pediatric cardiac arrest: an epidemiologic review and assessment of current knowledge. *Ann Emerg Med.* 2005;46:512–522.

31. Abella BS, Alvarado JP, Myklebust H, et al. Quality of cardiopulmonary resuscitation during in-hospital cardiac arrest. *JAMA.* 2005;293:363-365.

32. Fitzmaurice L, Gerardi MJ. Cardiovascular system. In: Gausche-Hill M, Fuchs S, Yamamoto L, eds. *APLS: The Pediatric Emergency Medicine Resource.* 4th ed. Sudbury, MA: American Academy of Pediatrics and American College of Emergency Physicians; 2007:106-145.

33. Samson RA, Atkins DL. Tachyarrhythmias and defibrillation. *Pediatr Clin North Am.* 2008;55:887-907.

34. Atkins DL, Everson-Stewart S, Sears GK, et al. Epidemiology and outcomes from out-of-hospital cardiac arrest in children: the Resuscitation Outcomes Consortium Epistry-Cardiac arrest. *Circulation.* 2009;119:1484-1491.

35. Samson RA, Nadkarni VM, Meaney PA, et al. Outcomes of in-hospital ventricular fibrillation in children. *N Engl J Med.* 2006;354:2328-2339.

36. Larsen MP, Eisenberg MS, Cummins RO, et al. Predicting survival from out-of-hospital cardiac arrest: a graphic model. *Ann Emerg Med.* 1993;22:1652-1658.

37. American College of Surgeons. *Advanced Trauma Life Support for Doctors.* 7th ed. Chicago, IL: American College of Surgeons; 2004.

38. Carcillo JA, Fields AI. Clinical practice parameters for hemodynamic support of pediatric and neonatal patients in septic shock. *Crit Care Med.* 2002;30:1365-1378.

39. Stoner MJ, Goodman DG, Cohen DM, et al. Rapid fluid resuscitation in pediatrics: testing the American College of Critical Care Medicine guideline. *Ann Emerg Med.* 2007;50:601-607.

40. Melendez E, Bachur R. Advances in the emergency management of pediatric sepsis. *Curr Opin Pediatr.* 2006;18:245-253.

41. De Caen RA, Reis A, Bhutta A. Vascular access and drug therapy in pediatric resuscitation. *Pediatr Clin North Am.* 2008;55:909-927.

42. Hickey RW, Kochanek PM, Ferimer H, et al. Hypothermia and hyperthermia in children after resuscitation from cardiac arrest. *Pediatrics.* 2000;106:118-122.

Pediatric Trauma Updates

Richard Amini and Dale P. Woolridge

IN THIS CHAPTER

Pediatric airway management

Pediatric ventilatory support

Pediatric circulatory support

Pediatric head trauma management

Pediatric thoracic trauma management

Pediatric abdominal trauma management

Pediatric trauma advancements

Introduction

Pediatric trauma is the leading cause of mortality in children, accounting for more than 45% of all deaths among children 1 to 14 years of age.[1] A total of 15,000 children die each year from trauma and another 150,000 become permanently disabled. Approximately half of the trauma in this age group is directly related to motor vehicle collisions. The mortality rate of hospitalized children after trauma is low; however, most pediatric trauma deaths occur while the patient is en route to the hospital. The most common form of pediatric trauma is blunt trauma, from either deceleration injuries or direct injury such as impact with a baseball or handle bar. The most common diagnosis is head injury, which can lead to permanent brain damage secondary to gray/white matter damage or herniation.[2]

Management of pediatric trauma is complicated by the fact that anatomy and physiology vary greatly with age. The initial evaluation can be difficult because of the limited ability to communicate with young children and their limited ability to cooperate with examination.[3] Moreover, the physiologic impulse to comfort a crying or injured child often interferes with taking appropriate stabilizing and therapeutic actions. Collaboration and communication among team members caring for the child are essential for appropriate stabilization and management. In addition, the concerned parents must be kept aware of what is happening to their child.

Airway

Assessing the airway is top priority in pediatric cases. An understanding of anatomic differences between adults and children will increase the likelihood of positive outcomes.

Children are obligate nose breathers. If the nasal passages are obstructed by blood clots, the child cannot easily compensate by oral ventilation. The tongue occupies a relatively greater portion of the airway, making intubation and ventilation techniques difficult. It is all too easy to obstruct the airway by pushing the tongue posteriorly. Head positioning with jaw thrust, chin lift, and neck extension is key to opening the airway.

The position of the patient is critical to successful airway management. Because of a child's large occiput, a supine patient's neck is in a passively flexed position. Placing a blanket under the shoulders helps to extend the neck and align the axes of intubation.[4]

Because of lack of frequent experience with the technique, many prehospital systems do not support pediatric intubation, and, for the same reason, there is a reluctance to undertake active airway management within the emergency department as well. The decision to intubate a child should be made for each individual situation, with the expertise and experience of the intubator playing a role in this choice.

Once the decision to intubate has been made, choosing the best endotracheal (ET) tube size is expedited by using length-based resuscitation tapes or the following formula:

ET tube size = age/4 + 4 uncuffed or age/4 + 3 cuffed

The pediatric airway is narrowest at the cricoid ring, which forms a natural anatomic seal around the ET tube and may eliminate the need for a cuffed tube, depending on the age and size of the child. When choosing uncuffed versus cuffed tubes, the general convention has been that children younger than 8 years require uncuffed tubes because of this anatomic seal. Children older than 8 years have larger, wider airways, similar to those of adults, and thus lack this anatomic seal, making a cuffed tube preferable.[4]

Update

Recent literature has discussed the benefit of routine use of cuffed ET tubes for all children. The primary argument for this shift in use is to allow a cuff to be in place and available in the event of a significant air leak.[5] The drawback of routine use of a cuffed tube is that it requires a reduction in tube size. This size reduction is considered more relevant when working with small ET tubes (<4F), since tube management and secretions are significantly more troublesome in the smaller sizes.[6] The clinician should therefore carefully scrutinize these benefits and drawbacks when choosing a cuffed tube in smaller children.

PEARLS

Pediatric airway

- Equipment needed for intubation
  - (SOAP ME) = suction, oxygen, airway equipment, pharmacy, mechanical equipment
- Consider a cuffed tube for all patients, particularly if an air leak is anticipated (eg, conditions requiring high peak pressures).
- Estimated ET tube size:
  - Tube size (uncuffed) = Age (in years)/4 + 4
  - Tube size (cuffed) = Age (in years)/4 + 3
- Centimeters of ET tube placement at the lip = 3 × normal tube size

Breathing/Ventilating

Anatomically, the chest wall of the pediatric patient is different from the adult thorax. Children have less chest wall rigidity and less intrinsic elasticity.[7] Their intercostal muscles are not fully developed (fewer slow-twitch type I muscle fibers), and their diaphragm is shorter and more flattened, which limits the ability to pull it down and further increase the negative force needed to expand the chest cavity for ventilation. These differences make the pediatric airway less capable of generating inspiratory force and more susceptible to fatigue. It is an indication for intubation and active ventilation when one can predict that the work of respiration will be increased and not tolerated by the child. Examples are shock; pulmonary contusion; chest wall trauma, as with a flail chest; and atelectasis and increased re-

spiratory rate, such as abdominal distention caused by the ileus that accompanies skeletal fractures, especially of the vertebrae.[4]

Pediatric patients have a smaller airway diameter, which increases resistance to the negative pressure of inspiratory effort. In addition, the smaller alveolar size increases the likelihood of atelectasis. More important, a child's basic metabolic rate is much greater than that of adults. This equates to increased oxygen consumption, which permits much less reserve than in the adult—another reason the child fatigues more easily.[4]

When providing positive-pressure ventilatory assistance, only enough pressure to create a chest wall rise should be used. Too much force will damage the already fragile respiratory system. Also, because of chest wall size, it is useful to minimize extrathoracic interference such as gastric distention by placing a nasogastric tube after intubation to evacuate the stomach and thereby improve ventilation (Table 24-1).

Circulation

When assessing the circulatory system of a child, it is important to examine both cardiac function and circulatory volume. The key components are evaluation of the pulse, capillary refill time, and blood pressure.

When evaluating cardiac function, place the child on the monitor and assess the extremities for pulses. A child's heart is less compliant than that of an adult and less able to increase contractility. Thus, to alter cardiac output, the pediatric patient relies almost entirely on adjustment in rate. Tachycardia is therefore the first sign of volume depletion.[2] Simple tachycardia may be caused by fear or pain. Furthermore, the younger the child, the faster the normal resting cardiac rate, leaving little ability to compensate for losses of volume. Children often develop a paradoxic bradycardia as they become hypoxic, and this

TABLE 24-1.
Pediatric mechanical ventilation

DOPE (trouble shooting): dislodged, obstructed tube, pneumothorax, equipment failure
Consider a pressure-limited mode if the patient weighs less than 10 kg
Rate: Start at 30 breaths per minute for neonates; otherwise, age appropriate
Inspiratory-to-expiratory (I:E) ratio: 1:2; 1:3–5 for patients with asthma
Avoid peak pressures >40 mm Hg
Peak inspiratory pressure: Start at 16 cm H_2O; increase by increments of 2 cm H_2O for adequate chest wall excursion
Tidal volume: 8–10 mL/kg
Positive end-expiratory pressure: 3–5 mm Hg
Obtain arterial blood gas measurement within 30 minutes of placing on mechanical ventilation

often confuses the picture of volume depletion. Finally, most institutions are unaccustomed to measuring blood pressures in small infants, leaving capillary refill and pulse rate as the only indicators of volume depletion.

Examining for capillary refill time is a helpful adjunct because it can provide information regarding arteriole vasoactivity. A child who is adequately perfusing will have relaxed peripheral vasculature that allows brisk capillary refill. However, when the patient is hypovolemic from dehydration, hemorrhage, or early sepsis, arterioles constrict and decrease capillary flow. A child's vasculature is more elastic than the stiff blood vessels of an atherosclerotic elderly patient, and the arterial vasoconstrictive forces are much more sensitive to catecholamine release. This allows children to constrict peripheral vessels more readily, decreasing capillary refill time. Typically, refill time longer than 2 seconds requires immediate intervention.[2]

Because of the elasticity and efficiency with which the pediatric vasculature compensates for decreased blood volume, the pediatric trauma patient will maintain blood pressure despite mild to moderate fluid loss. To address even the smallest deviation in the blood pressure, one must obtain an accurate reading. Accurate readings require appropriately sized blood pressure cuffs. The cuff diaphragm should be approximately 20% larger than the diameter of the arm and about two thirds of the length of the arm.

KEY POINT

Because of the elasticity and efficiency with which the pediatric vasculature compensates for decreased blood volume, the pediatric trauma patient will maintain blood pressure despite mild to moderate fluid loss.

To resuscitate a child, a fluid bolus of 20 mL/kg of normal saline should be given to increase blood flow to the vital organs. These organs should be assessed for lack of perfusion. Neurologic perfusion is assessed by determining the mental status; renal perfusion is assessed by measuring urine output, which should be approximately 1 mL/kg/hr; pulmonary perfusion is assessed by auscultation; and cardiovascular perfusion can be evaluated by monitoring blood pressure, heart rate, and capillary refill time.

Fluid resuscitation in the hypovolemic pediatric patient should be aggressive and should start with crystalloid replacement. If hypotension or tachycardia persists after the initial normal saline bolus, a second bolus of 20 mL/kg should be given. Persistent evidence of hypovolemia despite 40 mL/kg of crystalloid should prompt fluid resuscitation with blood products. This is done by administering a 10- to 20-mL/kg bolus of packed red blood cells.[2]

PEARLS
Pediatric circulation

- Hypotension = systolic blood pressure <70 mm Hg + (2 × age in years); neonates: systolic blood pressure <60 mm Hg
- Weight (kg) = (2 × years of age) + 8
- Drugs that can be given through an ET tube: NAVEL = naloxone, atropine, diazepam (Valium), epinephrine, lidocaine

Head Trauma

Traumatic brain injury is the most common cause of death and permanent injury in children and is the reason for more than 400,000 emergency department visits and nearly 3,000 deaths per year. Younger children are usually at greater risk for injury. Trauma is usually a result of a fall from standing.[8]

Although pediatric patients can be difficult to examine, signs and symptoms of increased intracranial pressure must be ruled out. These symptoms include full fontanels, split sutures, altered mental status, irritability, vomiting, headache, light sensitivity, focal neurologic signs, and, ultimately, papilledema. The goal is to prevent the secondary injuries that occur as a result of inflammation, which in turn can lead to cellular edema, brain herniation, and death. A few of the more common injuries are discussed below.

Skull fractures can be open, closed, linear, or depressed. The most common skull fractures are linear and are usually asymptomatic, except for tenderness over the fracture site. Depressed skull fractures are rare and often associated with brain injury.[8] Basilar skull fractures are indicated by physical findings such as periorbital or postauricular hematoma, temporal bone area subcutaneous hemorrhage, hemotympanum, and cerebrospinal fluid (CSF) rhinorrhea or otorrhea.

PEARLS
Basilar skull fractures

- Raccoon eyes – bilateral periorbital ecchymosis
- Battle sign – mastoid ecchymosis
- When CSF rhinorrhea or otorrhea is suspected, collect a fluid sample and send it for evaluation. When a drop of CSF fluid dries on paper, it creates a ring of blood and serum.

Epidural hematomas are rare, but they are critical life-threatening injuries. In the adult patient, the typical scenario involves injury to the middle meningeal artery and a lucid period followed by a decrease in mental status as the hemorrhage worsens. However, in children, the dura is more firmly attached to the skull and the groove for the middle meningeal artery is shallower. This combination creates a state allowing more mobility of the artery, thereby preventing injury.[8] The cause of a pediatric epidural hematoma is usually venous, and the clinical course is less obvious. The child may complain of ear or jaw pain, but not headache, and may develop a herniation syndrome while a mandible fracture is being sought. Arterial bleed epidural hematomas are less subtle and tend to produce focal findings earlier than those of venous origin.[9]

Subdural hematomas occur up to 10 times as often as an epidural bleed. They are more common in the neonatal population secondary to the weaker connective tissue and plasticity of the skull in this population. Subdural hematomas occur bilaterally in 80% of pediatric cases, whereas a subdural hematoma in adults is usually unilateral. A variation of subdural hematoma in children is a subdural hygroma, a collection of CSF in the subdural space, which can produce a mass effect like a hematoma.[10]

Unlike hematomas, cerebral contusions are caused by acute

deceleration forces that create shear stress injuries of the brain. These injuries are associated with cerebral edema and commonly occur at the tips of the frontal and temporal lobes. Damage to the parenchyma of the brain is most profound on the microscopic level. The resultant intracerebral edema can ultimately lead to herniation and death. Intracerebral hemorrhage contributes to severe permanent brain injury and a high mortality rate.

All of the above injuries can induce seizure activity, obtundation, nausea, and vomiting. Any head injury in a child can produce a short burst of seizure activity and one or two episodes of vomiting. For this reason, head injury precautions should include warning about new seizure activity and about vomiting that occurs more than two or three times. During hospitalization, the child can be checked every hour. When the child is at home, the parents should be advised to make sure the child can be awakened fully, including one time during the night, and to observe for seizure activity or episodes of vomiting.

A cerebral injury unique to the pediatric population is diffuse axonal injury, which is caused by shear forces created as the brain shifts inside the closed skull. In children younger than 1 year of age, the cause of this injury is usually not accidental. Accompanying injuries include torn bridging veins, petechial hemorrhages in the white matter, shearing of the myelin and axons, and the physical finding of retinal hemorrhages.[11]

Update

In late 2009, Kuppermann and associates completed a study designed to create and validate a decision rule intended to identify low-risk traumatic brain injuries in children.[12] From their study involving more than 42,000 pediatric trauma patients, they developed a decision rule that has a sensitivity of more than 98%, a specificity of more than 53%, and a negative predictive value of 100% (95% CI, 99.7–100). They concluded that a child can be discharged without further testing if he or she is less than 2 years old, has a Glasgow Coma Scale (GCS) score of 15, does not have an altered mental status, does not have a scalp hematoma, has not experienced loss of consciousness, has a mechanism of injury that is mild or moderate, is acting normally according to the parents, and has no physical finding suggestive of skull fracture. Older children (2–18 years of age) may be discharged without further testing if they have a GCS score of 15, no altered mental status, no loss of consciousness, no history of vomiting, a mild or moderate mechanism of injury, no clinical signs of basilar skull fracture, and no severe headache. The authors estimate that, with the use of their algorithm, 20% to 25% of computed tomography (CT) scans done on pediatric trauma patients can be avoided.[12]

Although the use of steroids for closed head injury was once accepted therapy, steroids are not useful and should not be used. The CRASH study demonstrated an increase in mortality among head-injured patients treated with steroids.[13] A Cochrane review updated on January 7, 2009, also recommends against the use of steroids.[14]

PEARL

Children with neurologic injuries recover remarkably well: 90% demonstrate significant improvement, and 60% have complete resolution of injuries.[8]

Leptomeningeal cysts are a complication of skull fractures that are unique to young children. These can occur in infants during the years of rapid brain growth and are rare after 3 years of age. Fractures associated with an underlying laceration of the dura can lead to herniation through the dural tear and prevent apposition and healing of the fracture. The CSF pressure and pulsations eventually widen the dural defect and expand the fracture margins. The term "growing fracture" is often used to refer to interval widening of the space between the fracture margins. It is therefore critical that children with known skull fractures return for repeat imaging, typically 2 to 3 months after the trauma event. If a leptomeningeal cyst is identified, surgical correction is warranted.

Cervical Spine Injuries

Cervical spine injuries are rare in the pediatric population, accounting for less than 10% of all cervical spine injuries. This is due, in part, to their lethality in children under the age of 3 years. Cervical injuries in patients younger than 8 years are typically higher in the cervical region (above C3). A child's larger head-to-body ratio mandates a higher pivot point, which is typically at C2-3, as opposed to C5-6 in adults. The larger head in children also creates greater torque in acceleration/deceleration injuries, which puts more stress on the cervical spine. In addition, the underdeveloped muscles and laxity of ligaments create a relatively unstable anatomy that is susceptible to spinal cord injuries. As a result of these differences, children with cervical spine injuries tend to have a higher mortality rate than adults.[8]

Cervical fractures represent only half of the spinal injuries among children. The thoracic and lumbar spine must not be overlooked, and it is especially important that the entire spine be immobilized during field management. The potential for thoracic and lumbar injury should be kept in mind when trying to comfort the child, so that serious spinal cord damage can be avoided.

The National Emergency X-Radiography Utilization Study (NEXUS) provided helpful guidelines on when to request imaging of the spine.[15] Based on records of more than 3,000 patients younger than 18 years, the study coordinators concluded that blunt trauma patients without the following conditions were at low risk of cervical spine injuries: midline cervical tenderness, altered mental status, evidence of intoxication, distracting injury, or evidence of neurologic abnormality. The NEXUS decision tool has a reported sensitivity of 100% and negative predictive value of 100%.

Update

The NEXUS did not involve sufficient numbers of children younger than 2 years to allow the decision tool regarding risk of cervical spine injury to be extended to them. In 2003, Lee and associates developed a clinical decision tool intended to increase the reliability of the NEXUS in the pediatric population. They reported that the cervical spine could be cleared if the physician could identify none of the following conditions in addition to the five NEXUS criteria: high-risk mechanism of injury, history of transient neurologic symptoms causing concern about spinal cord injury without radiographic abnormality (SCIWORA), physical signs of neck trauma, trauma to the head or face, or being inconsolable. The presence of any of these findings merits at least a plain film.[16]

Spinal Cord Injuries

Spinal cord injuries are rare among pediatric trauma patients. Just like other anatomic parts of children, the pediatric spine is very malleable. During a traumatic event, the spine may contort and twist and portions can separate without creating specific damage to the support system of the spinal column. However, the spinal cord is not as forgiving, and although the spinal column can stretch up to 5 cm before injury occurs, the spinal cord can be damaged with a 5- to 6-mm stretch.[12] In 1982, these injuries were defined as SCIWORA.[17] As the name implies, they are not evident on radiographs but may be demonstrated on magnetic resonance imaging. Symptoms can emerge up to 4 days after the trauma. Any child with persistent neck pain and neurologic complaints should be evaluated for SCIWORA. The treatment is immobilization ranging from 3 weeks to 3 months.

Update

Steroids have been used commonly for spinal cord injuries, with the hope of decreasing the inflammatory reaction and decreasing the production of oxygen free radicals. There has never been any evidence that this practice is useful in pediatric trauma. Recent prospective double-blind studies—the National Acute Spinal Cord Injury Studies (NASCIS I, II and III) performed in 1984, 1990, and 1997—demonstrated negative outcomes.[18–21] Current evidence indicates that steroids are not useful in any trauma patient, whether a child or an adult.

Chest Injuries

Blunt thoracic trauma is the leading cause of severe chest injuries. The mechanism of injury is typically a motor vehicle crash or a bicycle crash.[7] Because of their thoracic anatomy, children are prone to internal injuries without external manifestations. The child's thoracic wall is pliable, with cartilaginous ribs that tend to transmit energy forces. The flexible pediatric thorax transmits this energy to nearby organs, such as the lung, liver, spleen, and heart. Thus, significant internal injury can be present in the absence of rib fractures. If rib fractures are present, they are often an alarming sign of severe internal injuries.[7]

PEARL

If rib fractures are present, they are often an alarming sign of severe internal injuries.[7]

The most common cardiac injury is a myocardial contusion. The problem with this injury is that it is virtually impossible to diagnose. The variation known as "myocardial stunning" is a lethal injury, often seen after relatively minor blunt thoracic trauma in children younger than age 5. Sudden death is thought to be the result of an acute ventricular arrhythmia induced by a blow to the chest.[22]

Myocardial contusion does not cause specific physical findings or symptoms. It can be assumed to be present if the child has a sternal fracture or any acute arrhythmia (eg, atrial flutter) after thoracic blunt trauma. There are no diagnostic ECG changes, and cardiac enzymes do not rise in any useful fashion. Most of these patients require a few hours of monitoring for arrhythmia.

Occasionally, a myocardial contusion produces intense substernal chest pain 5 to 7 days after injury. Children who experience this pain need to be admitted and observed. They do not develop coronary arterial injury but behave like patients with myopericarditis and therefore need to be observed for pericardial effusions and treated with analgesia.

Any penetrating thoracic injury can cause a pericardial effusion and lead to the development of tamponade physiology. The best way to monitor children with this type of injury is with repeated transthoracic echocardiographic studies. A central pressure monitor is also useful, but it is probably unnecessary if ultrasonography is readily available. The physical findings of tamponade physiology are often absent because the child will get into trouble quickly when 100 to 200 mL of fluid has collected in the pericardial sac. An ECG will not usually show pulsus alternans or even low QRS amplitude because of the rapidity of development. There may well be pulsus paradoxus, but this is very hard to measure in a child. A drop in amplitude of the pulse with inspiration might be noticed, but the fastest way to discover the effusion will be with a sonogram.[23]

PEARL

The physical findings of tamponade physiology are often absent because the child will get into trouble quickly when 100 to 200 mL of fluid has collected in the pericardial sac.

The normal response to tamponade physiology is the development of tachycardia, which, as described above, is the only way a child can increase cardiac output. Immediately prior to arrest, however, a bradycardia will develop as a result of hypoxia. When such a compromised cardiac output is identified, thoracotomy must be performed or a pericardial window created to relieve the tamponade. This is a situation where pericardiocentesis is too slow and provides too minimal a volume relief from the pericardial sac to save the life. Usually the pericardial sac is so tense that it must be incised with a scalpel. Before tamponade physiology of this severity, as indicated by bradycardia, has developed, pericardiocentesis can be used to lower tamponade pressure. This is best performed by inserting a spinal needle into the left subxiphoid space, pointed toward the tip of the right scapula. It is possible to insert the needle on the right and move it toward the tip of the left scapula, but this approach carries a risk of injuring the right coronary artery. A direct anterior approach is also useful and can be performed safely while using the ultrasound probe to monitor the course of the needle.

Patients with pulmonary injuries are at risk for respiratory compromise. As mentioned earlier, the pediatric patient has immature intercostal muscles, muscle fibers that are easily fatigued, and less innate elasticity of the chest wall, which can be further compromised when the pliable chest wall transmits energy to the lungs and causes injury. Pulmonary injuries from thoracic trauma include pulmonary contusions, pneumothorax, and hemothorax, in descending order of occurrence.[7]

The two main mechanisms involved in the production of pulmonary contusion are compressive forces that are transmitted through the ribs and chest wall from a direct blow and shear forces from violent displacement such as in acceleration/deceleration injuries. The former cause local injury, whereas the latter can cause distal injuries to the tracheobronchial structures. These injuries can lead to edema, hemorrhage, and consolidation, which, if large enough, can compromise the patient's respiratory status. The imaging appearance of a pulmonary contusion is often deceiving. Large areas of white-out may not compromise ventilation, while seemingly innocuous chest films may be obtained from a patient with severe ventilatory impairment. The first clue to impairment of ventilation is an increase in respiratory rate. Unfortunately, this is one of the hardest vital signs to measure with regular accuracy in pediatric patients. The other clue to the onset of ventilatory impairment is a rising Pco_2. If either or both of these changes are noted, the child must be intubated to ensure ventilation. It is prudent to ventilate the left or right chest if this occurs, to prevent the development of a tension pneumothorax while the patient is on the ventilator. The symptoms consistent with ventilatory impairment are respiratory difficulty, auscultation abnormalities, and local tenderness. For most patients, supportive therapy is sufficient. Monitoring for respiratory compromise, pneumonia, and acute respiratory distress syndrome is critical during the hospital course. Fortunately, most pulmonary contusions resolve within a few days.[7]

Lung contusion and penetrating trauma can be complicated by air or blood escape from the parenchyma into the pleural space, creating pneumothorax or hemothorax, respectively. The symptoms associated with mild pneumothorax are tachypnea, mild to moderate distress, and oxygen desaturation. The physical examination is often confusing early after the pneumothorax develops, but over time, breath sounds on the side of the injury will decrease or become absent. Hyperresonance to percussion will become evident. Although all pneumothorax produces a drop in oxygen saturation as the first change following pleural penetration, tension pneumothorax is a life-threatening situation in which the pressure in the pleural space builds to a level higher than atmospheric pressure, with subsequent shifting of the mediastinum to the opposite side. This causes decreasing venous return, falling cardiac output, and worsening oxygenation and requires immediate decompression, which is performed by needle thoracotomy, placing the needle in the fourth intercostal space in the midaxillary line. In the past, an anterior approach was recommended, but problems are created by this approach. It is easy to injure the internal mammary artery, which does not always stay under the sternum, as would be predicted. Moreover, the needle must perforate the pectoralis major and minor, the serratus anterior, and the intercostal muscles. The needle chosen may not be long enough to enter the pleural cavity. Finally, high on the anterior chest wall, the intercostal vessels are doubled with a superior as well as an inferior branch, and it is easy to injure the superior branch with the anterior approach. Using the lateral approach, there is a window

between the pectoralis muscles and the latissimus dorsi, so the only muscles that need to be penetrated are the serratus and the intercostals. Therefore, the needle does not need to be so long. Only a small drop in the built-up pressure will reverse the tension. The needle thoracotomy should then be followed by a formal thoracostomy.[7]

A hemothorax can be difficult to diagnose depending on the quantity of blood in the pleural space. This is because the chest film will not reveal a hemothorax that is less than about 200 mL, but it can be visualized using ultrasonography. The patient may have only slightly diminished breath sounds and chest discomfort. A large hemothorax can manifest with dullness to percussion and respiratory distress. The hemothorax will require thoracostomy drainage to measure the volume of blood in the chest and to monitor for persistent or recurrent bleeding. Although some clinicians use the initial volume of blood in the chest as part of the decision for thoracotomy (see below), the length of time between the trauma and the thoracotomy should also be taken into consideration. More accurate indications for thoracotomy are persistent bleeding and recurrence of bleeding after the patient has been satisfactorily resuscitated.[7]

KEY POINTS

Indications for early thoracotomy

- Hematoma with volume >500 mL in the chest cavity
- Continued bleeding into the chest tube of 200 mL/hr for 4 consecutive hours
- Large air leak
- Large chest wall defect
- Recurrence of shock and new bleeding after successful resuscitation

Indications for delayed thoracotomy

- Persistent bleeding
- Persistent air leak
- Sepsis

PEARL

Nearly 21% of patients with pulmonary contusions develop pneumonia.

Abdominal Injuries

Pediatric abdominal trauma is the third most common traumatic injury in children. Approximately 10% to 22% of children with abdominal trauma have intraabdominal injuries.[1] The ratio of blunt to penetrating trauma is 85% to 15%. The two most common organs injured by blunt mechanisms are the liver and the spleen. In the past, spleen and liver injuries were most often managed surgically. It has become apparent over the years that it is prudent and possible to observe rather than operate on many of these children. The ability of these organs to heal without surgery was thought to be related to the muscular serosa of the spleen in children, causing contraction of the organ after the initial bleed and a much lower incidence of delayed or recurrent bleeding than in the adult. A primary motivation for the nonoperative strategy has been to maintain as much intrinsic splenic function as possible so as to maintain a normal immunogenic state. Similarly, it is becoming apparent that far fewer adults require immediate laparotomy for splenic injuries.[24,25] Nevertheless, a period of observation is critical to the safe management of these children.

PEARL

Approximately 10% to 22% of children with abdominal trauma have intraabdominal injuries.[1]

Another strategic change in the management of these children is the willingness to forgo imaging via CT scan. The scan exposes the child to a large dose of radiation, is not helpful for small bowel or pancreatic injuries, often overestimates the degree of solid organ injury, and gives little information about the physiologic status of the child. Careful observation of the child has led to far fewer CT scans and laparotomies being performed. If the child develops signs of deterioration, as described above, the trauma surgeon must decide whether to take the child to the operating room or the CT suite.

Objective evaluation of a child with abdominal trauma is still important in regard to initial management. The ultrasonographic FAST examination plays a useful role in identifying which children need extra careful observation. A positive FAST examination does not demonstrate anything more than blood or fluid in the abdomen, similar to diagnostic peritoneal lavage, but repeated FAST examinations can reveal active bleeding and explain a sudden deterioration.[25-27]

Diagnostic peritoneal lavage is rarely used in the evaluation of children with abdominal trauma. Nevertheless, in some children, the cause of deterioration cannot be identified within the abdomen, so an immediate decision must be made about whether these children should go to the operating room. In such cases, diagnostic peritoneal lavage may identify more occult injury and garner enough information to direct the surgeon to a likely region of exploration. It can assist in the identification of injury such as a ruptured bladder or a small bowel injury as the cause of deterioration. Diagnostic peritoneal lavage can reveal urine or fecal contents, elevated intraperitoneal white blood cell counts, or elevations in the alkaline phosphatase concentration to indicate a small bowel injury. Neither CT nor ultrasonography is especially accurate in identification of these injuries.[28]

Most other indications for surgery in patients with blunt abdominal injuries will appear over time, such as the onset of vomiting, abdominal distention, deterioration of vital signs, and increased respiratory difficulties with injuries such as a duodenal hematoma, pancreatic injury, or renal injury. As part of the observation of the child, it is often necessary to place a nasogastric tube to prevent gastric distention from ileus, which can cause severe hypotension and an acute abdomen. A Foley catheter is also necessary to monitor urinary output.

Certain types of trauma are related to the mechanism of injury. For example, sudden compressive forces exerted on the abdomen (such as from rapid deceleration while wearing a lap belt) can create intestinal rupture, traumatic diaphragmatic hernias, and vertebral blow-out fractures (Chance fractures). Clues to these injuries can be obtained by taking a careful history of the

mechanism of injury, ascertaining where the child was sitting in the vehicle that crashed and how the child was restrained, and performing an informed physical examination. An abdominal contusion in a child who was wearing a solitary lap belt is often a sign of small bowel injury, mesenteric contusion or tear, or a perforation of the antimesenteric wall. This injury is often accompanied by the vertebral burst fracture.[8]

Unfortunately, mesenteric and hollow viscus injuries resulting from blunt abdominal trauma are often insidious. CT scanning has an initial sensitivity of 50% to 75%.[28] As the mesenteric injury evolves, perforation can ensue, releasing infection into the peritoneum, or mesenteric hematomas could result in lumen narrowing and intestinal obstruction. These events often manifest 24 to 72 hours after the event as obstructive symptoms or peritonitis. For these reasons, pediatric patients with evidence of significant blunt abdominal trauma should be observed and should receive serial examinations or serial FAST screens, as mentioned above. If examination results are worsening, the patient can be taken to the operating room for exploratory laparotomy.

KEY POINT

Liver and spleen injuries can lead to hemorrhage; therefore, serial hemoglobin and hematocrit values should be obtained.

KEY POINTS

Indications for surgery

- Total volume required for resuscitation >50% of patient's total volume
- Continued hemodynamic instability
- Gunshot to abdomen or evisceration of bowel contents
- Signs of peritonitis
- Radiographic imaging demonstrating
  - Pneumoperitoneum
  - Intraperitoneal bladder rupture
  - Grade V renovascular injury

PEARL

Volume resuscitation with more than 40 mL/kg without resolution of tachycardia, hypoxemia, and hypotension requires administration of blood products.

KEY POINT

If a lap belt injury is evident, search for small bowel injuries and vertebral burst fractures.

Update

A recent study regarding the rate of CT-scan–induced malignancy estimated that, in pediatric patients who undergo an abdominal CT scan, the risk for malignancy can be as high as 1 in 550.[29] Less dangerous and equally efficacious studies are needed. Recent literature indicates that repeated FAST examinations in trauma patients appear to be beneficial. Chiu et al applied information from the FAST examination in addition to findings on the physical examination during the observational period and found that repeat evaluations with both can minimize the need for initial and repeat CT scans.[27] Before widespread acceptance of this strategy, additional pediatric studies are needed to confirm its application.

Conclusion

Although trauma is a leading cause of mortality in children, measures can be taken to decrease its lethality. An understanding of the physiologic differences between adults and children is vital to the effective management of the injured child. Advances in the diagnostic and therapeutic aspects of trauma are increasing the efficiency and effectiveness of the treatment of pediatric trauma.

References

1. Arias E, MacDorman MF, Strobino DM, Guyer B. Annual summary of vital statistics—2002. *Pediatrics.* 2003;112:1215-1230.

2. Schweer L. Pediatric trauma resuscitation: initial fluid management. *J Infus Nurs.* 2008;31:104-111.

3. Meyburg J, Bernhard M, Hoffmann GF, Motsch J. Principles of pediatric emergency care. *Dtsch Arztebl Int.* 2009;106:739-747.

4. Amini R. Pediatric airways are not just "little airways." In: Mattu A, Chanmugam AS, Swadron SP, et al, eds. *Avoiding Common Errors in the Emergency Department.* Baltimore, MD: Lippincott Williams & Wilkins; 2010:493-496.

5. Silver GM, Freiburg C, Halerz M, et al. A survey of airway and ventilator management strategies in North American pediatric burn units. *J Burn Care Rehabil.* 2004;25:435-440.

6. Pietrini D, Piastra M, Lamperti M, Ingelmo PM. New trends in pediatric anesthesia. *Minerva Anestesiol.* 2009;75:191-199.

7. Tovar JA. The lung and pediatric trauma. *Semin Pediatr Surg.* 2008;17:53-59.

8. Cakmakci H. Essentials of trauma: head and spine. *Pediatr Radiol.* 2009;39(suppl 3):391-405.

9. Thiessen ML, Woolridge DP. Pediatric minor closed head injury. *Pediatr Clin North Am.* 2006;53:1-26.

10. Lee KS. The pathogenesis and clinical significance of traumatic subdural hygroma. *Brain Inj.* 1998;12:595-603.

11. Wygnanski-Jaffe T, Morad Y, Levin AV. Pathology of retinal hemorrhage in abusive head trauma. *Forensic Sci Med Pathol.* 2009;5:291-297.

12. Kuppermann N, Holmes JF, Dayan PS, et al. Identification of children at very low risk of clinically-important brain injuries after head trauma: a prospective cohort study. *Lancet.* 2009;374:1160-1170.

13. Bracken MB. CRASH (Corticosteroid Randomization after Significant Head Injury Trial): landmark and storm warning. *Neurosurgery.* 2005;57:1300-1302.

14. Alderson P, Roberts I. Corticosteroids for acute traumatic brain injury. *Cochrane Database Syst Rev.* 2005;CD000196.

15. Hoffman JR, Wolfson AB, Todd K, Mower WR. Selective cervical spine radiography in blunt trauma: methodology of the National Emergency X-Radiography Utilization Study (NEXUS). *Ann Emerg Med.* 1998;32:461-469.

16. Lee SL, Sena M, Greenholz KS, Fledderman M. A multidisciplinary approach to the development of a cervical spine clearance protocol: process, rationale, and initial results. *J Pediatr Surg.* 2003;38:358-362.

17. Pang D. Spinal cord injury without radiographic abnormality in children, 2 decades later. *Neurosurgery.* 2004;55(6):1325-1342.

18. Bracken MB, Collins WF, Freeman DF, et al. Efficacy of methylprednisolone in acute spinal cord injury. *JAMA.* 1984;251:45-52.

19. Bracken MB, Shepard MJ, Hellenbrand KG, et al. Methylprednisolone and neurological function one year after spinal cord injury. *J Neurosurg.* 1985;63:704-713.

20. Bracken MB, Shepard MJ, Collins WF, et al. A randomized, controlled trial of methylprednisolone or naloxone in the treatment of acute spinal-cord injury. *N Engl J Med.* 1990;322:1405-1411.

21. Bracken MB, Shepard MJ, Holford TR, et al. Administration of methylprednisolone for 24 or 48 hours or tirilazad mesylate for 48 hours in the treatment of acute spinal cord injury. *JAMA.* 1997;277:1597-1604.

22. Abrunzo TJ. Commotio cordis: the single, most common cause of traumatic death in youth baseball. *Am J Dis Child.* 1991;145:1279-1282.

23. Levy JA, Bachur RG. Bedside ultrasound in the pediatric emergency department. *Curr Opin Pediatr.* 2008;20:235-242.

24. Lynn KN, Werder GM, Callaghan RM, et al. Pediatric blunt splenic trauma: a comprehensive review. *Pediatr Radiol.* 2009;39:904-916.

25. Eppich WJ, Zonfrillo MR. Emergency department evaluation and management of blunt abdominal trauma in children. *Curr Opin Pediatr.* 2007;19:265-269.

26. Blackbourne LH, Soffer D, McKenney M, et al. Secondary ultrasound examination increases the sensitivity of the FAST exam in blunt trauma. *J Trauma.* 2004;57:934-938.

27. Chiu WC, Wong-You-Cheong JJ, Rodriguez A, et al. Ultrasonography for interval assessment in the nonoperative management of hepatic trauma. *Am Surg.* 2005;71:841-846.

28. Killeen KL, Shanmuganathan K, Poletti PA, et al. Helical computed tomography of bowel and mesenteric injuries. *J Trauma.* 2001;51:26-36.

29. Brenner D, Elliston C, Hall E, Berdon W. Estimated risks of radiation-induced fatal cancer from pediatric CT. *AJR Am J Roentgenol* 2001;176:289-296.

Index

Page references followed by *f* indicate figure and by *t* indicate table.